Recent Advances in

Surgery 41

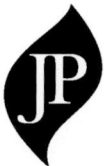

Recent Advances in Surgery 41

Michael Douek MB ChB MD FRCS(Eng)
FRCS (Gen) EBSQ (Breast)
Rosetrees Royal College of Surgeons of England Director of the Surgical Interventional Trials Unit and Professor of Surgical Sciences and Breast Cancer,
Nuffield Department of Surgical Sciences
University of Oxford, Oxford, UK

Rachel Hargest BSc MBBS FRCS MD FRCS(Gen)
Co-Director Global Surgery Policy Unit, Royal College of Surgeons of England & London School of Economics and Political Science
Co-Lead, World Health Organization Collaborating Centre for Health Policy and Impact in Emergency, Critical and Operative (ECO) Care
Clinical Senior Lecturer in Colorectal Surgery
Cardiff China Medical Research Collaborative and
Honorary Consultant Surgeon
University Hospital of Wales and Velindre Hospital
Cardiff, UK

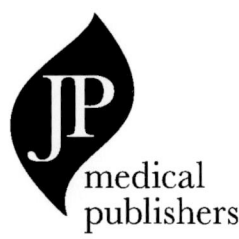

London • New Delhi

© 2026 JP Medical Ltd.

Published by JP Medical Ltd,
83 Victoria Street, London,
SW1H 0HW, UK
Tel: +44 (0)20 3170 8910
Email: info@jpmedpub.com
Web: www.jpmedpub.com

EU GPSR Authorised Representative
Logos Europe, 9 rue Nicolas Poussin
17000, La Rochelle, France
Phone: +33 (0) 6 67 93 73 78
E-mail: Contact@logoseurope.eu

The rights of Michael Douek and Rachel Hargest to be identified as the authors of this work have been asserted by them in accordance with the Copyright, Designs and Patents Act 1988.

All rights reserved. No part of this publication may be reproduced, stored or transmitted in any form or by any means, electronic, mechanical, photocopying, recording or otherwise, except as permitted by the UK Copyright, Designs and Patents Act 1988, without the prior permission in writing of the publishers. Permissions may be sought directly from JP Medical Ltd at the address printed above.

All brand names and product names used in this book are trade names, service marks, trademarks or registered trademarks of their respective owners. The publisher is not associated with any product or vendor mentioned in this book.

Medical knowledge and practice change constantly. This book is designed to provide accurate, authoritative information about the subject matter in question. However readers are advised to check the most current information available on procedures included and check information from the manufacturer of each product to be administered, to verify the recommended dose, formula, method and duration of administration, adverse effects and contraindications. It is the responsibility of the practitioner to take all appropriate safety precautions. Neither the publisher nor the authors assume any liability for any injury and/or damage to persons or property arising from or related to use of material in this book.

This book is sold on the understanding that the publisher is not engaged in providing professional medical services. If such advice or services are required, the services of a competent medical professional should be sought.

ISBN: 978-1-78779-197-8

British Library Cataloguing in Publication Data
A catalogue record for this book is available from the British Library

Library of Congress Cataloging in Publication Data
A catalog record for this book is available from the Library of Congress

Project Manager: Bhavana Sharma

Editorial Assistant: Keshav Kumar Baghel

Cover Design: Seema Dogra

Typeset, printed and bound in India.

Preface

We are delighted to present this volume of *Recent Advances in Surgery 41*. This book has a long history which has covered the history of surgical development across the world – for both technical developments and new concepts in the management of surgical cancers and other disorders. Multidisciplinary working is now the standard of care for many surgical conditions and we are grateful to our non-surgical colleagues for their role in shaping our thinking and contributing to much of the evidence cited in this edition.

We have included chapters on 'Sustainability in Surgery' and 'Human Factors in Surgery' for the first time. These cross-cutting topics influence surgical practice and their importance is now being recognised. The issues raised will stimulate further consideration and research.

Emergency surgery is a significant part of the workload for many surgeons and this edition includes several chapters on site-specific surgical emergencies including 'Management of Rectal Injuries, Modern Management of Aortic Dissection, Management of Acute Cholecystitis and Prevention and Management of Burst Abdomen', along with more general chapters on the use of 'Tranexamic Acid' to reduce bleeding and 'Improving Outcomes in Emergency Surgery'.

We are very grateful to all our chapter editors for their contributions and patience. Thank you for taking the time to prepare these chapters and we thank you for your efforts. We trust this book will prove useful to busy surgeons in front line practice across the globe, along with those studying for professional examinations.

Finally, we hope that each reader will find something of interest applicable to your daily practice.

Michael Douek
Rachel Hargest
September, 2025

Contents

Preface — v
Acknowledgements — ix

Section 1 Principles of general surgery

Chapter 1 Sustainability in surgery — 3
Ifeoluwa Osinkolu, Victoria Pegna

Chapter 2 Optimisation prior to surgery — 17
Gregory Warren, Scarlett McNally

Chapter 3 Recent advances in understanding the role of human factors in patient safety and surgical team performance — 35
Neil Mackenzie, Benjamin Whitworth, Rachel Oeppen, Peter Brennan

Section 2 Emergency surgery

Chapter 4 Improving outcomes in emergency surgery — 51
Sachal Safdar, Peter McCulloch, Giles Bond-Smith

Chapter 5 Management and prevention of burst abdomen — 57
Arunima Verma, Sunil Kumar

Section 3 Breast surgery

Chapter 6 Neoadjuvant endocrine therapy and agents for early breast cancer — 73
Aglaia Skolariki, Simon Lord, Ramsey I Cutress

Chapter 7 Percutaneous treatment for breast cancer — 103
Jenny Yijian Wang, Francesca Holt, Gloria Petralia, Gurdeep S Mannu

Section 4 Hepatobiliary surgery

Chapter 8 Contemporary management of incidentally detected gallstones — 117
Chiranjiva Khandelwal, Utpal Anand, Kislay Kant

Chapter 9   Recent advances in management of acute cholecystitis   123
Christian Macutkiewicz

Section 5   Intestinal surgery

Chapter 10   Management of rectal injuries   139
Deborah Keller, Richard Cohen, James J Crosbie

Chapter 11   Recent advances in intestinal transplantation   151
Jang I Moon, Kishore Iyer

Section 6   Vascular surgery

Chapter 12   Modern management of aortic dissection   165
Sven Tan, Richard White, W Rhodri Thomas,
Mohamad Bashir, Ian Williams

Chapter 13   The role of tranexamic acid in reducing surgical bleeding   179
John Houghton, Ian Roberts, Robert Sayers

Index   189

Acknowledgements

The authors wish to thank Ms Zoe Uttley for her administrative support and Dr Jane Lane for proofreading multiple chapters. We also wish to thank the staff at M/s Jaypee Brothers Medical Publishers (P) Ltd., New Delhi, India, for preparation and publishing of this edition of *'Recent Advances in Surgery 41'*.

Section 1

Principles of general surgery

Chapter 1

Sustainability in surgery

Ifeoluwa Osinkolu, Victoria Pegna

ABSTRACT

Addressing climate change has become a major priority for global public health. Healthcare delivery, in particular surgical care, contributes to the climate crisis. To address this, efforts are being made to embed sustainability into the way surgical care is delivered.

In this chapter, we have elaborated the link between climate change, healthcare, and surgery that suggest the principles of sustainable surgery as a guide to lower the environmental impact of clinical practice and outline a range of practical recommendations that can be applied to everyday practice. Finally, we have discussed the future of sustainability in surgery and the road to decarbonising the speciality.

INTRODUCTION: THE LINKS BETWEEN CLIMATE CHANGE AND HEALTHCARE

The accelerated release of greenhouse gasses into the atmosphere caused by the expansion of human activities has led to climate change. The most important greenhouse gas is carbon dioxide. As a result of land clearance for development of agricultural and urban societies around the world, and fossil fuel combustion, the global carbon cycle has been severely altered [1]. The level of carbon dioxide in atmosphere is increasing from approximately 280 ppm in preindustrial times to over 400 ppm in 2020 [1]. In 2021, the mean surface temperature globally was 1.1°C warmer than the preindustrial level average [2]. This resulting temperature rise has seen an increase in the frequency of extreme weather events, worsening air pollution, poorer food and water security, and changes in vector ecology [3]. These effects of climate change are affecting human health worldwide directly through increased exposure to extreme heat, wildfires, flooding, and pollution.

Ifeoluwa Osinkolu MBBS MRCS, Specialist Registrar, All Wales Higher Surgical Training Scheme, Sustainability Leadership Fellow, Health Education Improvement Wales (HEIW), Fellow at the Centre for Sustainable Healthcare (CSH), Oxford, UK
E-mail: Ifeoluwa.osinkolu@wales.nhs.uk (for correspondence)

Victoria Pegna MBBS MSc FRCS, Consultant Colorectal Surgeon, Worthing Hospital, University Hospitals Sussex, Sussex, UK
E-mail: VICTORIAPEGNA@hotmail.co.uk (for correspondence)

Indirectly, human health is affected when the systems and infrastructure on which health depends on are damaged.

The global healthcare industry contributes significantly to the climate crisis with an estimated annual carbon footprint of 2 billion tonnes of carbon dioxide equivalent [4]. This is approximately 4.4% of the global net carbon emissions [4]. The term 'carbon footprint' is defined as the estimated sum of direct and indirect greenhouse gas emissions which are attributable to a given process or product. If the health sector were a country, it would be the fifth largest carbon emitter [4]. The healthcare sectors in the US, China and countries of the European union are responsible for 56% of global healthcare's emissions [4]. In the USA, healthcare is responsible for 8–10% of all its greenhouse gas emissions [4]. The health sector directly and indirectly releases greenhouse gasses while delivering care. Through the production, transportation and disposal of pharmaceuticals, agricultural products, medical devices and equipment, the supply chain of healthcare is responsible for about 71% of its carbon footprint [4].

In 2021, the Intergovernmental Panel on Climate Change (IPCC) predicted that unless addressed, global surface temperatures are going to reach 1.5°C above preindustrial levels within the next decade [5]. This rise in temperature will have detrimental effects on natural and human systems. It is not surprising a climate emergency has been declared in 39 countries [6], and the World Health Organisation (WHO) is advocating for net-zero emission transmission of healthcare systems. Acknowledging healthcare's contribution to the climate crisis, in 2020 the National Health Service (NHS) in England became one of the few healthcare systems in the world to commit to achieving net zero carbon emissions by 2040 and published its decarbonisation strategy [7]. This has inspired 22 other countries to commit to lowering their emissions of their health systems to net zero [8].

The climate crisis is a healthcare crisis. Healthcare practitioners will need to participate in the innovation, adoption and embedding of sustainable healthcare principles which aim to deliver healthcare needs for today's generation without compromising the ability of the future generation to meet their needs [9]. This will be crucial in addressing this crisis and achieving the targets set in the United Nations climate change Paris agreement [10].

SURGERY'S CONTRIBUTION TO THE CLIMATE CHANGE

Surgical services, and in particular operating theatres, contribute significantly to the carbon footprint of healthcare. A systematic review looking at the carbon footprint of surgical operations showed a single operation could be responsible for as much as 814 kg CO_2e [11]. This is equivalent to driving 2,700 miles in an average petrol car [12]. Operating theatres are typically the most resource-intensive area in the hospital because of its high-energy demands, expensive equipment, anaesthetic gasses, and generation of excess amount of waste [13].

The energy required to run operating theatres can be six times more intensive than that required in the rest of the hospital [13]. Heating, ventilation, and air conditioning are to a great degree responsible for this energy intensity [13]. Although not totally under the control of surgical services, a significant amount of greenhouse gas emissions is associated with procurement. In England, the supply chain is responsible for 57% of the health and social care greenhouse gas emissions [14]. Medical instruments and equipment on their own are responsible for 13% of total healthcare-related emissions [14].

Inhaled anaesthetic gasses are greenhouse gasses which have varying global warming potentials, all of which are higher than carbon dioxide. Depending on the anaesthetic gas used, it can be responsible for as much as 63% of the carbon emissions of an operating theatre [13]. It is estimated that anaesthetic gasses are responsible for 2% of healthcare's carbon footprint in England [7]. Although waste only accounts for as little as 3% of healthcare's carbon footprint [4], operating theatres are responsible for 70% of hospital waste [15]. Not only does the manufacturing of single use plastic required for healthcare contribute to climate change, but inappropriate disposal is also leading to land fill and worsening ocean pollution [16].

A transformation of the way surgical care is delivered will be crucial for the decarbonisation of the healthcare sector. The surgical colleges in the UK have, therefore, made a climate emergency declaration [17], making effort to support sustainability within surgery by publishing peer reviewed evidence and guidance such as the intercollegiate green theatre checklist [18] to empower surgical teams to make changes in their practices.

PRINCIPLES OF SUSTAINABLE SURGERY

To embed sustainability into surgery, the value of surgical services must be redefined to consider patient and population outcomes against the environmental, social and financial costs of delivering care [9]. This is referred to as the *sustainable value* (**Equation 1.1**).

$$\text{Sustainable value} = \frac{\text{Outcomes for patients and populations}}{\text{Environmental + Social + Financial impacts (the 'triple bottom line')}}$$

Equation 1.1 Sustainable value in healthcare [9].

The principles of sustainable surgery have been developed as a guide to diminish the environmental impact of our clinical practice [19] (**Figure 1.1**). This transformation will require minimising demand, empowering patients, and designing surgical services in a way to prioritise low carbon treatment options, interventions that are resource efficient and maximise operational efficiency.

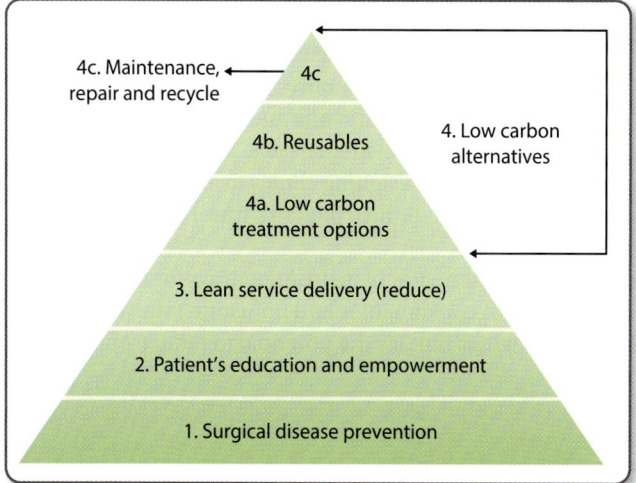

Figure 1.1 Principles of sustainable healthcare [19].

SURGICAL DISEASE PREVENTION

Primary prevention, which aims to intervene before surgical disease occurs, will ultimately decrease demand for surgical care. Primary prevention reduces population risks of surgical illness. These include developing public health measures to promote healthier living through increased physical exercise, healthier diet, alcohol moderation, smoking cessation and to address inequalities. Activities such as active travel not only to enhance individual physical and mental health but can also have environmental benefits by reducing pollution related to cars [20]. If surgical diseases can be avoided, there will be a reduction in the use of resources required for clinical assessment, investigation, operation and postoperative care of patients, therefore decreasing the environmental footprint of surgical care.

Secondary prevention to identify and treat diseases at the earliest stage is also essential. Preventing additional investigations and interventions associated with delayed diagnosis aids to optimise surgical resources.

Surgical organisations, societies and individual practitioners should be actively involved in primary prevention and health promotion campaigns at national and local level as prevention will have the highest impact on the decarbonisation of surgical care.

Patient's education and empowerment

Educating and empowering surgical patients to optimise their health and self-manage their health-needs, when appropriate, reduces the demand for surgery. This enables them to understand how to limit the progression of their condition and recognise exacerbation of their chronic illness, therefore reducing hospital visits and reliance on the service. Condition-specific education like dietary modification in patients known to have gallstones or pain-relieving exercises in patients with arthritis have the potential to reduce the need for surgery.

Patient-led disease optimisation is of particular importance given the increased waiting times for elective surgery seen globally as a result of the COVID-19 pandemic [21–23]. Patients having an active role in co-managing their health condition not only reduces demands on surgical services but has potential to improve patient's experience and outcomes.

Lean service delivery (reduce)

The way surgical care is delivered can be streamlined to optimise resource utilisation. Integrating activities with high impact and benefit to both patients and the environment into the design of surgical pathways can reduce waste of time, space, financial and workforce capacity [24]. Lean improvement methodologies used in the manufacturing industry have shown promise in the outpatient and perioperative setting to improve efficiency while reducing cost [25]. It is important that surgeons question routine practice and ensure surgical pathways are guided by the latest evidence base. For instance, integrating virtual clinics into surgical pathways or designing clinics to allow for patients to attend multiple specialities in one visit, can help to reduce patient's travel to hospital and patient's work disruption [20].

Operations can also be streamlined. Regular review of instrument trays for unused instruments will potentially reduce the use of consumables and unjustified waste. This is not only associated with significant cost savings but has the potential to reduce operation set up time [26].

Low carbon alternatives

This principle involves opting for lower carbon treatment options as well as choosing products and processes with lower carbon footprint.

Low carbon treatment options

When the most clinically effective treatment option is offered to patients, this helps to ensure that the environmental impact of any treatment is necessary, given that different treatment options may have varied greenhouse gas emissions associated with them [20].

For instance, choosing local or regional anaesthetic for operations such as knee arthroplasty or inguinal hernia has not only shown considerable clinical benefit [27,28], but by avoiding volatile anaesthetic gasses and intravenous medication required for general anaesthetic, it is associated with lower carbon footprint [29].

Conservative management of some acute surgical illnesses is associated with lower carbon footprint when compared to operative management. This treatment approach was widely adopted during the COVID-19 pandemic for early appendicitis with low failure and complication rates [30]. However, operative management of certain conditions is the low carbon treatment option. For example, consider the potential resource burden and patient's quality of life impact linked with non-operative management of a painful, non-obstructed and non-strangulated hernia long term.

The increased environmental impact of robotic surgery compared to laparoscopic surgery is important to note. Robotic procedures have up to 43.5% more greenhouse gas emissions and 24% more waste when compared to their laparoscopic alternative [31]. This makes it important to ensure that robotic surgery is used when there is sufficient clinical benefit to outweigh this increased environmental impact.

Reusable equipment

Procurement and medical instruments are significant carbon hotspots in surgery [11]. Single-use equipment is the largest culprit for this [32]. Even when sterilisation and packaging are factored in, the carbon footprint of reusable instruments is lower than their single-use alternative [11].

Historical concerns of the spread of prion infection led to the surge in uptake of single use medical products [33]. However, now that the standards of cleaning and sterilisation of instruments have risen, current evidence shows no difference in surgical site infection when comparing reusable instruments to their single use equivalent [34]. Hybrid surgical devices (reusable instruments with single-use components) also show significant carbon savings when compared to single-use instruments [35]. By swapping single-use products for their reusable or hybrid alternatives, significant environmental savings and financial savings can be achieved [35,36].

Maintenance, repair and recycle

A transition from the current linear *'take, make and dispose'* approach of consumption to a model that embeds circular economy principles which promotes reuse, repair and recycling is required to maximise finite resources. This provides a sustainable solution to waste and avoids the manufacturing processes involved in acquiring raw materials.

PRACTICAL RECOMMENDATIONS FOR SUSTAINABLE CLINICAL PRACTICE

Based on the current evidence, several interventions are available within clinical practice to aid transition to more sustainable surgery.

Travel

Patient and staff travel to and from hospital contributes significantly to the carbon emissions of healthcare. In the UK, patient and staff travel are responsible for about 10% of the NHS carbon footprint [7]. Embracing the use of technology to facilitate video or telephone consultations in the form of virtual/remote clinics in suitable patients can help to reduce this. For example, patients with chronic conditions who do not require physical examination and already know the surgeon may benefit from this.

Staff can adopt active travel, engaging in car sharing and using public transportation to commute to work. Attending meetings remotely when appropriate can also facilitate the reduction of this carbon footprint.

Anaesthesia

The use of local or regional anaesthetic should be optimised in surgical practice. Operations carried out using general anaesthetic have a higher environmental impact when compared to regional or local anaesthetic [29]. This is to do with the inhaled anaesthetic gasses and intravenous medications required for general anaesthetic.

For operations that must be carried out using general anaesthetic, the choice of inhaled anaesthetic gas is important. Different anaesthetic gasses possess their distinct greenhouse warming potential (GWP) with desflurane having the highest [37]. These gasses with high GWP should be avoided. The Association of Anaesthetists and the Royal College of Anaesthetists in the UK have committed to decommissioning desflurane by 2024 [38]. Limiting the use of nitrous oxide is also important as it also has a high GWP [39]. Hospital nitrous oxide manifolds for operating theatres should be decommissioned due to their high-leak rate [40]. They can be replaced with local cylinders, if deemed necessary.

Waterless hand scrub

Water is a resource which is used in large amounts when scrubbing for surgery. A single preoperative traditional scrub uses approximately 18.5 L of water [41]. The adoption of waterless hand scrubs can potentially save millions of litres of water yearly. There is no difference in the antiseptic efficacies of alcohol-based waterless hand scrub and traditional chlorhexidine and iodine-based hand scrubs [42]. This saving will reduce the energy required to deliver and treat the water, therefore, having both financial and environmental benefits.

The National Institute for Health and Care Excellence (NICE) recommends that after the first traditional hand scrub of the day, waterless hand scrubs can be used for subsequent cases [43].

Energy conservation

The air-conditioning, heating and ventilation systems account for 90% of operating theatre energy consumption [13]. Switching these systems off or putting them on standby when operating theatres are not in use have the potential to halve their energy consumption [13]. The use of ultra clean air ventilation technology (used to generate laminar flow of air) for all orthopaedic operations should be questioned. The NICE recommends its use primarily for joint replacement surgery [44]. The selective use of this technology could reduce energy consumption associated with orthopaedic surgery [45].

Reusable textiles

Ensuring that surgical textiles such as surgical gowns, drapes and hats are reusable can reduce the carbon emissions associated with surgery. Not only is the use of reusable surgical gowns associated with less consumption of energy, water and solid waste generation [46], but due to better water resistance and durability, they can offer better protection [47]. With regard to sterility, the use of reusable surgical hats, drapes, and gowns has demonstrated no difference in the rate of surgical site infection when compared to their single use counterparts [48,49].

Responsible waste disposal

As much as we try to avoid the generation of waste in the first place, surgery will always generate some waste. The environmental impact of disposal is, therefore, important. Although this may vary slightly internationally, high temperature incineration of waste is the disposal method with the highest carbon footprint while recycling of waste has the lowest [50].

Less than 50% of recyclable waste in operating theatre from, e.g., equipment packaging, is not recycled [51]. Ensuring that waste segregation occurs appropriately by separating clinical from non-clinical waste will minimise the high energy processes that goes into disposing of clinical waste.

Intraoperative equipment

The regular review of pre-prepared instrument trays/sets for unused instruments is required to reduce unjustified waste that has financial implications. This has been demonstrated in some centres where there was up to 70% reduction in the surgical instruments per set, leading to significant cost savings and no safety issues [52].

Using the reusable or hybrid version of a surgical instrument reduces the carbon footprint linked with that procedure and is associated with cost savings in almost every circumstance [35,36]. Minimising the use of single use instrument is vital.

Opting for sutures instead of skin clips is linked with reduced environmental impact [18]. Skin staplers are usually made of plastic, are of single use, and usually require contact with the healthcare service for removal with clip removers, that are also single use.

Medical device remanufacturing, a process that restores a used device to 'as new' performance specifications, can be an important solution for some single use equipment that does not have reusable alternatives. This circular economy solution has been widely adopted in the USA for energy devices and appears to have significant financial and environmental benefits [53].

Optimise clinical interventions

Asking patients to empty their bladders in the immediate preoperative period can avoid the use of catheters in short operations. The potential environmental savings from this should not be underestimated, given that the degradation of catheters is poor, and leads to non-biodegradable waste [54].

The NICE advises against the routine use of antibiotic prophylaxis for clean, non-prosthetic surgery [43]. The carbon intense processes used in the manufacturing of antibiotics, together with the ecological risks brought about by improper disposal methods [55] make it essential that their use is guided by the evidence base. This will not only help to combat antibiotic resistance but help to lower the 5% of global healthcare carbon footprint for which pharmaceuticals are responsible [4].

A recognised illustration of sustainable surgery put into practice can be seen at Aravind Eye Care Systems, a tertiary care centre in southern India. Cataract surgery performed in Aravind Eye Care Systems highlights how lean service delivery and low carbon alternatives can minimise the carbon footprint of a procedure without compromising the quality of care delivered [56]. A lifecycle analysis of cataracts surgery performed in Aravind showed how by optimising operating theatre capacity, reusing surgical instruments and gowns, and identifying instruments to be sterilised between cases using a shorter autoclave cycle, the carbon footprint of cataracts surgery performed in Aravind per case is 5% of the same procedure carried out in the UK [56]. This Aravind model serves as a practical example for sustainable surgery.

FUTURE OF SUSTAINABILITY IN SURGERY

Sustainability within surgery is an emerging field. The journey to minimise the environmental impact of surgical services is challenging, requiring research, innovation and collaboration between clinical and non-clinical professionals, industry, and policy makers. Barriers, such as the lack of awareness, limited quality research and poor support from senior leadership in healthcare are gradually being lifted to allow sustainability within surgery to become more of a priority.

Sustainability is now becoming embedded within surgical research, education and quality improvement activities. To aid the embedding of emerging data into clinical practice, surgical organisations, and societies need to recognise sustainability as a domain of quality for improvement. This has already been done by the Royal College of Physicians in the UK who have officially included sustainability to their quality improvement domains [57]. This approach will embed sustainability into quality improvement and empower surgical teams to embark on sustainable quality improvement projects that help to implement sustainable changes in their nuclear environment.

Education and training about sustainability and sustainable quality improvement approaches within healthcare will be crucial in achieving the culture change required to reduce the environmental impact of surgery. Introducing basic training in carbon foot printing, e.g., could allow surgical teams to better identify surgical equipment manufacturers who claim to be environmentally conscious for marketing purposes when they, in fact, fail to have environmentally sustainable processes (so-called greenwashing). Surgeons have an active role in choosing suppliers and, therefore, influence industry. By leveraging this purchasing power, industry can be hastened into decarbonising their manufacturing processes and be encouraged to invest in innovative sustainable solutions.

Surgical processes in low- and middle-income countries need to be recognised as a potential source of sustainable surgical innovation by surgical organisations in high-income countries. The sometimes extremely finite resources available to low- and middle-income countries have forced frugal innovation in the design of their surgical pathways and infrastructure leading to efficient and low-carbon services [58]. Services with high-quality patient outcomes should be recognised and studied as they can provide a roadmap to sustainable surgery.

Understanding the impact of the low-cost driven globalised supply chain of surgical instruments is important. USA, Mexico, China, Malaysia, Pakistan and Costa Rica are some of the leading suppliers of surgical instruments to Europe [59]. A surgical suture can be subject to 23,000 km of air travel across three continents before reaching a local supplier [19]. Complex supply chains are also difficult to regulate for adequate labour and employment standards. For instance, the Pakistan surgical instrument manufacturing industry has been associated with widespread child labour, unjust contractual obligations and poor health and safety protections [59]. The Malaysian glove manufacturing industry is also associated with similar labour and occupational health violations. Despite the development of the Labour Standards Assurance Systems (LSAS) by the UK in 2011 to regulate NHS suppliers, these issues are still reported in Pakistani surgical instrument factories and Malaysian gloves factories that supply the NHS [59]. Surgeons will need to work with industry and policy makers to address the ethical and environmental issues the global surgical supply chain poses.

The future of surgery is moving towards integrating innovative technologies to improve patient's care. It is important that sustainability is embedded into the implementation of these technologies to avoid negating outstanding clinical gains. Robotic surgery is linked with very high amounts of greenhouse gas emissions and solid waste because of large amounts of consumables and disposable instruments [31]. Reducing its environmental impact by, e.g., designing reusable drapes for robots, needs to be prioritised as robotic surgery becomes more mainstream.

Surgical societies and organisations must display strong and supportive leadership by playing a significant role in advocating, educating, promoting and guiding the surgical speciality into an environmentally sustainable future. The Surgical Royal Colleges in the UK have taken the first step in demonstrating this by publishing the intercollegiate green theatre checklist [18]. Award schemes that celebrate and showcase sustainable surgical innovations and successful sustainable quality improvement projects such as the Centre for Sustainable Healthcare's Green Surgery Challenge [60] and the Green Hospitals Asian Conference annual award [61] can also encourage innovation and teamwork to facilitate sustainable change. Actions like this from more surgical organisations will help to drive the much-needed transition to a future of sustainable surgery.

CONCLUSION

The climate crisis requires urgent action from the healthcare sector and surgery must play a key role in reducing its environmental impact. Adopting the principles of sustainable surgery leads to actions that minimising waste, optimising energy use, increase adoption of low carbon alternatives and prioritises prevention. These actions significantly lower the carbon footprint of surgical care. Embracing reusable instruments, lean service delivery and patient education further supports this transition. Collaboration among surgeons, hospital management, policy makers and industry is essential to bring about this change. Sustainability must become a core pillar of surgical quality improvement, ensuring that high standards of patient care is in line with our environmental responsibility. Through innovation and commitment, the surgical community can lead the way towards a future of sustainable healthcare.

> **Key points for clinical practice**
> - Stop/Reduce single use items where possible and/or advocate for procuring/researching reusables where possible
> - Adopt low-carbon alternatives in surgical and anaesthetic practices
> - Optimise resource use, reduce waste and segregate waste appropriately
> - Turn off electrical devices when not in use to improve energy efficiency in operating theatres
> - Promote primary prevention and empower patients with condition specific education
> - Streamline surgical pathways to reduce inefficiencies and minimise unnecessary interventions
> - Advocate for sustainable procurement and ethical supply chains

REFERENCES

1. Blunden J, Boyer T. State of the Climate in 2020. Bull Am Meteorol Soc 2021; 102:S1–S475.
2. World Meteorological Organization. (2021). 2021 one of the seven warmest years on record, WMO consolidated data shows. World Meteorological Society. Available from: https://public.wmo.int/en/media/press-release/2021-one-of-seven-warmest-years-record-wmo-consolidated-data-shows (Last accessed 15th July 2025).
3. Romanello M, Napoli CD, Drummond P, et al. The 2022 report of the Lancet countdown on Health and Climate Change: Health at the mercy of Fossil Fuels. Lancet 2022; 400:1619–1654.
4. Arup and Health Care Without Harm. (2019). Health care's climate footprint. How the health sector contributes to the global climate crisis and opportunities for action. Health Care Without Harm. Available from: https://noharm-global.org/sites/default/files/documents-files/5961/HealthCaresClimateFootprint_092319.pdf (Last accessed 15th July 2025).
5. Intergovernmental Panel on Climate Change. (2021). Climate change 2021, the physical science basis. Intergovernmental Panel on Climate Change. Available from: https://www.ipcc.ch/report/sixth-assessment-report-working-group-i/ (Last accessed 15th July 2025).
6. Climate Emergency Declaration and Mobilisation in Action. Climate emergency declarations. Climate Emergency Declaration and Mobilisation in action. Available from: https://www.cedamia.org/global/ (Last accessed 15th July 2025).
7. NHS England. (2022). Delivering a 'Net Zero' National Health Service. National health service England. Available from: https://www.england.nhs.uk/greenernhs/wp-content/uploads/sites/51/2022/07/B1728-delivering-a-net-zero-nhs-july-2022.pdf (Last accessed 15th July 2025).
8. World Health Organisation. Alliance for Transformative Action on Climate and Health (ATACH). Country commitments. World Health Organisation. Available from: https://www-who-int.abc.cardiff.ac.uk/initiatives/alliance-for-transformative-action-on-climate-and-health/country-commitments (Last accessed 15th July 2025).
9. Mortimer F, Isherwood J, Wilkinson A, et al. Sustainability in quality improvement: redefining value. Future Healthcare J 2018; 5:88–93.
10. United Nations Framework Convention on Climate change. (2015). Paris Agreement. United Nations. Available from: https//unfccc.int/sites/default/files/english_paris_agreement.pdf (Last accessed 15th July 2025).
11. Rizan C, Steinbach I, Nicholson R, et al. The carbon footprint of operating theatres: a systematic review. Ann Surg 2020; 272:986–985.
12. Department for business, energy and industrial strategy and the department for environment, food and rural affairs. (2022). UK government GHG conversion factors for company reporting. Available from: https://www.gov.uk/government/publications/greenhouse-gas-reporting-conversion-factors-2022 (Last accessed 15th July 2025).
13. MacNeill A, Lillywhite R, Brown C. The impact of surgery on global climate: a carbon foot printing study of operating theatres in three health systems. Lancet Planetary Health 2017; 1:e381–e388.

14. Sustainable Development Unit. (2018). Reducing the use of natural resources in health and social care. Faculty of Public Health. Available from: https://www.fph.org.uk/media/3126/k9-fph-sig-nhs-carbon-footprint-final.pdf (Last accessed 15th July 2025).
15. Rigante L, Moudrous W, De Vries J, et al. Operating room waste: disposable supply utilization in neurointerventional procedures. Acta Neurochir 2017; 159:2337–2340.
16. Borrelle SB, Ringma J, Law KL, et al. Predicted growth in plastic waste exceeds efforts to mitigate plastic pollution. Science 2020; 369:1515–1518.
17. Royal College of Surgeons of England. (2022). Intercollegiate climate emergency declaration. Available from: https://www.rcseng.ac.uk/news-and-events/news/archive/intercollegiate-climate-emergency-declaration/ (Last accessed 15th July 2025).
18. Royal college of surgeons of England. (2022). Intercollegiate Green theatre checklist. Available from: https://www.rcseng.ac.uk/about-the-rcs/about-our-mission/sustainability-in-surgery/ (Last accessed 15th July 2025).
19. Rizan CR, Mortimer F, Jones A, et al. Using surgical sustainability principles to improve planetary health and optimise surgical services following the COVID-19 pandemic. Bull R Coll Surg Engl 2020; 102:177–181.
20. Mortimer F. The sustainable Physician. Clin Med 2010; 10:10–11.
21. Uimonen M, Kuitunen I, Paloneva J, et al. The impact of the COVID-19 pandemic on waiting times for elective surgery patients: A multicenter study. PLoS One 2021; 16:e0253875.
22. The Lancet Rheumatology. Too long to wait: the impact of COVID-19 on elective surgery. Lancet Rheumatol 2021; 3:e83.
23. Fu SJ, George EL, Maggio PM, et al. The Consequences of Delaying Elective Surgery: Surgical Perspective. Ann Surg 2020; 272:e79–e80.
24. Baid H, Holland J, Pirro F. Environmentally sustainable orthopaedics and trauma: systems and behaviour change. Orthopaed Trauma 2022; 36:256–264.
25. Mason SE, Nicolay CR, Darzi A. The use of Lean and Six Sigma methodologies in surgery: a systematic review. Surgeon 2015; 13:91–100.
26. Farrokhi FR, Gunther M, Williams B, et al. Application of Lean Methodology for Improved Quality and Efficiency in Operating Room Instrument Availability. J Healthcare Qual 2015; 37:277–286.
27. Balentine CJ, Meier J, Berger M, et al. Using local rather than general anaesthesia for inguinal hernia repair is associated with shorter operative time and enhanced postoperative recovery. Am J Surg 2021; 221:902–907.
28. Memtsoudis SG, Cozowicz C, Bekeris J, et al. Anaesthetic care of patients undergoing primary hip and knee arthroplasty: consensus recommendations from the International Consensus on Anaesthesia-Related Outcomes after Surgery group (ICAROS) based on a systematic review and meta-analysis. Br J Anaesth 2019; 123:269–287.
29. Lopes R, Shelton C, Charlesworth M. Inhalational anaesthetics, ozone depletion, and greenhouse warming: the basics and status of our efforts in environmental mitigation. Curr Opin Anaesthesiol 2021; 34:415–420.
30. Emile SH, Hamid KS, Khan SM, et al. Rate of Application and Outcome of Non-operative Management of Acute Appendicitis in the Setting of COVID-19: Systematic Review and Meta-analysis. J Gastrointest Surg 2021; 25:1905–1915.
31. Papadopoulou A, Kumar SN, Vanhoestenberghe A, et al. Environmental sustainability in robotic and laparoscopic surgery: systematic review. Br J Surg 2022; 109:921–932.
32. Thiel CL, Woods NC, Bilec MM. Strategies to reduce greenhouse gas emissions from laparoscopic surgery. Am J Pub Health 2018; 108:S158–S164.
33. Bhutta MF. Our over-reliance on single-use equipment in the operating theatre is misguided, irrational and harming our planet. Ann R Coll Surg Engl 2021; 103:709–712.
34. Siu J, Hill AG, MacCormick AD. Systematic review of reusable versus disposable laparoscopic instruments: Costs and safety. ANZ J Surg 2018; 87:28–33.
35. Rizan C, Bhutta MF. Environmental impact and life cycle financial cost of hybrid (reusable/single-use) instruments versus single-use equivalents in laparoscopic cholecystectomy. Surg Endoscopy 2021; 36:4067–4078.
36. Drew J, Christie SD, Tyedmers P, et al. Operating in a Climate Crisis: A State-of-the-Science Review of Life Cycle Assessment within Surgical and Anesthetic Care. Environ Health Perspect 2021; 129:76001.
37. Ryan SM, Nielsen CJ. Global warming potential of inhaled anaesthetics: application to clinical use. Anesth Analg 2010; 111:92–98.

38. Association of Anaesthetists. (2023). Joint statement on NHSE's plan to decommission desflurane by early 2024. Available from: https://anaesthetists.org/Home/News-opinion/News/Joint-statement-on-NHSEs-plan-to-decommission-desflurane-by-early-2024 (Last accessed 15th July 2025).
39. Muret J, Fernandes TD, Gerlach H, et al. Environmental impacts of nitrous oxide: no laughing matter. Comment on Br J Anaesth 2019; 122:587–604. Br J Anaesth 2019;123:e481–e482.
40. Chakera A, Fannell-Wells A, Allen C. (2021). Piped Nitrous Oxide Waste Reduction Strategy. Association of Anaesthetists. Available from: https://anaesthetists.org/Home/Resources-publications/Environment/Nitrous-oxide-project (Last accessed 15th July 2025).
41. Wormer BA, Augenstein VA, Carpenter SL, et al. The green operating room: simple changes to reduce cost and our carbon footprint. Am Surg 2013; 79:666–671.
42. Ho YH, Wang YC, Loh EW, et al. Antiseptic efficacies of waterless hand rub, chlorhexidine scrub, and povidone-iodine scrub in surgical settings: a meta-analysis of randomized controlled trials. J Hosp Infect 2019; 101:370–379.
43. National Institute for Health and Clinical Excellence (NICE). (2019). Surgical Site Infections: prevention and treatment (NG125). National institute of Health and Clinical Excellence. Available from: https://www.nice.org.uk/guidance/ng125/resources/surgical-site-infections-prevention-and-treatment-pdf-66141660564421 (Last accessed 15th July 2025).
44. National Institute for Health and Clinical Excellence (NICE). (2019) Joint replacement (primary): hip, knee and shoulder. Evidence review for ultra clean-air. Available from: https://www.nice.org.uk/guidance/ng157/documents/evidence-review-9 (Last accessed 15th July 2025).
45. Jesudason EP. Pushing sustainability up the surgical agenda: practical steps towards sustainable orthopaedic care. Orthopaed Trauma 2022; 36:274–278.
46. Vozzola E, Overcash M, Griffing E. An Environmental Analysis of Reusable and Disposable Surgical Gowns. Aorn j 2020; 111:315–325.
47. McQuerry M, Easter E, Cao A. Disposable versus reusable medical gowns: A performance comparison. Am J Infect Control 2021; 49:563–570.
48. Overcash MR, Sehulster LM. Estimated incidence rate of healthcare-associated infections (HAIs) linked to laundered reusable healthcare textiles (HCTs) in the United States and United Kingdom over a 50-year period: Do the data support the efficacy of approved laundry practices? Infect Control Hosp Epidemiol 2021:1–2.
49. Haskins IN, Prabhu AS, Krpata DM, et al. Is there an association between surgeon hat type and 30-day wound events following ventral hernia repair? Hernia 2017; 21:495–503.
50. Rizan C, Bhutta MF, Reed M, et al. The carbon footprint of waste streams in a UK hospital. J Clean Prod 2021; 286:125446.
51. Pegg M, Rawson R, Okere U. Operating room waste management: A case study of primary hip operations at a leading national health service hospital in the United Kingdom. J Health Serv Res Policy 2022; 27:255–260.
52. Dekonenko C, Oyetunji TA, Rentea RM. Surgical tray reduction for cost saving in pediatric surgical cases: a qualitative systematic review. J Pediatr Surg 2020; 55:2435–2441.
53. Unger S, Landis A. Assessing the environmental, human health, and economic impacts of reprocessed medical devices in a Phoenix hospital's supply chain. J Clean Prod 2016; 112:1995–2003.
54. Sun AJ, Comiter CV, Elliott CS. The cost of a catheter: An environmental perspective on single use clean intermittent catheterization. Neurourol Urodyn 2018; 37:2204–2208.
55. Apreja M, Sharma A, Balda S, et al. Antibiotic residues in environment: antimicrobial resistance development, ecological risks, and bioremediation. Environ Sci Pollut Res Int 2022; 29:3355–3371.
56. Thiel CL, Schehlein E, Ravilla T, et al. Cataract surgery and environmental sustainability: Waste and lifecycle assessment of phacoemulsification at a private healthcare facility. J Cataract Refract Surg 2017; 43:1391–1398.
57. Royal College of Physicians. (2017). Defining the RCP's approach to quality. Royal College of Physicians. Available from: https://www-rcplondon-ac-uk.abc.cardiff.ac.uk/defining-rcp-s-approach-quality (Last accessed 15th July 2025).
58. Steyn A, Cassels-Brown A, Chang DF, et al. Frugal innovation for global surgery: leveraging lessons from low- and middle-income countries to optimise resource use and promote value-based care. Bull R Coll Surg Engl 2020; 150:198–200.
59. Trueba ML, Bhutta MF, Shahvisi A. Instruments of Health and harm: How the procurement of healthcare goods contributes to global health inequality. J Med Ethics 2020; 47:423–429.

60. Centre for sustainable healthcare. (2022). Green Surgery Challenge. Centre for Sustainable Healthcare. Available from: https://sustainablehealthcare.org.uk/what-we-do/green-surgery-challenge (Last accessed 15th July 2025).
61. Green Hospitals Asia Conference. (2022). Video competition. Green Hospitals Asia Conference. Available from: https://www.ghacindia2023.com/video-competition (Last accessed 15th July 2025).

Chapter 2

Optimisation prior to surgery

Gregory Warren, Scarlett McNally

ABSTRACT

There is overwhelming evidence that preoperative preparation can reduce complications of surgery by around 50% and length of stay by 1–2 days (including potential day surgery options).

Seven interventions are proven to reduce complications: Smoking cessation, exercise, nutrition, alcohol moderation, medication and senior clinician review, psychological preparation, and practical preparation.

An operation is a 'teachable moment'. All perioperative staff should learn motivational interviewing. Early screening helps to detect modifiable risk factors and target interventions. Functional capacity may be tested formally or simply.

Frailty, diabetes, anaemia and multiple comorbidities increase complication risk several-fold. Resources at www.cpoc.org.uk can assist management of these.

INTRODUCTION

In recent decades, surgical techniques have become ever more refined and data collection has contributed to improved outcomes, reducing unwarranted variation between surgeons and units. Within the population, however, there is increasing comorbidity and ill-health. These contribute greatly to the risks of surgery. The model of the patient as a passive recipient of care persists. While all patients have a form of preassessment before surgery, this can be focussed on documentation rather than optimisation. Many risks are modifiable. There is a finite number of options to improve outcomes. It is far better if the whole team contributes to optimisation of every patient. Every opportunity should be used for this. Complications occur in 10–15% of operations [1]. Up to 14% of patients express regret after surgery [2]. People living with frailty [3], or those who are physically inactive [4], have four times the rate of complications. Even in patients presenting for emergency or urgent surgery, there are factors which can be optimised. The concept of 'perioperative

---

Gregory Warren MBBS BSc PGCert FRCA, Consultant Anaesthetist, Torbay, UK
E-mail: Gregory.warren1@nhs.net

Scarlett McNally MB BChir, Consultant Orthopaedic surgeon, Eastbourne, UK
E-mail: scarlett.mcnally@nhs.net (for correspondence)

care' involves improving multiple small steps, akin to marginal gains in a 'Formula One racing car' team strategy. In the UK, the Centre for Perioperative Care (www.cpoc.org.uk) has evidence [5] that a perioperative approach reduces complications by 50%, length of stay by 1–2 days and critical care requirements. It also improves patient's satisfaction and staff morale. There are seven aspects of preoperative optimisation that can reduce complications by around 50%: Smoking cessation, nutrition, exercise, alcohol moderation, medication review with medical assessment, psychological preparedness with attention to mental health and physical preparedness.

Ten million surgical procedures occur every year in the UK [6]. Many complications are predictable and to some extent preventable. Over 250,000 of these patients are categorised as 'high risk', with a risk of death of over 5% [7]. In the UK, 50% of operations [7] that require a general or regional anaesthetic are performed in patients over the age of 65 years, a cohort where 41% are classified as completely physically inactive [8] and 62% have two or more long-term conditions [9]. The greatest reduction in risk occurs for people moving from completely inactive to moderately inactive, so every intervention is worth achieving.

Who is optimisation aimed at?

Every person who is contemplating surgery should ensure they are optimised physically and mentally for the surgery. The healthcare team and their family should support this. A screening assessment should be undertaken early, e.g. when the patient is referred to a surgeon. Some organisations collect screening information from the patient in the outpatient clinic. This allows time to prepare. The waiting list should be considered a preparation list [10].

Shared decision making (SDM) should be undertaken for every patient – especially where the risks and benefits are delicately balanced. This involves the patient discussing with a senior clinician the *B*enefits, *R*isks, *A*lternatives and do-*N*othing option, or 'BRAN' [11]. When older patients discuss their options with a senior geriatrician, 15% decide not to proceed with surgery [12]. This also reduces complications and regret.

Patients undergoing cancer treatment should also prepare – the Macmillan programme reported that patients found this empowering [13].

All patients should be offered general advice. Screening should identify those who would benefit from targeted advice. Improving fitness and readiness for surgery in all patients may also allow many to be considered for 'Day Case' surgery. There is currently a two-fold variation in between regions for similar procedures in whether a patient is admitted overnight or treated as a day case. More day surgery is better for patients and more efficient for the service.

How should optimisation be delivered?

Even patients on an emergency or urgent pathway can benefit from optimisation. This may involve organisations developing pathways to anticipate care needs. For example, pain management for patients with hip fractures can be optimised by having the facility to offer a fascia iliaca block preoperatively instead of opiates, to improve postoperative breathing and cognition.

For elective or planned patients, the preoperative assessment clinic (POAC) appointment can occur too late to maximise opportunities. Optimisation should be built into the pathways. Early screening of each patient should be monitored to identify how much intervention to start. Most patients should receive general advice, such as in a nurse-led service, supplemented by other resources [14]. Some organisations use a group 'surgery school' to advise and optimise patients, particularly for orthopaedic procedures. These are more effective when they are localised and personalised to the patient. Some use Apps or other services. Screening should identify patients who are at high-risk and they should be offered specialist medical review. This should include SDM – whether the operation should occur, which risk factors are fixed and which are modifiable, and what interventions to try for optimisation.

All staff should be taught motivational interviewing, using resources at www.movingmedicine.ac.uk or 'Making Every Contact Count.' This is part of a 'Trans-Disciplinary approach' [15] with all perioperative staff sharing simple skills, rather than a 'multidisciplinary team' approach which can mean patients wait for a specialist who may not be available.

SCREENING AND RISK ASSESSMENT

Screening uses a set of questions or investigations designed to have the discriminative quality to identify those at increased risk of adverse health outcomes, who may benefit from individualised risk assessment and optimisation. The earlier in the perioperative pathway this happens, the longer a patient has to address risk factors. The Australian and New Zealand College of Anaesthetists and the UK-based Centre for Perioperative Care (CPOC) have both set out standards for preoperative assessment [16,17] and optimisation, which recommend initial patient screening via an electronic questionnaire. Once validated by a POAC nurse, this will enable streaming of patients into a nurse led clinic (virtual or face to face), or toward a physician led clinic for high-risk patients.

Screening measures are also used to highlight those at risk of undiagnosed conditions such as anaemia, sleep disordered breathing, frailty, cognitive impairment, nutritional deficiencies and difficult to manage pain. If undiagnosed, or poorly controlled in the perioperative period, these contribute to an elevated perioperative risk profile.
All patients should have, and be informed about, an individualised risk assessment. For example, a risk model such as the 'Surgical Outcomes Risk Tool (SORT)' can be performed instantly on www.sortsurgery.com, in addition to experienced clinical judgement and an estimate of 30-day mortality can be calculated.

Patients who are at lower risk of complications, due to their preoperative status or the minor nature of surgery, can proceed with standard perioperative care involving generic advice.

FUNCTIONAL CAPACITY

A patient's functional capacity is the term used to describe their ability to perform daily tasks or exert themselves. Functional capacity is a surrogate marker of the aerobic capacity of a patient, or how well patients can match an increase in demand for oxygen, with an increased supply. This is reduced in many disease states and declines with age [18].

There is a focus on functional capacity because it has been shown to predict outcomes in terms of complications, length of stay and mortality and, therefore, plays an important role in identifying those patients at high risk, due to poor physiological reserve.

Functional capacity can be assessed subjectively via simple questionnaires, such as the DASI (Duke Activity Status Index). This is a validated measure of cardiopulmonary fitness and uses self-reported maximum activity levels to estimate a peak oxygen consumption in terms of 'metabolic equivalents' or METs. One MET is equal to basal metabolic rate at 3.5 mL/O_2/kg/min being consumed. The score has been shown to predict adverse outcomes such as mortality, myocardial ischaemia and complications [19].

A low score on the DASI questionnaire should prompt objective measurement of a patient's functional capacity, whereby a patient is asked to exercise in a monitored environment. The gold standard assessment method is cardiopulmonary exercise testing (CPET). Simpler measures may be used that do not require specialist equipment. These include the 6-minute walk test (6MWT), incremental shuttle walk test, timed up and go and 'sit to stand in 1 minute' test. They all involve repetitions of an activity within a time limit. Distance achieved, or number of repetitions can provide insight into fitness. Staff are encouraged to use these to help patients to set goals for prehabilitation.

Perioperative CPET has a number of indications and values derived from CPET have been shown to predict all-cause mortality [20], prolonged length of stay [21] and 5-year survival [22]. Along with its role in risk stratification to inform SDM and appropriate level of postoperative care, it can guide prehabilitation and rehabilitation programmes and diagnose occult cardiac or respiratory disease [23]. While a full review of CPET conduct and interpretation is beyond the scope of this chapter, the following is a brief description of the basic principles and indices obtained.

Cardiopulmonary exercise testing is a noninvasive assessment of the cardiopulmonary system at rest and exercise [24]. Most commonly, the patient sits on a cycle ergometer and standard monitoring is attached, along with a mouthpiece which measures inspired and expired oxygen and carbon dioxide, along with gas flow. This enables calculation of oxygen consumption (VO_2) and carbon dioxide production (VCO_2). The test lasts approximately 15 minutes and following a period of unloaded cycling, the patient pedals against a resistance, which ramps up with time, in order to achieve maximal effort around the 10-minute mark.

Monitoring enables tracking of the physiological response to exercise. During aerobic exercise, healthy individuals generate an increase in heart rate and stroke volume, which increases cardiac output linearly with oxygen demand. There is also a linear increase in carbon dioxide production which drives a rise in minute ventilation (VE), a product of respiratory rate and tidal volume. Plotting these variables over work, time or each other allows interpretation of physiological response to exercise. **Table 2.1** highlights three variables which are commonly used to assess risk. The patient is also monitored for the presence of any inducible ischaemia on ECG or fall in peripheral oxygen saturation, which may warrant further investigation.

An experienced clinician brings together information about a patient's comorbidities, magnitude of surgery and measures of functional capacity, with a subjective global assessment, to form the basis of individualised assessment of risk. This is usually expressed in terms of the likelihood of dying within 30 days of the proposed surgical procedure, or inability to get back to a preoperative functional baseline. This is then discussed with the patient in the context of their wishes, as part of SDM. It is also important to consider modifiable risk factors and fixed risk factors. Patients can improve their fitness with regular exercise and a medical review may help to optimise medical conditions. Earlier SDM conversations allow patients time to consider what their goals are.

Table 2.1 Overview of cardiopulmonary exercise testing (CPET) variables

CPET index	Explanation	Clinical use	Notable values
Peak VO_2 (mL/kg/min)	Peak rate of oxygen consumption (mL/kg/min) oxygen consumption at point test is terminated	May be unreliable – dependent on effort and engagement of true fitness	Peak VO_2 < 15 mL O_2/kg/min = greater risk of perioperative complications [21]
Anaerobic threshold (AT) (mL/kg/min)	• Oxygen consumption (mL/kg/min) (VO_2) when anaerobic metabolism takes over from aerobic metabolism • Anaerobic respiration produces lactic acid, buffered by bicarbonate, causes a step increase in CO_2 production	• AT occurs before peak VO_2 • AT is less effort dependent • After AT, CO_2 production increases more steeply than O_2 consumption (Aerobic, O_2 consumption = CO_2 production)	AT < 10.2 mL O_2/kg/min has greater risk of perioperative complications [25]
$VE/VECO_2$	• Ventilatory efficiency = Minute ventilation divided by CO_2 production • If a high-minute ventilation is required to breathe off a lower level of CO_2 production, this is inefficient and can highlight ventilatory insufficiency	*For example:* A patient with respiratory disease will have a higher minute ventilation for a given level of CO_2 production due to impaired gas exchange in lungs	$VE/VECO_2$ > 34 is associated with adverse perioperative outcomes [20]

EXERCISE

Major surgery represents a premeditated physiological stress which is comparable to running a marathon [26]. Surgical trauma elicits a proportionate cascade of homeostatic responses known collectively as the stress response. Impulses travelling along afferent nerves and release of cytokines from the site of trauma stimulate the hypothalamic-pituitary-adrenal (HPA) axis, leading to increased sympathetic tone and a range of haemodynamic, endocrine and immune responses. The body enters a state of hypercatabolism which mobilises stores of carbohydrate, fat and protein for use as energy and tissue repair substrate [27]. Upregulation of the immune system leads to local and systemic inflammation with activation of the innate and adaptive immune response. Overall, cell metabolic activity increases oxygen consumption within the tissues by 50% for several days after surgery [28]. Efforts to maintain an increased delivery of oxygen to tissues drives haemodynamic compensation via tachycardia, hypertension and water retention. Inability to meet this prolonged increase in oxygen demand may place organs or tissues into oxygen debt. Blood is redistributed towards muscles; splanchnic vasoconstriction further renders the gut and kidneys vulnerable to ischaemia, which may increase risk of anastomotic breakdown or kidney injury. Patients with coronary artery disease are at an increased risk of myocardial ischaemia, due to increased cardiac workload and blood viscosity.

How well this stress response is tolerated will depend on a patient's ability to withstand the catabolic nature of the stress response, without decompensating or losing the ability to perform activities of daily living and dipping into a more dependent state. This will largely be determined by preoperative physical reserve of the patient, i.e. how much muscle they can lose without impacting their functional capacity [29].

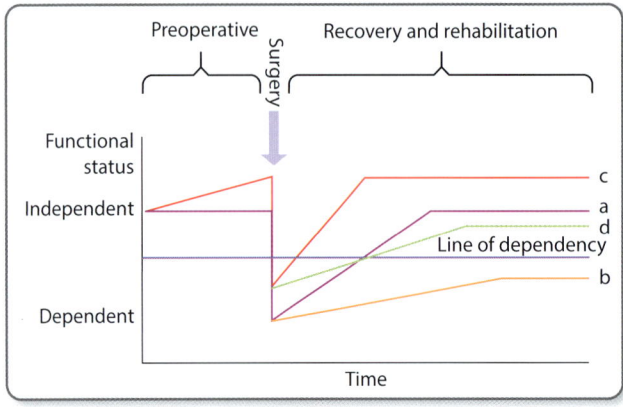

Figure 2.1 The prehabilitation concept. (a) All patients undergoing surgery experience a reduction in functional status postoperatively followed by a recovery period. (b) Patients suffering a complication may experience a slower and incomplete recovery threatening longer-term independence. (c) Prehabilitated patients are better placed to cope. (d) Should a complication occur, prehabilitation might be crucial to safeguarding longer-term functional status and independence [1].
Adapted from Durrand J, Singh SJ, Danjoux G. Prehabilitation. Clin Med 2019; 19:6.

Exercise programmes aim to prepare patients for this impending marathon by increasing both their physical reserve and metabolic capacity, i.e. their ability to keep up with metabolic demands. **Figure 2.1** represents the benefits of prehabilitation for patients in terms of functional status over the perioperative period.

Surgery presents an opportunity to support patients to make positive lifestyle changes. When discussed in the context of the potential for risk reduction and better recovery during the perioperative period, this added motivation can have positive effects on adherence to lifestyle changes leading up to surgery and beyond [30]. With one-third of adults in the UK classed as physically inactive [31], harnessing the power of the 'teachable moment' will form an important part of engaging them with exercise programmes.

Advice on exercise in line with the Chief Medical Officer's 2019 recommendations [32] should be given to all those undergoing surgery, along with information on the benefits of improved physical fitness on postoperative complications, length of hospital stay and quality of life (QoL) [17].

Targeted preoperative exercise training programmes should be offered to all patients undergoing elective major surgery. Where resources are limited, these services may be prioritised to those at high risk of complications, such as those with low cardiorespiratory fitness, those who have comorbidities that may be improved with exercise, those having preoperative chemo- or radiotherapy or patients over 70 years old [33]. Advancing age is associated with decreased physical activity, aerobic fitness and lean muscle mass (sarcopaenia), which is an independent risk factor for poor outcomes [34], and prevents postoperative mobilisation. Preoperative exercise training should be part of a multimodal approach to prehabilitation including medical optimisation, smoking cessation, psychological preparedness, nutrition and alcohol reduction as discussed further in this chapter. In order to track response to training and evaluate services, training programmes are bookended by pre- and postintervention assessment of fitness, e.g. CPET or 6MWT and QoL.

Healthcare professionals should have a basic understanding of the importance of exercise training and how to explore knowledge and beliefs to help an individual patient to get started, perhaps using resources at www.movingmedicine.ac.uk. Time should be taken to discuss the benefits of training programmes such as reduced complications [35], tumour regression [36] and improved QoL [33]. An exercise programme should be presented to the patient as an integral part of their perioperative pathway rather than an optional add-on.

Patients should have a simple screening for the few contraindications to exercise, including uncontrolled cardiovascular disease (aortic stenosis, hypertension, unstable angina and arrhythmias) or current acute illness. This can also provide an opportunity to assess and optimise medical comorbidities. Exercise training is recognised as a safe intervention, with no serious adverse events reported in a recent literature review [33]. It is advised that initial exercise sessions take place under supervision of professionals, with appropriate expertise due to improved adherence, which may be in a community facility. Simply encouraging patients to be active every day and add strength (e.g. sit to stand in 1 minute) may have value in motivated patients. Formal exercise plans tend to include a mixture of aerobic, resistance and inspiratory muscle training with the proportion of each modality tailored to an individual patient's preoperative status and risk profile.

- *Aerobic exercise* – increases cardiorespiratory fitness, typically 3–7 sessions per week. Variations include: 'Moderate continuous' (sustained below anaerobic threshold) or 'High-intensity interval training' includes exercising above their AT. Consider a target of maximum heart rate or level of exertion or breathlessness (rated numerically via the Borg scale). Examples: Cycle ergometer, treadmill or cross trainer.
- *Resistance training* – two to four times per week, develops lean muscle mass. This preserves strength, hence, reducing falls or decline in functional capacity [33]. Uses body weight, elastic resistance bands or fixed resistance machines focus on improving functional strength required to stand from sitting or climb stairs.
- *Inspiratory muscle training* – reduces postoperative pulmonary complications and morbidity [37]. Patients are trained to breathe against a fixed resistance with an inspiratory threshold device.

Exercise training should be commenced as early as possible in the patient journey for the greatest effect. Meaningful improvements in fitness can be attained in as little as 2 [38] to 4 [39] weeks, with the least fit patients making the most rapid improvements. Interval training has been shown to increase fitness in less time than moderate continuous training [40]. Evidence also suggests that exercise training can reverse the negative impacts of neoadjuvant chemoradiotherapy on physical fitness, in the short period between completion and surgery [41].

Supporting patients to set goals, keep an exercise diary, identify barriers to exercise and partake in supervised sessions, will improve motivation and compliance with exercise plans. Providing written information and signposting to exercise resources and support groups will also help. There is evidence to suggest that positive changes made in the perioperative period are more likely be sustained following recovery [26].

MEDICAL OPTIMISATION

The proportion of older people varies by country. Over half of emergency colorectal operations in the USA are performed on elderly patients [42] and by 2030, it is predicted that 20% of UK patients over the age of 75 years will undergo surgery each year [43]. Increased age is associated with inactivity, comorbidity and multisystem conditions such as frailty [44].

Patients will, therefore, present with the primary surgical problem accompanied by a range of long-term conditions, which will require optimisation and management throughout their surgical journey. In the UK, 62% of people over 65 have multiple medical conditions [9], which is an independent risk factor for poor surgical outcomes, including complications after surgery. Frailty alone is associated with a five-fold increase in complications [3]. Elderly patients, therefore, comprise the majority of patients classified as 'high risk'.

The components of effective medical optimisation include recognition of comorbidities, assessment of disease control, holistic review of the patient, medication review and management of specific comorbidities. This process includes the multidisciplinary perioperative team and should commence in primary care, as soon as surgery is contemplated [17]. When completing a surgical referral, primary care practitioners will ideally include a minimum level of information including BMI, cardiovascular observations, recent haemoglobin (Hb), glycosylated haemoglobin (HbA1c) and an assessment of frailty, e.g. Rockwood clinical frailty score [45]. This should prompt pre-emptive review and optimisation of any poorly controlled comorbidities in the community.

Patients with mutimorbidity, old age or associated conditions such as frailty and cognitive impairment, require a holistic review of their medical, functional and psychosocial domains and benefit from referral to a specialist multidisciplinary geriatric service [e.g. POPS (46)]. This is achieved via methodologies such as comprehensive geriatric assessment (CGA) during which investigations and discussion can occur at a single clinic visit. These services are well placed to facilitate high-quality SDM which leads to 15% of older people deciding against surgery following discussion [12]. Output from CGA ranges from new diagnoses, rationalisation of polypharmacy, lifestyle advice and therapeutic interventions [12]. CGA also aligns well with multimodal prehabilitation programmes and, when integrated into perioperative pathways, can reduce duplication of work.

Poorly controlled comorbidities increase perioperative risk by contributing to inactivity, poor physical fitness and functional status. A common health belief in patients with long-term conditions is that their condition precludes them from exercise. On the contrary, exercise can reduce dementia, diabetes, bowel cancer and depression by over 30% and improve health in these and almost all other long-term conditions [47].

Some conditions will predispose patients to specific risks and require appropriate management plans for the perioperative period, such as those listed in **Table 2.2** along with obstructive sleep apnoea and those at increased risk of poor perioperative pain control [17]. It is important to integrate best practice guidelines for standardised management of these conditions into perioperative pathways, to ensure timely detection and management by teams with appropriate expertise.

Nutrition

Preoperative malnutrition is common and is present in up to 65% of patients undergoing general surgery [51]. It is important to detect, manage and prevent malnutrition throughout the perioperative pathway. Poor preoperative nutritional state is an independent risk factor for infection, mortality, length of stay and increased healthcare costs [52].

As discussed previously, the stress response to surgery leads to a catabolic state, where proteins are broken down into constituent amino acids for synthesis of glucose, inflammatory proteins and immune factors leading to loss of mass from skeletal muscle, respiratory and gut tissues [53]. This catabolic state may remain elevated for

Table 2.2 Medical optimisation of anaemia, diabetes and frailty

Comorbidity	Rationale for optimisation	Key principles for preoperative optimisation
Anaemia *Source:* CPOC anaemia guideline [48]	• >1/3 having major surgery are anaemic preoperatively • <3 times rate of complications • As an independent risk factor, anaemia causes 20% more complications • Poorer wound healing, slower mobilisation and an increased risk of death • Blood transfusion itself carries risks	Use 'patient blood management': *Detection/management of anaemia:* • Diagnose early, investigate cause • Consider oral iron. Works in 4 weeks but is poorly absorbed from the gut in inflammation • Nutritional advice and patient's information • Consider IV iron when oral iron is ineffective, contraindicated or not tolerated or if the procedure is within 4 weeks *Minimisation of blood loss:* • Manage anticoagulants and antiplatelets • Consider tranexamic acid or cell salvage Optimise the patient's physiological tolerance of anaemia
Diabetes *Source:* CPOC [49]	• 15% of all operative procedures are in patients with diabetes • Diabetes can increase length of stay by 3 days postoperatively • HbA1c > 69 mmol/mol is associated infections, poor wound healing and increased length of stay • Patients must have access to day surgery and not be presumed to be high risk	*Standardised referral form including:* • HbA1c within 3 months of referral • Control comorbidities and medications If HbA1c > 69 mmol/mol (8.5%) refer for optimisation *Individualised plan:* • Pre- and postsurgery medication changes • Day surgery if possible *On admission:* • Ensure medicines reconciliation • Use preoperative plan • Maintain CBG at 6–12 mmol/L • Minimise fasting period
Frailty *Source:* CPOC and BGS Frailty Guidelines [50]	• 300,000 older people living with frailty undergo surgery each year • Frailty leads to increased rates of postoperative hospital acquired geriatric syndromes, complications, mortality and adverse patient reported outcomes such as quality of life and loss of independence • Perioperative complications common with frailty (e.g. delirium, falls, hospital acquired deconditioning and complex discharge issues)	*Primary care referral:* • Start SDM including nonsurgical options • Make Every Contact Count; medical and lifestyle optimisation • Referral to include frailty score, presence, severity and management of comorbidities. Presence of advance directives or power of attorney for health and welfare *Surgical and preoperative assessment outpatient services:* • Use information from primary care • Reassess and document frailty • Refer to perioperative frailty team/other services for optimisation • Discuss patient's wishes and agree treatment escalation plan • Undertake SDM including discussion about nonsurgical and palliative surgical options • Plan admission and discharge

months following surgery. Malnourished patients and those with sarcopaenia are less able to cope with the multifactorial reduction in lean muscle mass and clinically, this may manifest in falls, loss of independence and delayed discharge from hospital due to social concerns.

Early detection of malnutrition requires routine screening for risk factors that predispose a patient to poor nutritional status. Available clinical tools include the Malnutrition

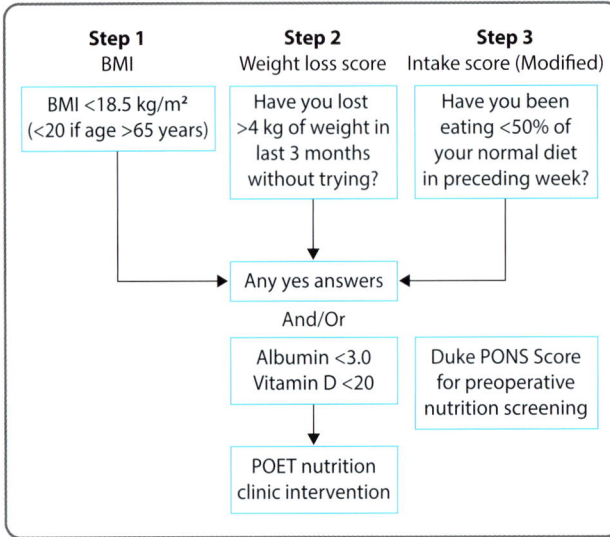

Figure 2.2 Duke university preoperative nutrition score (PONS). Any score ≥1 signifies malnutrition risk, and the patient should receive preoperative nutrition therapy before undergoing surgery. (POET) Perioperative enhancement team [54]; Albumin 3.0 is in units of g/dL, which equates to 30 g/L, vitamin D units of ng/mL.
Adapted from Gillis C, Wischmeyer PE. Pre-operative nutrition and the elective surgical patient: why, how and what? Anaesthesia 2019; 74(S1):27–35.

Universal Screening Tool and the Perioperative nutrition score which is based on MUST but adapted for perioperative use including serum albumin (**Figure 2.2**) [54].

If possible, patients with or at risk of malnutrition should be referred to a dietician for a comprehensive nutrition assessment, which includes a personalised approach to nutrition. Surgical patients will have a variety of reasons for inadequate nutrition such as inflammation, low absorption, difficulty swallowing, nausea and mechanical obstruction. A personalised management plan, which aims to overcome barriers to nutrition, may include high-protein diet, oral nutritional supplements and fortified foods or enteral/parenteral nutrition [54].

Recovery from surgery depends on adequate preoperative nutritional reserve to support stress induced catabolism. Transitioning from a protein deficit to an overall increase in body protein facilitates protein anabolism, which is essential in maintaining lean mass. This can be achieved by optimising dietary protein intake in line with recommendations of 1.2–1.6 g/kg/day which will stimulate muscle growth on its own. Pairing this with a resistance training programme exerts an independent and additive effect on protein anabolism [54].

Obese patients should not be assumed to be well-nourished and their assessment and management should take a multidisciplinary approach. Obesity-related sarcopaenia exists and confers its own challenges, leading to increased morbidity and mortality. Fat infiltration into muscle (myosteatosis) is a marker of muscle quality and predicts a longer length of admission [55].

Smoking cessation

Smoking cessation remains the single most important intervention in terms of perioperative risk reduction. One quarter of surgical patients smoke [56] and the behaviours of those who remain active smokers, despite widely publicised adverse effects, may be harder to change [57]. Smoking has been consistently linked to increased risk of poor wound healing, surgical site infection postoperative pulmonary and cardiovascular complications [58].

Smoking has well-documented adverse effects on both respiratory and cardiovascular physiology and immune response, which limit a patient's ability to meet metabolic demands in the perioperative period and underpin complications secondary to impaired oxygen delivery, immune function and sputum clearance. Evidence suggests that cessation 4 weeks prior to surgery leads to a reduction in complications. However, even smoking cessation 24 hours prior to surgery will increase oxygen carrying capacity of the blood and reduce cardiac workload [58].

All healthcare workers have a responsibility to engage with patients on the risks of smoking and offer appropriate support for cessation. This should remain a key message from contemplation of surgery throughout the patient journey. Ideally, prehabilitation services will include a smoking cessation support team, or have formed links with community initiatives. Behaviour changes in the perioperative period can lead to sustained abstinence from smoking [58].

Interventions to affect change in behaviour in smokers usually include advice, support and nicotine replacement therapy. Programmes classified as either low or high intensity, with the latter including weekly contact with patients, both have evidence supporting an effect on cessation [58]. The introduction of devices for monitoring exhaled carbon monoxide has shown increases in willingness to quit and referral to smoking cessation services [59]. Carbon monoxide monitors can be easily integrated into preoperative assessment services and used as a fulcrum around which to base smoking cessation efforts.

Alcohol reduction

Hazardous levels of alcohol intake cover a broad spectrum, ranging from drinking more than the recommended limit of 14 units a week, referred to as 'increased risk' drinking, to complex alcohol dependence with end-organ disease, hallucinations and withdrawal. Around one in five elective surgical patient show features of alcohol dependency [60].

Alcohol-related harm increases in a dose-dependent manner, rendering patients at the severe end of the spectrum at the highest risk of individual harm. Perioperative interventions primarily target those who drink more than the recommended limits but who are not dependent, as larger patient numbers in this group lead to higher levels of population harm [61].

Even in those without evidence of alcohol related liver, pancreas or neurological dysfunction, excess alcohol has adverse effects on immune response, coagulation, cardiovascular system and endocrine response to surgery [62]. Consuming two or more drinks a day is enough to place a patient at increased risk of experiencing related complications, such as increased rates of infection, arrhythmia and blood loss [63].

As with most optimisation strategies, detecting those at increased risk is a key first step in their management. Validated screening tools such as AUDIT (Alcohol Use Disorders Identification Test) questionnaire increase detection of alcohol misuse when compared to subjective clinician assessment [61].

Interventions described in the literature can be broadly classified into either 'intensive' or 'brief' interventions. Intensive interventions take place over 4–8 weeks and aim to achieve complete abstinence from alcohol. They include patient's empowerment, support, education and may involve the use of pharmacological adjuncts such as disulfiram. Intensive interventions can reduce the number of postoperative complications, increase the number successfully quitting, and reduce postoperative alcohol consumption after the intervention [62].

Brief interventions are based around motivational interviewing techniques, advice and patient's empowerment and last for 5–30 minutes. They aim to reduce alcohol intake through goal setting. With the evidence base for reduced alcohol consumption mainly in primary care [61], these less resource intensive programmes are well suited for integration into perioperative care pathways.

THEORIES OF BEHAVIOUR CHANGE

There are many theories of behaviour change. The COM-B system includes Capability, Motivation and Opportunity to change Behaviour [64]. Changing behaviour requires knowledge, motivation, often a trigger, easily available opportunities and the skills needed to make a change, feeling empowered or supported (e.g. by friends), a physical environment that facilitates the change and a plan to cope with future potential failure and persevere [47].

Different barriers are experienced by people from different backgrounds. There is a distinction between interventions (such as behavioural support for smoking cessation) and policies (such as taxation or fines). Environments can be adjusted to 'nudge' people to make the best choice an easier choice [65].

The brain reward pathways can be harnessed, with different neurotransmitters involved [66]. Dopamine is stimulated with rewards, so progress needs a series of goals and rewards; serotonin increases with sunlight or group activity, such as signing up for a charity event; oxytocin increases with physical contact and doing a good deed; and endorphins are released with exercise but this takes 20 minutes to work, so a commitment in advance and practical preparation can help to prevent the resolution failing.

Behaviour is often determined by the norms or expectations of a person's culture. It can be helpful to include family members in commitments to change behaviour. Many people with long-term conditions are fearful of worsening their condition by making changes [67]. Healthcare professionals have a powerful role [67] in individualising and simplifying messages with each patient, e.g. 'go for a brisk walk every day' or 'have days without alcohol'. Creating new habits requires activities to be fitted into everyday life, such as active travel or alcohol-free days.

'Motivational interviewing' involves engaging with the patient, agreeing a focus and then evoking the patient's own motivation to change, followed by planning [47]. This skill is the basis of the 'Making Every Contact Count' programme for all healthcare workers [68]. This encourages staff to listen for and amplify a patient's 'change talk' and refocus their inertia to verbalise the reasons for change. Brief interventions can be highly effective, especially at a 'teachable moment', before surgery is where an individual is primed to make healthier decisions. The website www.movingmedicine.ac.uk has clear resources for patients and simple education for healthcare staff, on how to include promoting exercise in a 1-minute consultation. The critical point is that every member of staff gives the same message and has basic skills in supporting patients. The Centre for Perioperative Care www.cpoc.org.uk has a repository of electronic resources for patients and educational materials for all staff.

SURGERY SCHOOLS

Helping patients to understand what to expect throughout their journey is an established standard in perioperative care, which enables patients to feel more prepared and less anxious about surgery. The course a patient takes, and specific aspects of their preparation, will vary depending on hospital, specialty and complexity of operation. Group education strategies aim to inform, manage expectations and teach specific skills required in the postoperative period such as crutch use, breathing exercises or stoma care. They also represent an opportunity to provide lifestyle advice, support behavioural change and provide a platform for prehabilitation. These group initiatives, commonly referred to as 'Surgery schools' are predominantly delivered face to face, as a one-off session over a few hours, with a group of patients on a waiting list with a family member, learning and discussing together as a peer group with staff giving advice and information. There is a growing number of web or app-based resources [69]. Evaluations have demonstrated high levels of patient's satisfaction, improved recovery and change in behaviours [70]. On the other hand, it is recognised that one size does not fit all, with poorer uptake among those from deprived areas, who may have the most to gain in terms of modifiable risk factors. Barriers to attending face-to-face programmes may include poor mobility, travel costs and lack of confidence. Harnessing technology to provide alternative means of participation via virtual surgery schools may overcome these barriers and increase uptake.

CONCLUSION

The multiple opportunities for optimisation prior to surgery for every patient are often missed. Most patients undergoing major surgery have multiple comorbidities and are physically inactive or frail – all of which increase length of stay and the risks of complications several-fold. There are seven key interventions that reduce complications – some by half: smoking cessation, nutrition, exercise, alcohol moderation, medication review with medical assessment, psychological preparedness with attention to mental health and physical preparedness. All staff should learn about motivational interviewing and give clear messages. Giving general advice is safe and screening should identify those who need specific advice. Senior clinicians should be involved in risk assessments, comprehensive geriatric assessment and Shared Decision Making (SDM). Such considerations help many patients decide against unwarranted surgery, which reduces complications and regret. Prehabilitation services or surgery schools deliver excellent results, but where these do not exist, every member of the team should contribute to patient optimisation. A culture change is needed so that the physiological insult of surgery is recognised as similar to undertaking a marathon. Optimisation is possible – and simple education and resources from www.cpoc.org.uk could help patients and all staff to feel confident.

Key points for clinical practice

- Complications occur in 10–15% of operations – several-fold higher if frail or physically inactive; 14% of patients express regret
- Good perioperative care can reduce complications by around 50% and length of stay by 1–2 days

- 'Shared Decision Making' involves the patient and a senior clinician understanding the patient's values and discussing the Benefits, Risks, Alternatives and doing Nothing (BRAN)
- Over half the patients for major surgery have multiple comorbidities. Following comprehensive geriatric assessment (CGA), 15% of patients decline surgery
- *Seven interventions are proven to reduce complications:* Smoking cessation, exercise, nutrition, alcohol moderation, medication review with senior clinician review, psychological preparation with attention to mental health and practical preparation
- Meaningful improvements in fitness can occur rapidly preoperatively through exercise programmes and optimising nutrition, reducing muscle loss from the surgical stress response
- Surgery is a 'teachable moment' and interventions can have a rapid improvement
- Clear pathways help to plan standardised nurse-led advice for most patients and identify complex patients for senior clinical optimisation (see www.cpoc.org.uk)
- All perioperative staff should learn to do motivational interviewing to help behaviour change

REFERENCES

1. PQIP. (2018). Perioperative Quality Improvement Programme 2017/18 Annual Report. Available from https://pqip.org.uk/FilesUploaded/PQIP%20Annual%20Report%202017-18.pdf. (Last accessed 18 July 2025.)
2. Wilson A, Ronnekleiv-Kelly SM, Pawlik TM. Regret in Surgical Decision Making: A Systematic Review of Patient and Physician Perspectives. World J Surg 2017; 41:1454–1465.
3. Hewitt J, Long S, Carter B, et al. The prevalence of frailty and its association with clinical outcomes in general surgery: a systematic review and meta-analysis. Age Ageing 2018; 47:793–800.
4. Tatematsu N, Park M, Tanaka E, et al. Association between physical activity and postoperative complications after esophagectomy for cancer: a prospective observational study. Asian Pacific J Cancer Prevent 2013; 14:47–51.
5. Centre for Perioperative Care. (2020). The impact of perioperative care on healthcare resource use—rapid research review. Available from https://cpoc.org.uk/about-cpoc-cpoc-policy/proving-case-perioperative-care. (Last accessed 18 July 2025.)
6. NHS Digital. (2022). Hospital Episode Statistics for England. Admitted Patient Care statistics, 2021-2. Available from https://digital.nhs.uk/data-and-information/publications/statistical/hospital-admitted-patient-care-activity/2021-22#. (Last accessed 18 July 2025.)
7. Snowden C, Swart M. Anaesthesia and perioperative medicine: GIRFT Programme national specialty report. Getting It Right First Time, NHS England and NHS Improvement, London, UK. Published online 2022. Available from https://gettingitrightfirsttime.co.uk/medical_specialties/apom/. (Last accessed 18 July 2025.)
8. Sport England. (2022). Active Lives Adult Survey November 2020-21 Report. Available from https://www.sportengland.org/research-and-data/data/active-lives/active-lives-data-tables. (Last accessed 18 July 2025.)
9. Barnett K, Mercer SW, Norbury M, et al. Epidemiology of multimorbidity and implications for health care, research, and medical education: a cross-sectional study. Lancet 2012; 380:37–43.
10. Levy N, Selwyn DA, Lobo DN. Turning waiting lists for elective surgery into preparation lists. Br J Anaesth 2021; 126:1–5.
11. Santhirapala R, Fleisher LA, Grocott MPW. Choosing Wisely: just because we can, does it mean we should? Br J Anaesth 2019; 122:306–310.
12. Shahab R, Lochrie N, Moppett IK, et al. A Description of Interventions Prompted by Preoperative Comprehensive Geriatric Assessment and Optimization in Older Elective Noncardiac Surgical Patients. J Am Med Dir Assoc 2022; 23:1948–1954.

13. Macmillan. (2015). The Importance of Physical Activity for People Living with and beyond Cancer. A Concise Evidence Review. Available from https://be.macmillan.org.uk/Downloads/CancerInformation/LivingWithAndAfterCancer/MAC138200415PhysicalActivityevidencereviewDIGITAL.pdf. (Last accessed 18 July 2025.)
14. McNally SA, El-Boghdadly K, Kua J, et al. Preoperative assessment and optimisation: the key to good outcomes after the pandemic. Br J Hosp Med 2021; 82:1–6.
15. Academy of Medical Royal Colleges. (2020). Developing Professional Identity in Multi-Disciplinary Teams. Available from https://www.aomrc.org.uk/wp-content/uploads/2020/05/Developing_professional_identity_in_multi-professional_teams_0520.pdf. (Last accessed 18 July 2025.)
16. Australian and New Zealand College of Anaesthetists. (2021). A Framework for Perioperative Care in Australia and New Zealand. Available from https://www.anzca.edu.au/getattachment/6651a581-9308-4363-bf07-65de1ef2802b/The-Perioperative-Care-Framework-document. (Last accessed 18 July 2025.)
17. Centre for Perioperative Care. (2021). Preoperative Assessment and Optimisation for Adult Surgery, including consideration of COVID-19 and its implications. Available from https://cpoc.org.uk/guidance-preoperative-assessment-and-optimisation-adult-surgery-published. (Last accessed 18 July 2025.)
18. Durrand J, Singh SJ, Danjoux G. Prehabilitation. Clin Med 2019; 19:458–464.
19. Wijeysundera DN, Beattie WS, Hillis GS, et al. Integration of the Duke Activity Status Index into preoperative risk evaluation: a multicentre prospective cohort study. Br J Anaesth 2020; 124:261–270.
20. Wilson RJT, Davies S, Yates D, et al. Impaired functional capacity is associated with all-cause mortality after major elective intra-abdominal surgery. Br J Anaesth 2010; 105:297–303.
21. Moran J, Wilson F, Guinan E, et al. Role of cardiopulmonary exercise testing as a risk-assessment method in patients undergoing intra-abdominal surgery: a systematic review. Br J Anaesth 2016; 116:177–191.
22. Colson M, Baglin J, Bolsin S, et al. Cardiopulmonary exercise testing predicts 5 yr survival after major surgery. Br J Anaesth 2012; 109:735–741.
23. Levett DZH, Jack S, Swart M, et al. Perioperative cardiopulmonary exercise testing (CPET): consensus clinical guidelines on indications, organization, conduct, and physiological interpretation. Br J Anaesth 2018; 120:484–500.
24. Chambers DJ, Wisely NA. Cardiopulmonary exercise testing; a beginners guide to the nine-panel plot. BJA Educ. 2019; 19:158–164.
25. Hartley RA, Pichel AC, Grant SW, et al. Preoperative cardiopulmonary exercise testing and risk of early mortality following abdominal aortic aneurysm repair. J Br Surg 2012; 99:1539–1546.
26. Wynter-Blyth V, Moorthy K. Prehabilitation: preparing patients for surgery. BMJ 2017; 358:j3702.
27. Cusack B, Buggy DJ. Anaesthesia, analgesia, and the surgical stress response. BJA Educ 2020; 20:321–328.
28. Minto G, Biccard B. Assessment of the high-risk perioperative patient. Cont Edu Anaesth Crit Care Pain 2014; 14:12–17.
29. Gillis C, Ljungqvist O, Carli F. Prehabilitation, enhanced recovery after surgery, or both? A narrative review. Br J Anaesth 2022; 128:434–448.
30. Flocke SA, Clark E, Antognoli E, et al. Teachable moments for health behavior change and intermediate patient outcomes. Patient Educ Couns 2014; 96:43–49.
31. Richardson K, Levett DZH, Jack S, et al. Fit for surgery? Perspectives on preoperative exercise testing and training. Br J Anaesth 2017; 119:i34–i43.
32. UK GOV. (2019). UK Chief Medical Officers' physical activity guidelines. Available from https://assets.publishing.service.gov.uk/government/uploads/system/uploads/attachment_data/file/832868/uk-chief-medical-officers-physical-activity-guidelines.pdf. (Last accessed 18 July 2025.)
33. Tew GA, Ayyash R, Durrand J, et al. Clinical guideline and recommendations on pre-operative exercise training in patients awaiting major non-cardiac surgery. Anaesthesia 2018; 73:750–768.
34. Friedman J, Lussiez A, Sullivan J, et al. Implications of sarcopenia in major surgery. Nutr Clin Pract 2015; 30:175–179.
35. Barberan-Garcia A, Ubré M, Roca J, et al. Personalised Prehabilitation in High-risk Patients Undergoing Elective Major Abdominal Surgery: A Randomized Blinded Controlled Trial. Ann Surg 2018; 267:50–56.
36. West MA, Astin R, Moyses HE, et al. Exercise prehabilitation may lead to augmented tumor regression following neoadjuvant chemoradiotherapy in locally advanced rectal cancer. Acta Oncol (Madr) 2019; 58:588–595.
37. Miskovic A, Lumb AB. Postoperative pulmonary complications. Br J Anaesth 2017; 118:317–334.
38. Moran J, Guinan E, McCormick P, et al. The ability of prehabilitation to influence postoperative outcome after intra-abdominal operation: A systematic review and meta-analysis. Surgery 2016; 160:1189–1201.

39. Chen BP, Awasthi R, Sweet SN, et al. Four-week prehabilitation program is sufficient to modify exercise behaviors and improve preoperative functional walking capacity in patients with colorectal cancer. Support Care Cancer 2017; 25:33–40.
40. Weston M, Weston KL, Prentis JM, et al. High-intensity interval training (HIT) for effective and time-efficient pre-surgical exercise interventions. Perioperative Med 2016; 5:2.
41. West MA, Loughney L, Lythgoe D, et al. Effect of prehabilitation on objectively measured physical fitness after neoadjuvant treatment in preoperative rectal cancer patients: a blinded interventional pilot study. Br J Anaesth 2015; 114:244–251.
42. Simon HL, Paula T, Luz MM, et al. Frailty in older patients undergoing emergency colorectal surgery: USA National Surgical Quality Improvement Program analysis. Br J Surg 2020; 107:1363–1371.
43. Fowler AJ, Abbott TEF, Prowle J, et al. Age of patients undergoing surgery. J Br Surg 2019; 106:1012–1018.
44. Stewart JJ, Partridge JSL, Dhesi JK. Perioperative medicine for Older People undergoing Surgery (POPS): Comprehensive Geriatric Assessment (CGA) and optimization in the perioperative setting. Int Anesthesiol Clin 2023; 61:62–69.
45. Rockwood K, Song X, MacKnight C, et al. A global clinical measure of fitness and frailty in elderly people. Cmaj 2005; 173:489–495.
46. Partridge JSL, Moonesinghe SR, Lees N, et al. Perioperative care for older people. Age Ageing 2022; 51:afac194.
47. Academy of Medical Royal Colleges. (2015). Exercise: The miracle cure and the role of the doctor in promoting it. Available from https://www.aomrc.org.uk/reports-guidance/exercise-the-miracle-cure/. (Last accessed 18 July 2025.)
48. Centre for Perioperative Care. (2022). Guideline for the Management of Anaemia in the Perioperative Pathway. Available from https://cpoc.org.uk/guidelines-resources-guidelines/anaemia-perioperative-pathway. (Last accessed 18 July 2025.)
49. Centre for Perioperative Care. (2021). Guideline for perioperative care for people with diabetes mellitus undergoing elective and emergency surgery. Available from https://cpoc.org.uk/guidelines-resources-guidelines-resources/guideline-diabetes. (Last accessed 18 July 2025.)
50. Centre for Perioperative Care. (2021). Guideline for perioperative care for people living with frailty undergoing elective and emergency surgery. Available from https://cpoc.org.uk/guidelines-resources-guidelines/perioperative-care-people-living-frailty. (Last accessed 18 July 2025.)
51. Wischmeyer PE, Carli F, Evans DC, et al. American society for enhanced recovery and perioperative quality initiative joint consensus statement on nutrition screening and therapy within a surgical enhanced recovery pathway. Anesth Analg 2018; 126:1883–1895.
52. Weimann A, Braga M, Carli F, et al. ESPEN guideline: clinical nutrition in surgery. Clin nutr 2017; 36:623–650.
53. Gillis C, Carli F. Promoting Perioperative Metabolic and Nutritional Care. Anesthesiology 2015; 123:1455–1472.
54. Gillis C, Wischmeyer PE. Pre-operative nutrition and the elective surgical patient: why, how and what? Anaesthesia 2019; 74:27–35.
55. Malietzis G, Currie AC, Athanasiou T, et al. Influence of body composition profile on outcomes following colorectal cancer surgery. Br J Surg 2016; 103:572–580.
56. Schmid M, Sood A, Campbell L, et al. Impact of smoking on perioperative outcomes after major surgery. Am J Surg 2015; 210:221–229.
57. McDonald S, Yates D, Durrand JW, et al. Exploring patient attitudes to behaviour change before surgery to reduce peri-operative risk: preferences for short- vs. long-term behaviour change. Anaesthesia 2019; 74:1580–1588.
58. Thomsen T, Tønnesen H, Møller AM. Effect of preoperative smoking cessation interventions on postoperative complications and smoking cessation. Br J Surg 2009; 96:451–461.
59. Matuszewski PE, Comadoll SM, Costales T, et al. Novel Application of Exhaled Carbon Monoxide Monitors: Smoking Cessation in Orthopaedic Trauma Patients. J Orthop Trauma 2019; 33:e433–e438.
60. Budworth L, Prestwich A, Lawton R, et al. Preoperative Interventions for Alcohol and Other Recreational Substance Use: A Systematic Review and Meta-Analysis. Front Psychol 2019; 10:34.
61. Snowden C, Lynch E, Avery L, et al. Preoperative behavioural intervention to reduce drinking before elective orthopaedic surgery: the PRE-OP BIRDS feasibility RCT. Health Technol Assess. 2020; 24:1–176.
62. Egholm JWM, Pedersen B, Møller AM, et al. Perioperative alcohol cessation intervention for postoperative complications. Cochrane Database Syst Rev 2018; 11:CD008343.
63. Shabanzadeh DM, Sørensen LT. Alcohol consumption increases post-operative infection but not mortality: a systematic review and meta-analysis. Surg Infect (Larchmt) 2015; 16:657–668.

64. Michie S, van Stralen MM, West R. The behaviour change wheel: A new method for characterising and designing behaviour change interventions. Implement Sci 2011; 6:42.
65. Thaler RH, Sunstein CR. Nudge: improving decisions about health. Wealth Happiness 2008; 6:14–38.
66. Breuning LG. Habits of a Happy Brain: Retrain Your Brain to Boost Your Serotonin, Dopamine, Oxytocin, and Endorphin Levels. Avon, Massachusetts : Adams Media, 2015.
67. Reid H, Ridout AJ, Tomaz SA, et al. Benefits outweigh the risks: a consensus statement on the risks of physical activity for people living with long-term conditions. Br J Sports Med 2022; 56:427–438.
68. Public Health England. (2016). Making every contact count (MECC): consensus statement. Available from https://www.england.nhs.uk/wp-content/uploads/2016/04/making-every-contact-count.pdf. (Last accessed 18 July 2025.)
69. Fecher-Jones I, Grimmett C, Carter FJ, et al. Surgery school—who, what, when, and how: results of a national survey of multidisciplinary teams delivering group preoperative education. Periop Med 2021; 10:20.
70. Fecher-Jones I, Grimmett C, Edwards MR, et al. Development and evaluation of a novel pre-operative surgery school and behavioural change intervention for patients undergoing elective major surgery: Fit-4-Surgery School. Anaesthesia 2021; 76:1207–1211.

Chapter 3

Recent advances in understanding the role of human factors in patient safety and surgical team performance

Neil Mackenzie, Benjamin Whitworth, Rachel Oeppen, Peter Brennan

ABSTRACT

Human error is ubiquitous and occurs regularly in our personal and professional lives. Human factors are a broad term that relates to how individuals and teams perform and interact with each other, as well as with the environment and technology. In this chapter, we consider the scale of medical error and various factors and techniques that can be adopted to help reduce it, thereby improving patient safety and team working. We also discuss the importance of optimising performance, effective communication, situational awareness (SA) and decision making.

WHAT ARE HUMAN FACTORS?

'Human factors (HFs) refer to environmental, organisational and job factors and human and individual characteristics, which influence behaviour at work in a way which can affect health and safety.' This definition includes three interrelated factors that need to be considered – the individual, the organisation and the job.
1. *The individual*: Including their personality, skills, competence (including cognitive and physical ability), motivation and risk perception. The relationship between behaviour

---

Neil Mackenzie MA FRCS FDS, Programme Manager at NHS National Services Scotland, The University of Edinburgh, Edinburgh, Scotland, UK
E-mail: Neil.Mackenzie@NHS.Net (for correspondence)

Benjamin Whitworth MSc, Director, Synergy Human Factors, Chippenham, Wiltshire, UK
E-mail: ben@synergyhumanfactors.com (for correspondence)

Rachel Oeppen MRCP FRCR, Consultant Radiologist, Department of Clinical Radiology, University Hospital Southampton, UK
E-mail: Rachel.oeppen@uhs.nhs.uk (for correspondence)

Peter Brennan OBE PhD FRCS, Consultant Surgeon Maxillofacial Unit, Portsmouth Hospitals NHS Trust, Portsmouth, UK
E-mail: Peter.Brennan4@NHS.Net (for correspondence)

and individual characteristics is complex with some characteristics such as personality being innate while others such as attitudes and skills being adaptable.
2. *The organisation*: Including the workplace culture, leadership, methods of communication, shift patterns and availability of resources. These factors have a significant influence over both individual and group behaviour.
3. *The job:* Including the specific task, process and procedure design, the working environment, the volume of work, the ergonomics and the degree of autonomy. The physical and the mental requirements of the job can vary significantly.

In summary, HF is concerned with what people are being asked to do, who is doing it and where they are working – all of which are influenced by wider social constructs. HF can, and should, be included within a good safety management system and the application of HF in healthcare can lead to improved patient safety, better team working and improved staff morale.

Human performance is variable, and we all make mistakes such as forgetting a mobile phone or wallet. On average, these simple errors occur 5–7 times a day and are generally accepted as inconvenient and inconsequential. However, we often fail to appreciate that highly consequential errors in our work, which may lead to patient harm and mortality, happen for the same reasons.

Just as we cannot prevent all day-to-day errors, we can never eliminate error in our professional work. As surgeon and medical author Atul Gwande comments: '*No matter what measures are taken, doctors will sometimes falter, and it isn't reasonable to ask that we achieve perfection. What is reasonable is to ask that we never cease to aim for it.*'

Learning from mistakes and sharing lessons widely is one of the most important factors in improving patient safety across healthcare. Furthermore, changes in ways of working, procedure and policy design, ergonomics and attitudes toward HF can have a significant influence over outcomes and potential error.

ERROR IN HEALTHCARE

The complex interactions between HF and human error in clinical incidents are progressively becoming more widely understood. This includes the many factors that have their origins in the hospitals and organisations where we work. There is often more than one issue, or layer, that leads to error and this is readily represented by the well-known Swiss cheese model (**Figure 3.1**) [1]. Collaborating factors are often multifactorial and take place concurrently. Appreciating this fact is of fundamental importance in appreciating the application of HF to surgery. These multifactorial issues include ones that affect us as individuals such as tiredness, stress, repetition, distraction and multitasking. Other factors which can impact and influence team working include loss of SA, steep or flat authority gradients and poor communication or leadership. The introduction of the World Health Organisation (WHO) surgical checklist has improved attitudes toward presurgery briefing and patient safety, and the benefits of recognising and applying these HF principles to surgery are well known [2].

Several studies have demonstrated that approximately one in 20 hospital admissions results in some form of error and of these, one in 20, equating to one in 400 admissions, is serious. The operating theatre is known to be one of the most high-risk areas in the hospital due to high patient turnover, staff diversity, unfamiliar teams and a multiplicity of procedures [3].

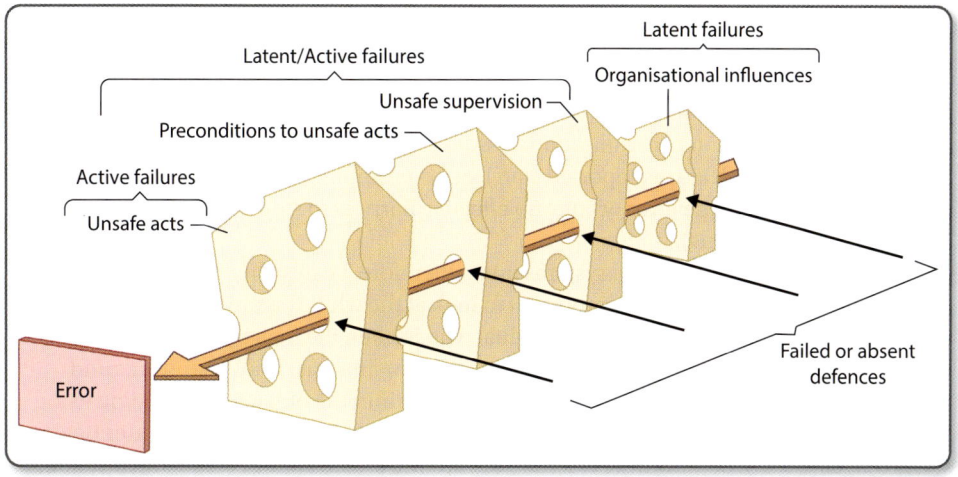

Figure 3.1 The Swiss cheese model of human error. Each slice can act as a barrier.

NEVER EVENTS

Never events are defined by NHS England as 'serious incidents that are entirely preventable because guidance or safety recommendations providing strong systemic protective barriers are available at a national level and should have been implemented by all healthcare providers.' Despite this, never events continue to happen and surgical procedures continue to be a significant contributor with three categories on the list:
1. Wrong site surgery
2. Wrong implant or prosthesis
3. Retained foreign object postprocedure

According to the NHS Improvement website in the period April 2021 to March 2022, there were a total of 407 never events, including 171 wrong site surgery, 98 retained foreign object and 47 wrong implant or prosthesis. Therefore, surgical never events represented 77% of all reported never events and clearly represent a significant contributor to these adverse patient safety events.

WHAT ARE THE DIFFERENT TYPES OF ERROR AND FAILURE?

The Human Factors Analysis and Classification System (HFACS) categorises failure across four broad domains in line with James Reason's Swiss cheese theory (**Figure 3.1**) [1]. These are:
1. Organisational influences
2. Unsafe supervision
3. Preconditions to unsafe acts
4. Unsafe acts

The theory is that in ideal situations, single errors or unsafe acts rarely happen and even when they do, they are mitigated and there is no ensuing harm. However, occasionally, a combination of problems at each level accumulates and interacts resulting in a 'perfect storm' of conditions which result in a serious error or accident. In the Swiss cheese metaphor, such a combination is represented by a hole in each cheese slice perfectly aligning to allow the accident or error trajectory to pass through (**Figure 3.1**). This equates to a combination of organisational issues (such as a demoralised workforce), poor supervision (such as unsupported staff), error-promoting conditions (such as poor equipment) and, once the error occurs, no effective barriers to stop it causing damage (such as warning systems).

Error and accident prevention systems must, therefore, be designed to address this multifactorial causation and it is important to look at the whole organisation rather than simply analysing and criticising the individual who is often the final point of failure in a poorly designed system. Root cause and causal factor analysis of adverse events and incidents events frequently reveal a chain of events within the organisation leading to a remote point of failure at an individual level. In aviation, the aircraft manufacturer Boeing states that 80–90% of contributing error factors are within the control of the organisation, with just 10–20% within the control of individual operators, further justifying the exploration of system wide causal influences, rather than simply focusing on individual performance [4].

Examples of failures in the clinical setting that can have their origin in the employing organisation include pressures from overbooked clinics or operating theatre sessions, meeting clinical and hospital targets and prolonged working hours without adequate breaks. Medical error can begin to evolve well before the actual event itself because of organisational failure. The exciting challenge is to design systems that accurately identify and prevent the terminal point of failure which ultimately leads to patient harm.

WHAT HUMAN FACTORS IN SURGERY SHOULD WE BE THINKING ABOUT?

Box 3.1 summarises some important HF that can contribute to and ultimately lead to surgical error as categorised by the HFACS. These include factors which can affect us as individuals such as tiredness and fatigue, hydration and nutritional status, emotional states including anger and stress, multitasking and loss of SA. These will now be considered further.

Impact of tiredness and fatigue

Commercial and military aviation both recognise how tiredness and fatigue impact on personal performance and increase the likelihood of accidents. As a result, there are strict rules in place for the maximum duration of work that can be undertaken without a break.

Tiredness and fatigue are both commonly found in surgical team members. Tiredness is a state that can only be reversed by sleep. Fatigue is a more complex condition and incorporates both physical and mental fatigue. Physical fatigue results from muscle fatigue brought about by intense physical activity. Mental fatigue results from prolonged periods of cognitive activity which impairs cognitive ability and can also impair physical performance. Complex cognitive tasks, decision-making and SA all become impaired and errors become more likely [5].

Taking regular short breaks, for example, during a long and complex 8-hour operation, is not only beneficial to individuals and teams but it may also prevent errors from occurring.

> **Box 3.1 Simplified Human Factors Analysis and Classification System (HFACS) relevant to surgery**
>
> *Organisational influences within the hospital:*
> - Hospital targets and pressures to deliver results (either perceived or real)
> - Climate, process and resource management within the hospital
> - Communication, training and recognition by the senior management of human factors responsible for possible error
>
> *Unsafe supervision:*
> - Inadequate supervision of trainees or other healthcare staff
> - Failure of briefings/complacency with WHO checklist
> - Failure of the team to know what to do when things go wrong
> - Loss of situation awareness, especially if not recognised by the theatre team
>
> *Preconditions to unsafe acts:*
> - Fatigue, hunger and nutritional status
> - Emotional influences (anger, personal issues) and running late
> - Tiredness, boredom and communication issues remember *HALT*
> - *Environmental factors*: Background noise, distractions, lighting, ambient temperature and humidity
> - Panic
>
> *Unsafe acts (less likely):*
> - Unfamiliar with changes from what is seen as a 'normal event'
> - Distracting and multitasking
> - Operating outside of one's area of expertise or following a long period of no operating (surgical currency)

Most people would not drive continuously for 8 hours without a break so why should it be deemed safe to do so during surgery? A useful fact to remember is that our cognitive function after being awake for 18 hours is equivalent to being twice over the UK legal alcohol limit for driving. Paradoxically, taking a break can speed up the eventual finishing time of the operation as continuing to operate when tired will lead to a progressive degradation in cognition, performance, manual dexterity and ultimately the finishing time. Hospitals are increasingly recognising that tired clinicians are more likely to make mistakes and legislation such as the European working time directive (EWTD) has set limits on maximum shift length and working week.

No one else appreciates how an individual feels if they have been operating on an emergency throughout the night and are expected to work the following day. The simple statement '*I don't feel safe*' is extremely powerful when discussing options with managers and colleagues.

Importance of hydration and nutritional status

Hydration, nutrition and individual recovery are seen as important parameters in sport, but their importance is often overlooked in the operating theatre to maintain performance [6–8]. Even small deficits in total body water can have a significant impact on cognitive function resulting in poor decision making, tiredness, lethargy, headaches and impatience, a relatively modest 1–2 kg loss in body water in an average build individual has been shown to reduce cognitive function by 15–20%. This tends to develop slowly and insidiously so that the individual is not aware that their performance is gradually deteriorating. Good hydration is particularly important if personal protective equipment (PPE) is being worn, as this can increase the rate of perspiration and loss of body water. Water requirements are unique to individuals and while a multitude of factors including body mass, ambient temperature, pregnancy and diet play a role, the minimal requirement is approximately 2 L/day. Caffeine was previously thought to be a mild diuretic but recent studies have indicated that moderate consumption does not contribute to dehydration as the water content of the tea or coffee contributes to the total water intake and any counteracts any diuretic effect.

Good and balanced nutrition distributed over a sensible time also helps optimise personal performance and supports complex mental and physical tasks over a sustained period. A well-balanced, small-portioned meal every 3–4 hours consisting of complex carbohydrates, protein, healthy fats and dietary fibre is the optimal approach. In contrast, erratic consumption of large meals, consisting of simple sugars or processed foods, is more likely to produce fluctuating energy levels which can have a detrimental effect on physical and mental performance. This is the approach taken by elite and aspiring athletes with top performers even employing a nutritional expert to complement their physical and psychological coaches. Preplanned breaks during long operating lists, clinics and on-call periods should be adopted to ensure all team members have to opportunity to benefit from this strategy.

Effect of emotion and stress

Stress and emotion are well known to affect physical performance and can have an adverse effect on patient outcomes. Mental resilience and its impact on surgical performance need to be acknowledged. Powerful emotions such as anxiety, anger or disappointment can easily interfere with decision making, especially when trying to perform a task that requires intense concentration and meticulous attention to detail. The atmosphere in the operating theatre can be stressful for the whole surgical team, many will have heard colleagues raise their voices or indeed shout. One of the reasons for this is the accumulation of minor stressors or other factors accumulating. Most team members have an envelope of comfort within which they can function well, but the accumulation of minor stressors can cause them to be outside their comfort zone and become emotionally labile. During such times, error is far more likely, not to mention the potential effect the loss of civility has on wider team dynamics, which can lead to respect and confidence being lost.

Pausing during an operation, if it is safe to so do, to address these underlying issues is a useful strategy that may reduce the likelihood of error. We recommend taking a short break, again if it is safe to do so. The easily remembered pneumonic *HALT* – Hungry, Anxious/Angry, Late (or lonely) and Tired – brings the above considerations together. It is a powerful reminder of the factors that can lead to surgical error in addition to recognising the importance and value of stopping when one or more of these elements arise. Acknowledging the impact of stress and emotion not only helps reduce risk of error but also benefits surgical training. It leads to a more effective and happier team working which will ultimately improve overall patient experience and management. 'Lonely' has also been included as this word introduces the idea of remembering the value of involving colleagues for complex cases or after a prolonged period of no operating (during COVID, for example). Dual surgeon operating can be very useful in this regard [9]. Not only can this give surgeons confidence, but it can also improve patient outcomes. The adage of 'a problem shared is a problem halved' is entirely relevant as the emotional burden of making a difficult decision is shared and has the additional benefit of adding a degree of medicolegal robustness.

Performance shaping factors

Various factors can influence or shape human performance. While some may be outside of direct surgeon control, they are worthy of consideration during task planning and briefings. For example, time shortage is suggested to carry a risk factor of x11 which can manifest, or be visible to individuals or other team members, as rushing to complete a task, or attempting to do too many things within a small-time window. Task unfamiliarity comes with a risk factor of x17, which can be easily understood when relating to completing a task for the first time [10]. However, this can also form the foundation of a briefing-based discussion if a task within the team has not been completed recently or is unfamiliar.

SITUATIONAL AWARENESS

A simple definition of SA is being aware of what is going on around us now, and what might affect us in the future. An awareness and appreciation of several factors that raise the risk of medical error (summarised in **Box 3.2**) can be used to our advantage to help improve SA for individuals and the whole team. SA is a dynamic concept and can change quickly [11-13]. It is important to appreciate that SA can change or degrade over time in different circumstances as does our ability (or not) to adapt to it. Scenarios in which a surgeon may become fixated on a task, develops tunnel vision and becomes blind to other factors that may readily occur. In such cases, surgeons can lose wider SA. This can result in working and thinking in the here and now, rather than considering threats and potential errors that exist in the future. This can be further exacerbated by confirmational bias in which they overweigh indications or information that confirms the direction they are already following. These include convincing themselves that an anatomical structure or location is indeed what they were expecting when it is something entirely different. Numerous errors have occurred as a result including cut ureters, bile ducts, vessels and important nerves.

Box 3.2 Situations that might raise the chance of error situations in the operating theatre environment. Being aware of these can help improve situational awareness

- High physical or mental workloads
- Interruptions and distractions during key parts of an operation
- Tasks requiring an 'out of normal' response and/or unanticipated new tasks
- Multitasking
- Changes in physical environment

An appreciation of the value of SA alongside a well-briefed team, who feel empowered to voice their concerns, provides the optimal environment to reduce the risk of medical error taking place. Team members are constantly looking out for each other, thereby improving patient safety and optimising the working environment. By actively thinking ahead and effectively anticipating hopefully errors can be avoided or mitigated. The best drivers are those who anticipate problems early and predict behaviour thereby avoiding potentially hazardous situations. In a similar way, thinking and discussing with the team about any potential 'what if?' scenarios before an operation commences can reduce the likelihood of a startle reaction, and ensures the team is effectively prepared.

The concept of PPP – patient, procedure, people (team)–has recently been introduced as a useful way of prompting oneself to regain wider SA when something does not seem quite right [14]. In some circumstances, it may be the procedure that needs rediscussing first to help regain SA. In most instances, stepping back from the acute situation, if it is safe to do so, and discussing with the team is the best way to understand the problem. This introduces a pause for reflection and helps to decide the best course of action. This tool has been adapted from the aviation pneumonic – aviate, navigate, communicate (ANC).

TEAM BRIEF AND DEBRIEF

Surgery is a team sport and patient care is rarely, if ever, performed in isolation from other team members. The introduction of the WHO checklist and team brief has brought significant improvements to patient safety in the operating theatre environment. An appreciation of team working, understanding and valuing individuals' contributions and reduced hierarchy all contribute toward safer patient outcomes and a more enjoyable experience for the whole team. The way in which a briefing is conducted is paramount. It should not be rushed and all team members should feel equally valued and empowered to speak up if they have any concerns, without fear of retribution [15–17]. **Box 3.3** provides a summary of items that may be included in both briefing and debriefing sessions. The team brief should also emphasise the importance of looking out for each other to reduce the likelihood of losing SA and the importance of highlighting concerns when they see negative factors such as tiredness and stress being expressed in others. During periods of intense concentration, surgeons can experience attentional tunnelling, and rapidly lose track of time. Several hours can pass, and the reliance on others to keep an eye on the clock and suggest a short break, after perhaps 3 hours, should be considered good practice.

Most surgical procedures have a critical time when full attention must be applied to the task in hand. During these, safety critical times distractions must be minimised as time away from the primary task can be detrimental to performance at a time when full concentration is required [18–22]. These should be raised at the team brief and predictable distractions kept to a minimum. The sterile cockpit approach (where pilots focus only on flying below 10,000 ft with no distractions) is a valuable technique to apply in the operating theatre (**Figure 3.2**).

A simple distraction such as a telephone call asking for advice during a complex part of an operation significantly raises the risk of error. It is far better to either limit predictable distractions (including noise) during these times or stop and focus on one task at a time rather than trying to multitask. Some surgeons are happy to have background music playing or for background chat during most of the procedure but will request absolute

> **Box 3.3 Items to consider during a team briefing. A debrief is a powerful way to develop and enhance team working for future operating sessions**
>
> A well-prepared team is advantageous in that every member knows their role and looks out for their colleagues. It can also help team members to feel valued.
>
> *Briefing*:
> - Introductions, open culture, 'please speak up if concerned'
> - Leadership, team working and decision-making
> - Think about the 'what if?' scenarios that might occur during a procedure
> - Identify the major steps and who will be doing what
> - Ask 'What am/expected to do if and when something goes wrong?'
> - Situational awareness – how to intervene and communicate effectively and timely when something does not seem right
>
> *Debriefing*:
> Consider debriefing for learning:
> - What went well?
> - What should we do differently next time?
> - What do you think about my performance today?
> - Saying 'Thank you' to the team!

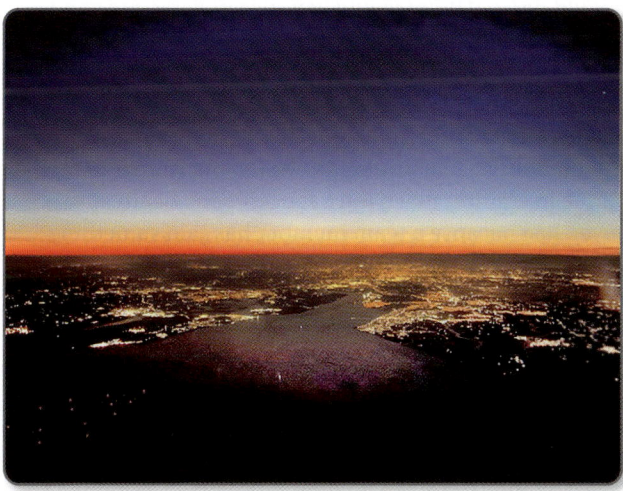

Figure 3.2 An 'office view' descending to London Heathrow Airport. Below 10,000 ft, pilots focus purely on flying with no distractions. The same practice should be adopted in the operating theatre during safety critical times.

quiet during the critical stages of a procedure to ensure maximum concentration on the task in hand.

At the end of the operating list, it is good practice to conduct a short debrief session. This does not necessarily have to be formal, but it gives the team an opportunity to discuss what went well, and what could be improved the next time. The power of saying thank you to the team cannot be overemphasised. The opportunity to ask for feedback from other team members on our own performance is also valuable and builds practice and non-technical skills.

LOWERING AUTHORITY GRADIENTS AND ENHANCING COMMUNICATION

In aviation, the most junior airline pilot is actively encouraged to question the most senior captain without fear [15,16]. Similarly empowering all members of the surgical team including medical students, trainees, nurses and non-clinical staff to voice their concerns ensures a safe working environment for everyone. It is vital to appreciate that everyone will see the procedure from a different perspective and will have a contribution to make. This must be managed within reason by each individual and the team leader recognised as they are ultimately responsibility for the collective decisions. A flat hierarchy is as dangerous as a steep one as it can lead to a situation where no one knows what anyone is doing or the leader being unable to undertake their fundamental responsibilities. However, what is most important to appreciate is that any team member can speak up when concerned, without fear of retribution, with the expectation that their concern will be listened to.

Effective communication between team members is a fundamental element of good team working and interaction and for this, four elements are required – the sender, receiver, message and feedback. If one of these elements is missing, or suboptimal in some manner, communication can fail or be less effective. For example, simply 'sending' a message to someone cognitively engaged in a task may appear appropriate, but without consideration for whether the receiver is 'ready' to receive, or without any feedback, effective communication has failed [23,24]. The regular use of open questions such as '*What do you think we should do?*' or '*What would you suggest here?*' are good at bringing the team together, and ensuring the person responding is cognitively engaged in the response, and not simply responding with an answer they feel is correct. As a rule, the use of pronouns such as '*pass me it or that*' should be avoided, especially at safety critical times. It is preferable to issue clear and unambiguous instructions and instead use the correct names of the individual surgical instruments. Asking the runner to repeat back the details is a useful technique to confirm that a message has been heard and interpreted correctly by the receiver. Just because a team member has said something does not automatically mean that others have heard and understood the message or instruction. This is especially important if a runner is being sent to another theatre, department or storeroom to collect an essential instrument or person, as otherwise valuable time is wasted when they return with the wrong instrument or individual.

Intervention can be operationalised using a tool, with one such example described using the mnemonic *PACE*. This stands for *P*robing, *A*lerting, *C*hallenge and *E*mergency. This tool can be discussed within the team briefing, and its use encouraged to ensure that suitable and timely intervention takes place if required. Probing is commonly known as hinting and tipping and takes place many times throughout the day. Alerting is directly stating that a problem exists, and challenge describes the problem with a potential solution. Emergency is when 'stop' would be called if appropriate, or suitable prevention of a negative event progressing enacted. Where somebody would enter the PACE model would depend entirely upon time available – there is little point hinting and tipping, or probing, when a threat to patient safety is immediate. However, if one had more time – then this could be a suitable method of commencing intervention.

DECISION MAKING

We make tens of thousands of remotely conscious decisions each day, and it is reasonable to state that some decisions are more important than others. However, the process and concept of decision making are often influenced by multiple factors, and individuals may have significant confidence in their ability to make 'good' decisions [24,25]. However, our decisions are not based upon what we do not know, but instead consider the information we do know [26]. This means that decisions are often based on incomplete or imperfect information, or influenced by how information is perceived or recalled from memory.

The process of arriving at a suitable decision will often utilise information that is readily available, with the decision maker applying greater validity to that information. This is known as the availability heuristic. Further heuristics, described as mental rule of thumb strategies, include representativeness where decisions are based upon known pieces of information, or mental stereotypes and transferring that known information and knowledge to alternative questions. For example, assuming a surgeon is good because he or she is busy or making a judgement about a hospital department because it is clean and tidy. Lastly, anchoring, where our decisions are adapted, or 'anchored' to an initially received piece of information, influencing our decisions.

Biases can also influence decision making. These can include framing where decisions are based upon the presentation of how information is presented or 'framed', or confirmatory bias where information that opposes a held belief is discounted in favour of information that supports the initial position. Furthermore, the Dunning–Kruger effect describes one's inability to recognise one's own incompetence or believing one is more proficient at a task than in reality. Lastly, outcome/hindsight bias where a judgement is made based upon the information that is available post event, failing to consider information that was available at the time, within the context.

Much of decision making can be described by systems 1 and 2 thinking, conceptualised by Kahneman:

- System 1 decision making can be described as quick, autonomous, intuitive and easy. Sometimes, it is entirely appropriate to utilise this form of decision making, e.g. when the brake must be suddenly applied in the car on the way home from work. However, when attempting to solve complex problems, system 1 may be subjected to some systematic errors.
- System 2 thinking is described as generally more conscious, logical and deliberate in nature, but does take more cognitive effort to engage, and generally takes longer to perform. However, it may challenge 'feel right' responses, that may be influenced by the environment, our knowledge, our experience and biases and heuristics.

To ensure decision making challenges our intuition and activate a system 2 response, it can be helpful to enact a formal process. At the start of any such process, a consideration for how long to complete the decision-making process should be considered. Then the problem statement must be identified, prior to an evaluation of options, before determining which option might be the most suitable. What follows then is a clear delegation of responsibility and task allocation, prior to an effective review to establish whether new information has come to light and confirm that the decision addresses the problem statement as defined.

In summary, HF application is essential to ensure both individuals and teams are optimised to care for patients. Some elements are just common sense, just as stopping for a short break regularly while driving a long distance, using the bathroom regularly and eating our meals at consistent times. However, it can be all too easy to leave common sense at the front door of the hospital when we come to work and adopt a different persona who works to an artificial set of strange rules while undertaking surgical procedures.

CONCLUSION

This chapter serves as an introduction and update regarding the importance of human factors in the healthcare setting. Errors are inevitable but a thorough understanding of HF can help to prevent, significantly mitigate, and reduce the seriousness of these adverse events.

> **Key points for clinical practice**
> - Human performance is variable and we all regularly make mistakes
> - Approximately 1 in 20 hospital admissions has some form of preventable error – the operating theatre is one of the highest risk places in healthcare
> - Most preventable error is multifactorial, often beginning at an organisational level
> - Tiredness and fatigue are commonly found in surgical teams and contribute to the chances of increased error
> - Situational awareness can degrade over time. Individuals and whole teams can lose SA
> - Good communication is vital and the importance of a good team briefing cannot be overemphasised; all team members should be empowered to speak up if they have any concerns

REFERENCES

1. Reason J. Human error: Models and management. BMJ 2000; 320:768–770.
2. Allard J, Bleakley A, Hobbs A, et al. Pre-surgery briefings and safety climate in the operating theatre. BMJ Qual Saf 2011; 20:711–717.
3. Panagioti M, Khan K, Keers RN, et al. Prevalence, severity, and nature of preventable patient harm across medical care settings: systematic review and meta-analysis. Br Med J 2019; 366:l4185.
4. Boeing. (2016). Maintenance Error Decision Aid, Users Guide. Available from https://sassofia.com/wp-content/uploads/2022/12/MEDA-Users-Guide-rev_January-2016_v2.pdf [Last accessed 23 July 2025]
5. Sugden C, Athanasiou T, Darzi A. What are the effects of sleep deprivation and fatigue in surgical practice? Semin Thorac Cardiovasc Surg 2012; 24:166–175.
6. Brennan PA, Oeppen R, Knighton J, et al. Looking after ourselves at work: The importance of being hydrated and fed. BMJ 2019; 364:l528.
7. Riebl SK, Davy BM. The Hydration Equation: Update on Water Balance and Cognitive Performance. ACSMs Health Fit J 2013; 17:21–28.
8. Winston J, Johnson C, Wilson S. Barriers to healthy eating by national health service (NHS) hospital doctors in the hospital setting: Results of a cross-sectional survey. BMC Res Notes 2008; 1:69.

References

9. Ellis R, Hardie J, Summerton DJ, et al. Dual surgeon operating to improve patient safety. Br J Oral Maxillofac Surg 2021; 59:752–756.
10. Swain AD, Guttmann HE. (1983). Handbook of human-reliability analysis with emphasis on nuclear power plant applications. Final report. Available from https://www.nrc.gov/docs/ML0712/ML071210299.pdf [Last accessed 23 July 2025].
11. Brennan PA, Holden C, Shaw G, et al. Leading article: What can we do to improve individual and team situational awareness to benefit patient safety? Br J Oral Maxillofac Surg 2020; 58:404–408.
12. Green B, Parry D, Oeppen RS, et al. Situational awareness - what it means for clinicians, its recognition and importance in patient safety. Oral Dis 2017; 23:721–725.
13. Green B, Mitchell DA, Stevenson P, et al. Leading article: how can I optimise my role as a leader within the surgical team? Br J Oral Maxillofac Surg 2016; 54:847–850.
14. Hardie J, Hunn D, Mitchell T, et al. Patient, Procedure, People (PPP): Recognising & responding to intra-operative critical events. Ann Roy Coll Surg Eng 2022; 109:409–413.
15. Brennan PA, Davidson M. Improving patient safety. We need to reduce hierarchy and empower junior doctors to speak up. Br Med J 2019; 366:l1441.
16. Green B, Oeppen RS, Smith DW, et al. Challenging hierarchy in healthcare teams - ways to flatten gradients to improve teamwork and patient care. Br J Oral Maxillofac Surg 2017; 55:449–453.
17. Quine L. Workplace bullying in NHS community trust: staff questionnaire survey. BMJ 1999; 318:228–232.
18. Mentis HM, Chellali A, Manser K, et al. A systematic review of the effect of distraction on surgeon performance: directions for operating room policy and surgical training. Surg Endosc 2016; 30:1713–1724.
19. Sevdalis N, Undre S, McDermott J, et al. Impact of intraoperative distractions on patient safety: a prospective descriptive study using validated instruments. World J Surg 2014; 38:751–758.
20. Mahadevan K, Cowan E, Kalsi N, et al. Distractions in the cardiac catheterisation laboratory: impact for cardiologists and patient safety. Open Heart 2020; 7:e001260.
21. Healey AN, Primus CP, Koutantji M. Quantifying distraction and interruption in urological surgery. Qual Saf Health Care 2007; 16:135–139.
22. Westbrook JI, Raban MZ, Walter SR, et al. Task errors by emergency physicians are associated with interruptions, multitasking, fatigue and working memory capacity: a prospective, direct observation study. BMJ Qual Saf 2018; 27:655–663.
23. Hardie J, Oeppen RS, Shaw G, et al. You Have Control: aviation communication application for safety-critical times in surgery. BJOMS 2020; 58:1073–1077.
24. Rabol LI, McPhail A, Ostergaard D, et al. Promoters and barriers in hospital team communication. A focus group study. J Commun Health 2012; 5:129–139.
25. Gillespie BM, Harbeck E, Kang E, et al. Correlates of non-technical skills in surgery: a prospective study. BMJ Open 2017; 30:e014480.
26. Kahneman D, Lovallo D, Sibony O. Before you make that big decision. Harv Bus Rev 2011; 89:50–60.

Section 2

Emergency surgery

Chapter 4

Improving outcomes in emergency surgery

Sachal Safdar, Peter McCulloch, Giles Bond-Smith

ABSTRACT

The outcomes of emergency abdominal surgery are significantly worse than those of equivalent elective operations. Part of this disparity is due to the poorer systems available for managing these patients. Improving outcomes, therefore, requires a focus on system improvement.

Management should optimise rapid diagnosis and decision making by involving experienced clinicians in manning ambulatory assessment units, with point-of-care testing and rapid imaging. Preoperative assessment and preparation should involve anaesthetists and physicians, using standardised protocols. Teamwork training can enhance staff co-operation and reduce intrateam barriers.

Timely access to theatre and postoperative intensive care are essential. Surgery should be conducted by appropriately skilled operators and systems should encourage seeking senior help early. Standardised intraoperative care and pain relief protocols should be designed by anaesthetists within the multidisciplinary team.

Early mobilisation programmes can minimise hospital stay. Detection and effective management of complications is facilitated by 'resilient' escalation processes, and standardised communication tools.

BACKGROUND

The impact of emergencies on hospital workload can be judged by the fact that, at any one given time, half of all beds in the UK are occupied by patients admitted as an emergency [1], with this proportion still increasing [2]. Emergency surgery outcomes are invariably much worse than for equivalent elective surgery [3] and up to 15% of patients who undergo emergency surgery are readmitted within 30 days of discharge [4]. Part of this is because

---

Sachal Safdar MSc MBBS, Clinical Research Fellow, King's College London, UK
E-mail: sachal.safdar@kcl.ac.uk (for correspondence)

Peter McCulloch MD, Consultant Surgeon, Nuffield Department of Surgical Science, University of Oxford, UK
E-mail: Peter.mcculloch@nds.ox.ac.uk (for correspondence)

Giles Bond-Smith MBBS, BSc, FRCS, Consultant Surgeon, Directorate of General and Emergency Surgery, Oxford University Hospitals NHS Foundation Trust, Oxford, UK
E-mail: Giles.bond-smith@ouh.nhs.uk (for correspondence)

of the nature of the patient population – often, these patients have advanced disease and acute decompensation, and tend to be older and in poorer general health than elective surgery patients [5]. Resource allocation also tends to be structured around predictable elective surgery and the extent to which accommodation is made for emergencies is variable and frequently inadequate. Not surprisingly, round-the-clock access availability of emergency surgeons and nurses is linked to better outcomes.

Urgency, along with prioritisation of elective work, combines to ensure processes for emergency surgery is often substandard compared to elective work – unfamiliar teams with less experienced surgeons, often fatigued and with much less support than for elective surgery in terms of imaging, laboratory services, intensive care, physiotherapy, etc. Emergency surgery volume for each surgeon is also linked to better outcomes – demonstrating the need for better clinical pathways for more inexperienced surgeons.

Systems analyses and audits of critical incidents [e.g. The National Confidential Enquiry on Perioperative Deaths (NCEPOD)] illustrate numerous ways in which systems of care for emergencies are deficient, and, therefore, make the argument that emergency surgery outcomes could potentially be improved substantially. This chapter will look at the problem through a human factors lens, analysing the work system to detect areas for potential improvement. It will also highlight valid scientific evidence for interventions which could improve outcomes where this exists, and will augment this with advice, based on practice in a large busy teaching hospital Surgical Emergency Unit, which has adopted and developed a set of practices based on these two sources.

PREOPERATIVE CARE

There should be no barrier to review by the surgical team. The emergency department, general practitioners, paramedics or tertiary services should all be able to refer a patient to an acute surgical unit with no resistance. It is quicker, more efficient and kinder to the patient to accept these patients and exclude a surgical pathology than send them 'round the houses' in an effort to reduce surgical workload at the expense of other departments.

In dealing with acute emergencies, the principal tool for improving outcomes is speed. Evidence from extensive investigation of speed of response has found that in-hospital delays (IHDs) are linked directly to surgical mortality. This should make us suspicious of the idea of 'acceptable delay', which might well be the window during which subsequent complications could have been avoided.

Speed will be improved if we optimise preoperative diagnosis and assessment. Here, it may be useful to think in terms of the enhanced recovery after surgery (ERAS) guidelines for preoperative optimisation. These can be summarised as the following:
- Early identification of physiological derangement and intervention
- Screen and monitor for sepsis – then, early imaging and surgery in cases of sepsis
- Risk assessment for surgery
- Age-related evaluation of frailty and cognitive assessment
- Reversal of antithrombotic medication – then, assessment of thromboembolism risk
- Preanaesthetic medication, including analgesia
- Preoperative glucose and electrolyte management; carbohydrate loading
- Nasogastric intubation
- Patient and family shared decision making

Rapid blood analysis is essential for correction of abnormalities. It is obviously important to be aware of abnormalities, such as anaemia, to then better manage them intraoperatively.

One way to achieve a rapid test is to have point-of-care testing (POCT) machines. A similar POCT approach has been designed for imaging, particularly ultrasound [point-of-care ultrasound (POCUS)]. Lack of resource, especially for out of hours imaging, is an important barrier to optimal emergency care. Acute surgery units should ideally have the same access to X-ray, CT scans, ultrasound, MRI, etc., as the emergency department.

Rapid access to observations, blood tests (POCT machines) and ultrasound scans in an acute surgical unit triage can allow the clinician to have all the results inside 15 minutes of arrival. This massively improves time to a definitive decision, which should be under 60 minutes from time of arriving in a surgical emergency unit triage. Access to endoscopy is another major factor in improving speed and service quality as it ensures rapid diagnosis and management for the substantial percentage of patients requiring flexible-sigmoidoscopy, oesophagogastroduodenoscopy (OGD) and endoscopic retrograde cholangiopancreatography (ERCP).

Delegation of initial assessment to inexperienced staff, with inadequate close support, is a common factor in poor outcomes. Inefficient work systems often impose excessive workload on these staff, and inadequate systems for communication and cooperation between departments mean that juniors may be unable to reach the right person, or different departmental priorities may prevent other specialities providing the right timely help.

Preoperative optimisation should be based on both:
1. The patient's condition – meaning the physiological derangements such as fluids and electrolytes, blood loss, treatment of sepsis, etc.
2. The care pathway – ensuring a timely response in terms of key components such as antibiotic administration, CT scanning, scheduling of surgery, etc.

There is evidence for multidisciplinary teams (MDTs) resulting in better outcomes, and qualitative evidence that useful nursing input is not adequately integrated. Lack of systems for communicating critical information can be somewhat remedied by standardisation of a 'shared language'; e.g. there is moderate improvement in patient outcomes when 'situation, background, assessment, recommendation' (SBAR) is used.

Emergency surgery work is disorganised or delayed when decision-making is structured around the convenience of the senior team members – deferring planning and execution until a morning ward round, for example. Restructuring of work systems to match expertise and manpower to need, and to eliminate avoidable delays is obviously likely to be helpful. Similarly, it is important to understand when the peaks and troughs are throughout the day, week and year – to ensure rota management that optimises staffing for workload. The use of a prospective registry to collect relevant system and process data alongside outcomes has been proposed and may help to point out areas for system improvement.

Preoperative pain relief and counselling are important in optimising recovery. Similarly, early interaction with the operative team can help prevent unnecessary delays. Early consultation with anaesthetic teams and intensive care teams is essential in planning preoperative/postoperative care: Medical team consultation may be required for complex and frail patients. There should also be clarity about level of care and priority for surgery needs; an early discussion between senior clinical staff can smooth this process.

Standardisation of protocols for perioperative care, and escalation of concerns, can be helpful in ensuring all aspects of preparation are considered in a timely fashion. Teamwork between doctors and nurses can be enhanced by specific teamwork training and this increases engagement with process improvement exercises – this is the so-called concept of 'shared decision making'.

Transfer logistics are another common problem delaying emergency surgery in many hospitals. Porters are usually disempowered and unable to restart stalled efforts at transfer. A standard handover, ID and transfer protocol with the responsibilities of all parties made clear help to standardise all sorts of handover, to streamline and improve results.

Finally, access to an ambulatory unit so that patients are not admitted to hospital just for investigation, or to reassure the surgeon rather than the patient, greatly improves efficiency and patient experience. However, this can only be achieved if experienced surgeons are the 'gatekeepers' who rapidly decide on which patients to manage on an outpatient basis.

ACCESS TO THEATRE AND INTRAOPERATIVE CARE

Unlike medicine, acute surgical treatment is in theatre. Without access to theatre, the patient cannot get their definitive treatment and so stay in hospital longer, not only before but after treatment, e.g. laparoscopic cholecystectomy patients operated on within 24 hours of admission can usually go home the same day or within 24 hours.

Major savings in time, and improved outcomes, are likely to be brought about by having standard operating procedures (SOPs) for common conditions such as abscesses, acute pancreatitis, cholecystitis, gallstone-related jaundice, intractable biliary colic, diverticulitis, rectal bleeding, pancreatitis, etc. Education is required for anaesthetic and nursing teams as part of these SOPs, to neutralise common but inaccurate beliefs. All over the UK, e.g., hot laparoscopic cholecystectomy is still seen as a nonemergent pathology, despite the evidence that the quicker a symptomatic gallbladder is treated, the less it costs the NHS and the quicker the patient returns to work.

The WHO checklist compliance should ensure that ID checks, antibiotics, deep vein thrombosis (DVT) prophylaxis, allergy and other safety checks are undertaken before surgery commences. Safety checklists have the additional benefit of actually improving team communication. Briefing the team on the plan and possible problems with their solutions is probably the most valuable part of the checklist process but is one of the aspects most commonly omitted or inadequately done.

Responsibility for intraoperative supportive care rests with the anaesthetist but should be discussed with the senior surgeon. One way to pre-empt untoward events is to have better intraoperative communication tools to increase shared situational awareness. Control of fluid balance and cardiac output by transoesophageal echo, the use of epidurals and nerve blocks all require team awareness and response.

Surgery should be conducted rapidly, and more experienced help requested promptly if it seems likely to be required. There are strong cultural barriers to asking for help early, which are deep seated and international. These cannot be overcome by exhortation but require the introduction of systems which make such escalation mandatory in specific circumstances. Novel analgesia methods, such as rectus sheath catheters, can improve recovery and encourage early mobilisation of patients. Intraoperative analgesia is evidenced as being better than postoperative analgesia alone.

POSTOPERATIVE CARE

Adequate monitoring and skilled nursing are essential in the first 12–24 hours after major emergency surgery. Lack of resource for tertiary level care needs to be balanced against the risks of delay. Inappropriate delay should be avoided by early liaison between senior clinicians and managers. In terms of the team looking after patients postoperatively, surgical residents, who can provide round-the-clock care, have been shown to improve outcomes overall for patients (alone or in conjunction with other teams).

Analgesia, early mobilisation and re-establishment of enteral nutrition and physiotherapy should be part of the standard postoperative protocol. Physiotherapy is a low-cost, postoperative intervention to reduce complications after emergency surgery. There is also reduced mortality when early enteral nutrition is established. Delayed mobilisation increases the risk of readmission and of death, especially in the old and frail. ERAS programmes in the acute setting ensure patients eat and drink and mobilise quicker. Perioperative input, before and after the operation, can speed this process up, as well as good patient education before the operation.

Managing complications is also a crucial part of the postoperative care of the patient. There is some suggestion that SBAR is better implemented if used in conjunction with other interventions [5]. The human factors interventions of a shared language for communication about critically ill patients, and of 'resilient' escalation procedures, (which strengthen rescue processes by making them more agile in adapting to rapidly evolving situations) are currently under evaluation and are showing promise in improving the speed and quality of escalation and treatment. The concept of 'failure to rescue' may be a better measure of service quality than simple operative mortality, whose use needs to be contextualised.

If MDTs are involved, as they should be, they should also be part of discharge planning. This would bring about a more co-ordinated discharge effort and would reduce unnecessary stalling while awaiting input from multiple specialities, who may have visited the patient during the current admission.

Key points for clinical practice

- Systems analyses and audits of critical incidents (e.g., NCEPOD) illustrate numerous ways in which systems of care for emergencies are deficient and, therefore, make the argument that emergency surgery outcomes could potentially be improved
- In dealing with acute emergencies, the principal tool for improving outcomes is speed
- Lack of resource, especially for out of hours imaging, is an important barrier to optimal emergency care
- Delegation of initial assessment to inexperienced staff, with inadequate close support, is a common factor in poor outcomes and escalation to senior staff should be mandatory in specific circumstances
- Early consultation with anaesthetic teams and intensive care teams is essential in planning preoperative/postoperative care: medical team consultation may be required for complex and frail patients
- Major savings in time, and improved outcomes, are likely to be brought about by having SOPs for common conditions
- The human factors interventions of a shared language for communication about critically ill patients, and of 'resilient' escalation procedures, are currently under evaluation and are showing promise in improving the speed and quality of escalation and treatment

ACKNOWLEDGEMENT

This work was funded in part by the National Institute for Health Research (NIHR) (Programme Grant for Applied Research NIHR200868).

REFERENCES

1. Watson R, Crump H, Imison C, et al. Emergency General Surgery: Challenges and Opportunities Research Report. London: Nuff Trust, 2016.
2. Wohlgemut JM, Ramsay G, Jansen JO. The Changing Face of Emergency General Surgery: A 20-year Analysis of Secular Trends in Demographics, Diagnoses, Operations, and Outcomes. Ann Surg 2020; 271:581–589.
3. Thompson AM, Stonebridge PA. Building a framework for trust: critical event analysis of deaths in surgical care. BMJ 2005; 330:1139–1142.
4. Havens JM, Olufajo OA, Cooper ZR, et al. Defining Rates and Risk Factors for Readmissions Following Emergency General Surgery. JAMA Surg 2016; 151:330–336.
5. Lo L, Rotteau L, Shojania K. Can SBAR be implemented with high fidelity and does it improve communication between healthcare workers? A systematic review. BMJ Open 2021; 11:e055247.

Chapter 5

Management and prevention of burst abdomen

Arunima Verma, Sunil Kumar

ABSTRACT

Burst abdomen (BA), also known as 'evisceration' or 'fascial dehiscence', occurs as a postoperative complication of a laparotomy. Presentation of BA may range from 1 to >23 days, most commonly around 7 days postoperatively. The rate of occurrence has been reported to be 0.2–5.0% in elective surgery and 3.8–28.0% in emergency laparotomies. BA is associated with increased length of hospital stay and morbidity, a mortality rate of 10–30% and risk of incisional hernias of up to 33%. Various factors affect the occurrence of BA and they are patient related, technique related and depend on the pathology for which the surgery was done. BA is considered a preventable condition, if due care is taken in both patient selection and technical surgical skills. BA presents with a complex spectrum of symptoms which makes the surgical repair challenging. Research has focussed on placement of incisions, choice of suture material, suturing technique and use of adjuncts such as meshes or negative pressure devices. No single protocol is available for management of BA. The group of patients with BA is heterogenous so that individual patient factors need to be considered and the guidelines available can be used as a basis for decision making, when considering different therapeutic approaches.

INTRODUCTION

The simplest definition of a burst abdomen (BA) is spontaneous opening of a surgical wound after an abdominal operation. BA is also known as 'evisceration' or 'fascial dehiscence'. A more detailed description of BA would be an unintended acute wound failure at the level of the fascia, which presents as a postoperative complication of a laparotomy, after primary closure of the incision [1]. Another clinical entity, with similar challenges as the BA, is an open abdomen (OA). However, OA is formed as a result of

---

Arunima Verma MS FRCS FACS, Chief Medical Superintendent and Head of Surgery, Tata Motors Hospital, Jamshedpur, Jharkhand, India
E-mail: vermaarunima@yahoo.co.in (for correspondence)

Sunil Kumar MS FRCS(Edinburgh) FRCS(England) FACS FFST(Edinburgh) Professor and Ex-Head Consultant Surgeon, Tata Main Hospital, Jamshedpur, Jharkhand, India
E-mail: vermaarunima@yahoo.co.in (for correspondence)

a deliberate decision not to close the fascia at the end of laparotomy and is used in the management of critically ill patients with serious intra-abdominal conditions, such as in damage control surgery for abdominal trauma, or in conditions causing abdominal compartment syndrome.

A BA rate of 0.2–5.0% [2–4] in elective surgery and 3.8–28.0% [5–7] in emergency laparotomies has been reported. The accuracy of reporting is uncertain due to different populations and different standards or technique for fascial closure and is probably under reported. BA is associated with increased length of hospital stay, morbidity, mortality 10–30% [8–10] and risk of incisional hernias of up to 33% [11].

RISK FACTORS

There is no single cause for BA. Various factors affect the occurrence of BA and they are patient related, technique related and depend on the pathology for which the surgery was done, as listed in **Table 5.1**.

PATHOPHYSIOLOGY

Drainage of serosanguinous fluid from the incision precedes dehiscence in up to 84% of cases. BA may occur during the first 24 hours after surgery, but presentation may range from 1 to >23 days, most commonly around 7 days postoperatively. Fascial healing is a complex process which completes over a period of 1 year. Rapid gain in strength occurs from the 8th postoperative day, which is the beginning of the proliferative phase, and continues up to the 2nd month, which marks the end of collagen synthesis. After 2 months, the fascia regains almost 50% of its original strength. Two basic events seen in wound dehiscence are decreased, wound strength and increased collagenolysis, most commonly due to infection. As a result of infection, there is hypoperfusion of the healing linea alba, which leads to inhibition of collagen synthesis which requires adequate oxygen supply. Nutritional elements such as ascorbic acid and ferrous ions are also required for this process. Degradation of collagen exceeds the synthesis of collagen in wounds of patients with BA. Examples are shown in **Figures 5.1 to 5.3**.

Table 5.1 Risk factors for burst abdomen			
Patient factors	**Intraoperative factors**	**Postoperative factors**	**Primary disease**
• Age >55 years • Male gender • Intraperitoneal sepsis • Malnourishment • Obesity • Jaundice • Cirrhosis • Uraemia • Steroids • Anaemia • Smoking • Diabetes mellitus • Sarcopenia	• Emergency surgery • Surgical technique for closure • Suturing • Knotting • Suture material	• Prolonged ventilation • Postoperative blood transfusion • Poor tissue perfusion – e.g. postoperative hypotension • Postoperative ileus • Chest complications • Wound infection • Radiotherapy	• Peritonitis • Intestinal obstruction • Blunt abdominal trauma • Gastrointestinal malignancy

Pathophysiology

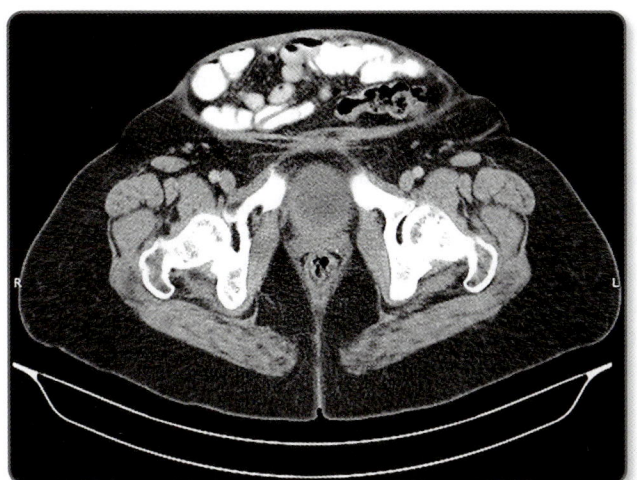

Figure 5.1 Burst abdomen with herniation of intestinal contents through a pfannenstiel incision.

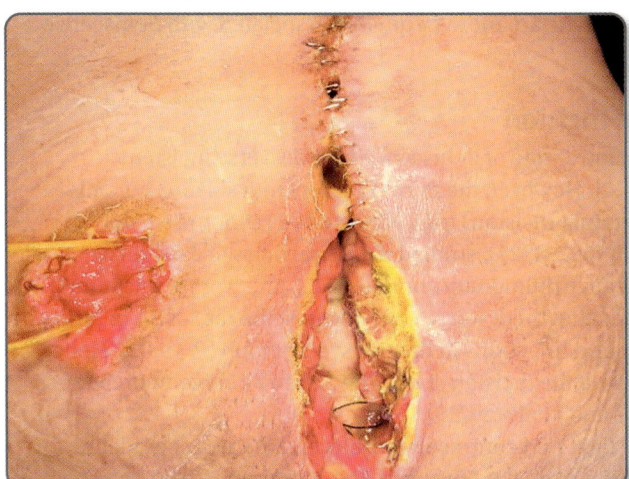

Figure 5.2 Burst abdomen in a case of exploratory laparotomy with temporary stoma.

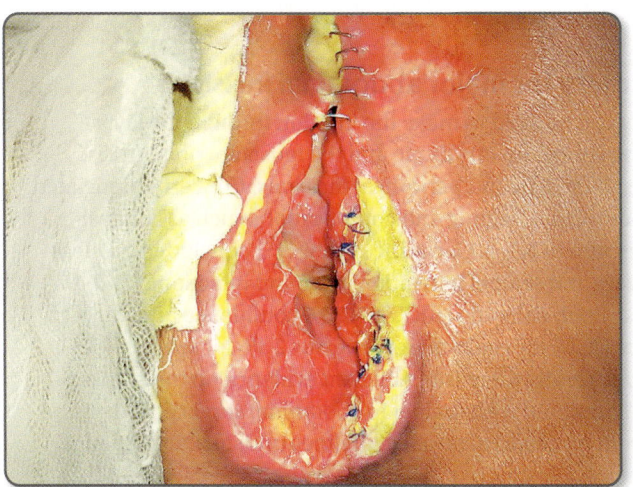

Figure 5.3 Burst abdomen with visible bowel loops, surgical site infection and broken fascial sutures.

PREVENTION AND MANAGEMENT OF BURST ABDOMEN

Burst abdomen is considered a preventable condition, if due care is taken in both patient selection and technical surgical skills.

For elective surgery, patient condition should be optimised by correcting anaemia and malnutrition and ensuring optimal control of comorbidities, such as hypertension and diabetes. In emergency situations, these factors cannot be altered and, hence, excellent surgical technique and good postoperative care assume even greater importance.

There are many different opinions on the optimum surgical technique for closing the abdomen to prevent the complication of BA. Hence, this chapter will consider various options and the supporting evidence. Research has focussed on placement of incisions, choice of suture material, suturing technique, use of adjuncts such as meshes or negative pressure devices.

Abdominal incisions
Many different incisions will allow access to the abdominal cavity and some are preferred for specific conditions. However, some are more frequently associated with dehiscence and BA.

Midline versus transverse incision
There are studies which report a lower rate of dehiscence for transverse incisions compared to vertical incisions [12]. However, the POVATI (Postsurgical Pain Outcome of Vertical and Transverse Abdominal Incision) trial, which was a randomised, double-blinded equivalence trial (ISRCTN60734227), studied the frequencies of early onset of complications (e.g. BA, postoperative pulmonary complications and wound infections) as its primary endpoint and found that there was no difference in the rate of BA in both groups. It also reported more wound infections in the transverse group ($P = 0.02$). Hence, it concluded that the decision about the incision should be driven by surgeon preference considering the patient's disease and anatomy [13].

However, other studies have suggested contrasting results and the recent guideline for closure of abdominal wall incisions, from the European and American Hernia Societies, has proposed that avoiding midline incision for laparotomies and specimen extraction sites may reduce the risk of incisional hernia [14].

Scalpel versus electrosurgery for major abdominal incisions
Both scalpel and electrosurgery can be used to make the incision through the layers of the abdominal wall, including subcutaneous tissue and the musculoaponeurosis, irrespective of the technique used for skin and peritoneal incisions. Concerns associated with electrosurgery include poor wound healing and complications such as surgical site infection, which may predispose to BA. A Cochrane review [15] concluded no clear difference between electrosurgery and scalpel in relation to wound infections [7.7% for electrosurgery versus 7.4% for scalpel; risk ratio (RR) 1.07; 95% confidence interval (CI) 0.74–1.54] or wound dehiscence (2.7% for electrosurgery versus 2.4% for scalpel; RR 1.21; 95% CI 0.58–2.50). Hence, currently there is insufficient evidence on the relative effectiveness of electrosurgery compared with scalpel in abdominal surgery, so decision makers are likely to follow current local and national guidelines until further evidence becomes available.

Choice of suture material

Burst abdomen, after a laparotomy, is associated with both an increased mortality rate and complications including incisional hernias. Several trials have been carried out to identify the ideal suture material to be used, or the type of abdominal closure to be performed (see below), to avoid these complications. Most of the available evidence is of low quality due to the limitations of study designs and number of patients included. High-quality trials are needed to address this clinical challenge.

The first step in the pathophysiology of wound healing is the migration of inflammatory cells to the wound. In the case of laparotomy, fascial closure is of utmost importance for preventing BA. Fascial healing starts after inflammatory cell recruitment, which starts to produce collagen after 2–5 days. Thereafter, the proliferation phase lasts for 3 weeks during which type III collagen, consisting of thin weak fibres, is produced. This is followed by the maturation phase where type III collagen is replaced by type I collagen, which is strong and thick. The maturation phase is then followed by remodelling or realignment of collagen fibres along tension lines and this can take up to a year. With this background, we can see that the suture material chosen should have a half-life tensile strength long enough to provide support to the healing fascia.

A meta-analysis [16], including 23 randomised controlled trials (RCTs), found no significant differences on incisional hernia rate when comparing nonabsorbable, slowly absorbable and fast-absorbable sutures, using the same suturing technique. No significant difference was seen in the occurrence of incisional hernia and BA, between slowly absorbable and nonabsorbable sutures. However, nonabsorbable sutures were associated with prolonged wound pain and suture sinus formation [17]. The RCT [18] compared the incidence of wound dehiscence with a delayed absorbable and a nonabsorbable suture material, in the mass closure of vertical laparotomy wounds. It reported an overall incidence of wound dehiscence to be 11.5% and found a significant difference in the incidence of wound dehiscence between the two groups – 6% with Prolene and 17% with Vicryl ($X^2 = 05.944$, 1 DF, $P = 00.0148$). Based on this, they recommended Prolene to be a better and more economical suture material for closure of vertical laparotomy wounds.

There is no universal guideline for the best suture material and the ISSAAC-Trial [19], which was a prospective multicentre historically controlled trial, was designed to evaluate the clinical safety and efficacy of MonoMax, which is a long-term absorbable monofilament *suture*, which was also used in the INSECT trial. However, it concluded that MonoMax was a safe suture for abdominal wall closure after primary midline laparotomy, but the RCT, including a larger number of patients, would be necessary to evaluate its efficiency in terms of incisional hernia development. However, using slowly absorbable suture material, as it retains its strength until the fascial tissue is healed, seems prudent.

Suturing technique

A Cochrane review [17], including 55 RCTs with a total of 19,174 participants, concluded that the risk of wound dehiscence was not reduced or altered by suture absorption (absorbable versus nonabsorbable sutures, RR 0.78; 95% CI 0.55–1.10, moderate-quality evidence; or slow versus fast absorbable sutures, RR 1.55; 95% CI 0.92–2.61, moderate-quality evidence), or closure method (mass versus layered, RR 0.69; 95% CI 0.31–1.52, moderate-quality evidence) or closure technique (continuous versus interrupted, RR 1.21; 95% CI 0.90–1.64, moderate-quality evidence).

The STITCH trial [20] (small bites versus large bites for closure of abdominal midline incisions), which was a double-blind, multicentre, RCT, compared large bites suture technique with the small bites technique for fascial closure of midline laparotomy incisions. They concluded that the small bites suture technique was more effective than the traditional large bites technique, for prevention of incisional hernia (1-year incisional hernia in small bite technique 13% and large bite technique 21%; $p = 0.0220$) in midline incisions and also it was not associated with a higher rate of adverse events.

Current practice guidelines suggest continuous small-bites suturing technique, with a slowly absorbable suture, should be used for closure of elective midline incisions [19]. The suture length (SL) to wound length (WL) (SL:WL) ratio of 4:1 is recommended [1]. The rationale for this is that continuous suturing distributes tension better along the suture line, leaves less foreign body in the wound and takes less time to complete. The small bite technique constitutes tissue bites of 5–9 mm from the wound edges to incorporate aponeurosis only, with the stitches placed 5 mm apart to ensure adequate distribution of tension. A slowly absorbable monofilament suture, that has more than half of the tensile strength remaining after 6 weeks and absorption completed after 6–8 months, is recommended.

Continuous versus interrupted sutures for prevention of burst abdomen

The multicentre INSECT (Interrupted or Continuous Slowly Absorbable Sutures for Closure of Primary Elective Midline Abdominal Incisions) trial [21] found no difference between continuous and interrupted fascial closure in elective cases but the debate regarding the most effective strategy of abdominal wall closure in emergency laparotomies still continues. To find further evidence to recommend optimal suturing technique in emergency laparotomies, a single-centre RCT, the CONIAC (continuous and interrupted abdominal-wall closure after primary emergency midline laparotomy) trial [22], has been registered, the results of which may impact emergency laparotomy closure techniques.

Although the INSECT trial results were considered to be highly generalizable to hospitals of all categories in developed countries treating mainly a Caucasian population, concern existed regarding its relevance to the Asian population. The rationale for possibly having a different technique for the Asian population is that, while the western world patients are usually well nourished and present to surgeon within a few hours of acute abdomen, with a risk of 2–4% for wound dehiscence, the Asian population has a very high incidence of BA in the range of 10% or more, possibly due to high prevalence of protein calorie malnutrition, significant incidence of tuberculosis and typhoid and delayed presentation to the surgeon for laparotomy [23].

A multicentre RCT from India [23] looked at the advantages of interrupted X sutures for fascial closure, while an experimental study from Spain [24] discussed the 'double-diabolo' suturing method for better outcome in abdominal closure. The rationale of such interrupted suturing method to be superior to continuous suture is that the continuous suture has a Gigli saw effect when there is abdominal wall movement on breathing, coughing, sneezing, micturition and defecation, as the suture moves 'to and fro'. All the forces exerted on a thread, fixed at two points, can be described according to parameters such as direction, angulation and the intersection of threads. Ideally, the tension is equally distributed across the whole length of a continuous suture between the two fixed points, making it better for withstanding forces. However, the tearing stress, separation stress and

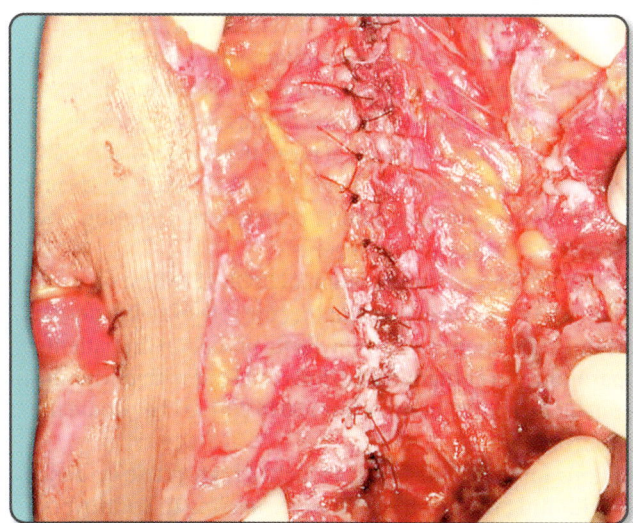

Figure 5.4 Primary fascial closure done with interrupted sutures complicated by burst abdomen.

breaking stress were calculated to be highest with a double application of 'X' like suture configuration called 'double diabolo.' Based on this, the 'cut out or cut through force' of 'X' suture was expected to be low. It is also argued that wound dehiscence occurs due to suture cutting through fascia and, in a continuous suture, the integrity of the entire wound is placed on a single suture thus, if there is a cut through at a single point, the entire suture can slacken. Despite the better results for interrupted sutures, BA can still occur **(Figure 5.4)**. Keeping these factors in mind, an emergency surgeon should be aware of the risk factors of BA and should decide on the type of suturing technique accordingly.

Role of mesh augmentation in abdominal wall closure

At times after laparotomy, or in BA, it is not possible to reapproximate the fascia without tension and closure under tension is doomed to failure. This leads to the requirement for a fascial substitute. Many different methods have been used to close the abdomen, ranging from simple closure of the skin over the defect, leaving the fascia and peritoneum wide open, to doing relaxing incisions of both fascia and skin well away from the wound, or closing the primary wound and skin grafting the resulting defect. Alternatively, mesh augmentation has also been used and numerous meshes have been developed and marketed for this indication. There is low-quality evidence to recommend the use of prophylactic mesh augmentation, after elective midline laparotomy, to reduce incidence of incisional hernia, with limited data on the occurrence of BA or mesh infection and surgical site occurrences (SSO). An American cost-utility analysis [25] found prophylactic mesh augmentation after suture closure of the midline in high-risk patients to be more effective and less costly and, overall, more cost-effective than primary suture closure.

An RCT [26] conducted on 100 patients, using a supra-aponeurotic polypropylene mesh in the primary closure of laparotomies with a high risk of incisional hernia, found that no incisional hernia was detected in the group in which closure was done using the mesh ($P = 0.02$). However, there is very little evidence to suggest use of permanent synthetic mesh for prophylactic mesh augmentation, as some studies found biological mesh with better results in terms of incisional hernias and mesh explantation.

The ROCSS trial [27] (prophylactic biological mesh reinforcement versus standard closure of stoma site), which was an RCT carried out in 37 hospitals across three European countries, including patients above 18 years of age, compared the reinforcement of the abdominal wall with a biological mesh at the time of stoma closure with standard closure technique. This study supported the use of biological mesh in stoma closure site reinforcement to reduce the early formation of incisional hernias, as it showed significant reduction of hernia by use of mesh without significant difference in wound infection rate, seroma rate, quality of life, pain scores or serious adverse events.

Another multicentric RCT [28], PROPHYlactic Implantation of BIOlogic Mesh in peritonitis (PROPHYBIOM), is in phase IV. This trial is evaluating the role of swine dermal collagen prosthesis in the preperitoneal position, as a prophylactic procedure in patients undergoing urgent/emergent laparotomy, in contaminated/infected field with peritonitis, with the objective to reduce the rate of incisional hernias from 50 to 20% and evaluate the morbidity and mortality in this group.

Just as debates over the indications for use of mesh due to lack of high-grade evidence persist, the evidence regarding positioning the mesh is also weak, leading to controversy over the precise placement of the mesh with respect to the layers of the abdominal wall. The ROCSS trial, based on consensus meeting with clinicians, used the biological mesh in the intra-abdominal position (deep to the abdominal wall). This position was less technically complex, had lower seroma formation rate and was not associated with any increase in pain.

The PRIMA trial [29] (prevention of incisional hernia with prophylactic onlay and sublay mesh reinforcement versus primary sutures only in midline laparotomies), a multicentre, double-blind, RCT including 480 patients, used the polypropylene mesh and recommended use of onlay mesh reinforcement, as they reported a significant reduction in incidence of incisional hernia with onlay mesh reinforcement compared with sublay mesh reinforcement ($P = 0.05$) and primary suture only ($P = 0.0016$). Although there was higher seroma formation in the onlay group, the incidence of wound infection did not differ in the groups in this trial.

The guidelines do not advise synthetic mesh prophylactically in the intraperitoneal space, due to the increased risk of adhesive complications. Retromuscular mesh placement has the lowest incidence of wound infection compared to other sites such as onlay mesh, although surgical skill for retromuscular placement may not be available. Therefore, although the onlay implantation is associated with an increased risk of SSO, it is still recommended as it is easy to perform and, if in future incisional hernia repair is required, the retromuscular plane remains intact.

The potential benefits of mesh augmentation in an emergency setting are considered very minimal, due to the various indications for emergency laparotomies and types and position of mesh used. Therefore, the final decision to use a mesh, the type of mesh and the mesh position should be taken by the surgeon in charge, taking into account the patient's condition and availability of resources and technique [1,14].

Role of component separation/relaxing incisions/myoplasties in abdominal wall closure

Component separation is an elective technique for closing abdominal wall defects, resulting from previous surgery or trauma or for large complex abdominal wall hernia. There are some reports favouring it as an early technique (within 6 days) for closure of the OA following emergency laparotomy for penetrating trauma, or in patients suffering severe burns requiring a decompressive laparotomy [30,31]. The abdominal wall of patients with a BA does not present the same characteristics as an abdominal wall of an individual who undergoes an elective hernia surgery, in terms of rigidity and oedema. Use of the component separation technique may add potential complexity to future hernia repair in the same patient. A small study [32] used the incision of transversus abdominus and internal oblique muscles (TI incision), with incision including the external oblique muscle (TIE incision) in addition, or incision involving the Scarpa's fascia (TIES incision) and reported good results in BA. However, guidelines suggest a careful and judicious evaluation of the patient's condition and requirements before using the technique, to avoid potential harm for future abdominal wall surgical treatment [1].

Dynamic and static abdominal wall closure

Dynamic closure techniques should be used in BA for patients who do not have intestinal fistula and in whom definitive (primary) fascial closure is likely, within the initial hospitalisation period. Some novel techniques for dynamic abdominal wall closure, such as the delayed dynamic abdominal closure (DDAC) device (abdominal retraction anchor – ABRA system), Wittmann patch, ABRA system+ negative pressure wound therapy (NPWT), fascial traction (mesh or other) + NPWT or innovative techniques with punctate holes made in the longitudinal axis of the surgical wound and transfixing all layers of the abdominal wall, have also claimed good results and alleviate the need for a prosthetic mesh, or vascularised flaps or skin graft, providing good cosmetic results [33,34].

A novel device (Fasciotens Abdomen; Essen, Germany) **(Figure 5.5)**, which works on the principle of a dynamic vertical traction force on the fascia, was successfully implemented in a series of 20 patients. This achieved early primary fascial closure within at a mean of 3 days (0–14 days), without mesh augmentation or component separation in all cases and without any severe complications [35]. However, early application of dynamic closure devices is not possible if there is haemodynamic instability, persistent abdominal peritonitis, uncontrolled source of infection or increased intra-abdominal volume due to visceral oedema.

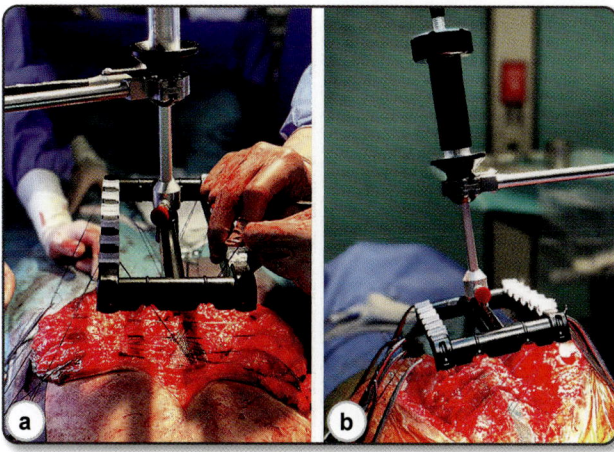

Figure 5.5 (a) Vertical traction device (Fasciotens Abdomen; Essen, Germany). (b) The main principle of the device is the application of dynamic vertical traction along both fascial margins over a clamping system.

Where dynamic closure is not available, static closure technique needs to be considered. Such static closure techniques include the Bogota bag, NPWT **(Figure 5.6)** (commercial and noncommercial) and Mesh bridging (inlay). Low-quality evidence from multiple studies reported fascial closure rates of approximately 28.5% with Bogota Bag, 36.9% with mesh bridging and 52.1% with NPWT [1]. However, there is higher incidence of fistula formation in the mesh group with more SSO. Hence, NPWT appears to be the most effective static closure technique.

A combination of a dynamic closure device with NPWT shows a higher primary fascial closure rate in OA but the role in BA has not been defined due to low quality of evidence.

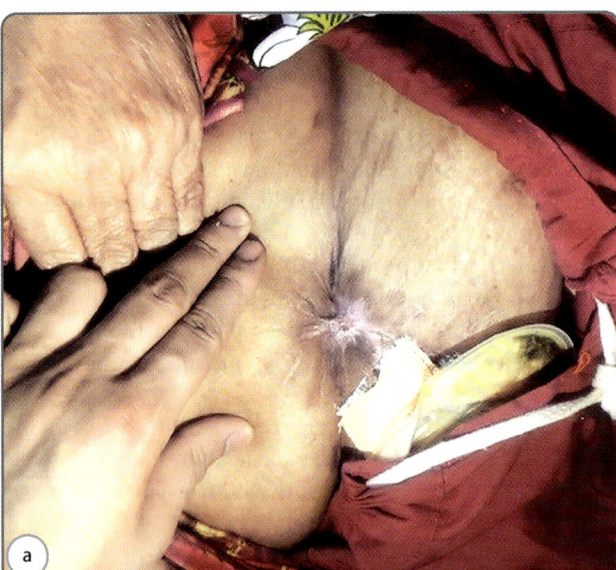

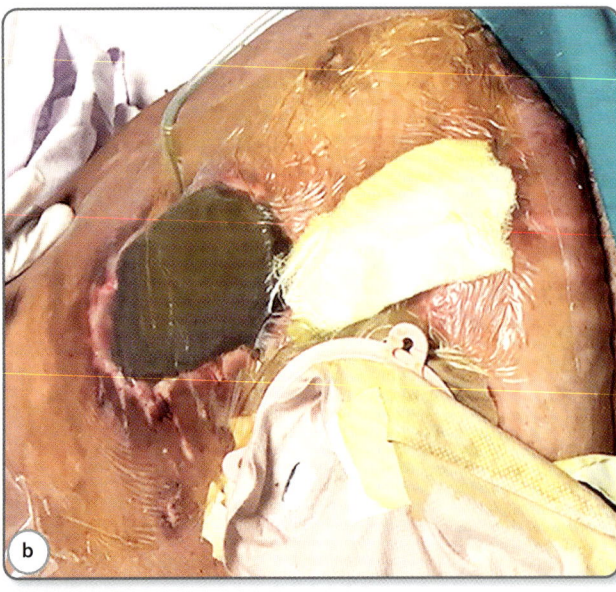

Figure 5.6 Noncommercial NPWT used in BA, followed by abdominal closure. (a) NWPT device applied. (b) Skin and subcutaneous tissue dehiscence needing secondary suturing. (c) Healed wound with closure of abdominal wall post NPWT and secondary suturing. BA, burst abdomen; NPWT, negative pressure wound therapy. *Continues opposite.*

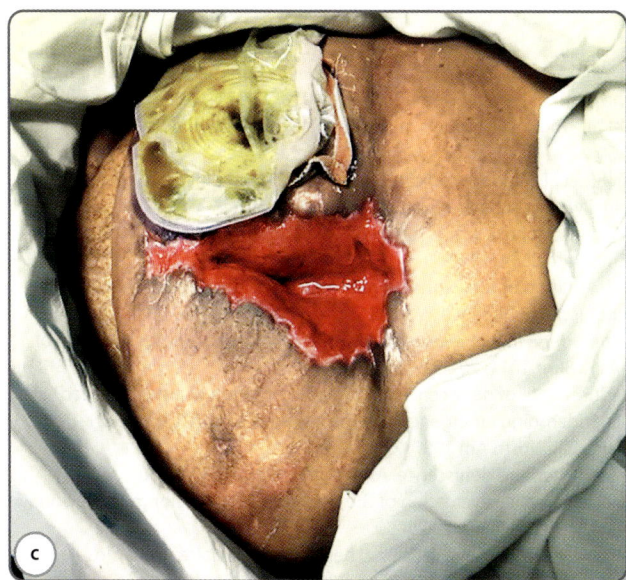

Figure 5.6 *Continued.*

CONCLUSION

The BA presents with a complex spectrum of symptoms which makes surgical repair challenging. Patient selection, careful planning of the incision and optimal closure technique are all important in preventing BA. Dynamic closure techniques may be better for abdominal wall closure once BA occurs, to prevent complications such as intra-abdominal hypertension, abdominal compartment syndrome or enteroatmospheric fistulas, the aim being early primary fascial closure. However, the group of patients with BA are so heterogenous that individual patient factors need to be considered, using the guidelines available as a basis for decision making, when considering different therapeutic approaches.

Key points for clinical practice

- Burst abdomen is spontaneous opening of a surgical wound after an abdominal operation and is associated with high morbidity and mortality
- Risk factors for BA are multifactorial and are patient related, technique related and dependent on the pathology for which the surgery was done
- Burst abdomen is a preventable condition, if due care is taken in the suturing technique and certain precautionary measures taken in patients with risk factors for BA
- Current practice guidelines suggest continuous small-bites suturing technique, with a slowly absorbable suture for closure of elective midline incisions with SL:WL ratio of 4:1
- Mesh augmentation for abdominal wall closure, the type of mesh and the mesh position should be balanced by the surgeon taking into account the patient's condition and the availability of resources and familiarity with the technique
- Component separation should be used judiciously in emergency procedures to avoid potential harm for future abdominal wall surgical treatment

REFERENCES

1. López-Cano M, García-Alamino JM, Antoniou SA, et al. EHS clinical guidelines on the management of the abdominal wall in the context of the open or burst abdomen. Hernia 2018; 22:921–939.
2. Webster C, Neumayer L, Smout R, et al. Prognostic models of abdominal wound dehiscence after laparotomy. J Surg Res 2003; 109:130–137.
3. Bloemen A, van Dooren P, Huizinga BF, et al. Randomized clinical trial comparing polypropylene or polydioxanone for midline abdominal wall closure. Br J Surg 2011; 98:633–639.
4. Kenig J, Richter P, Lasek A, et al. The efficacy of risk scores for predicting abdominal wound dehiscence: a case-controlled validation study. BMC Surg 2014; 14:65.
5. Marwah S, Marwah N, Singh M, et al. Addition of rectus sheath relaxation incisions to emergency midline laparotomy for peritonitis to prevent fascial dehiscence. World J Surg 2005; 29:235–239.
6. Kim JJ, Liang MK, Subramanian A, et al. Predictors of relaparotomy after nontrauma emergency general surgery with initial fascial closure. Am J Surg 2011; 202:549–552.
7. Tolstrup MB, Watt SK, Gögenur I. Reduced rate of dehiscence after implementation of a standardized fascial closure technique in patients undergoing emergency laparotomy. Ann Surg 2017; 265:821–826.
8. Carlson MA. Acute wound failure. Surg Clin North Am 1997; 77:607–636.
9. Johnson H, Cohen JR. Factors influencing wound dehiscence. Am J Surg 1992; 163:324–330.
10. Yilmaz KB, Akinci M, Doğan L, et al. A prospective evaluation of the risk factors for development of wound dehiscence and incisional hernia. Turkish J Surg 2013; 29:25–30.
11. Korgaard Jensen T, Gögenur I, Tolstrup MB. High rate of incisional hernia observed after mass closure of burst abdomen. Hernia 2021; 26:1–8.
12. Seiler CM, Bruckner T, Diener MK, et al. Interrupted or continuous slowly absorbable sutures for closure of primary elective midline abdominal incisions: a multicenter randomized trial (INSECT: ISRCTN24023541). Ann Surg 2009; 249(4):576–582.
13. Begum B, Zaman R, Ahmed M, et al. Burst abdomen-A preventable morbidity. Mymensingh Med J 2008; 17(1):63–66.
14. Seiler CM, Deckert A, Diener MK, et al. Midline Versus Transverse Incision in Major Abdominal Surgery: A Randomized, Double-Blind Equivalence Trial (POVATI: ISRCTN60734227). Ann Surg 2009; 249(6):913–920.
15. Deerenberg EB, Henriksen NA, Antoniou GA, et al. Updated Guideline for Closure of Abdominal Wall Incisions from the European and American Hernia Societies. Brit J Surg 2022; 109(12):1239–1250.
16. Charoenkwan K, Iheozor-Ejiofor Z, Rerkasem K, et al. Scalpel versus electrosurgery for major abdominal incisions. Cochrane Database Syst Rev 2017; (6):CD005987.
17. Henriksen NA, Deerenberg EB, Venclauskas L, et al. Meta-Analysis on Materials and Techniques for Laparotomy Closure: The MATCH Review. World J Surg 2018; 42(6):1666–1678.
18. Patel SV, Paskar DD, Nelson RL, et al. Closure methods for laparotomy incisions for preventing incisional hernias and other wound complications. Cochrane Database Syst Rev 2017; (11):CD005661.
19. Pandey S, Singh M, Singh K, et al. A Prospective Randomized Study Comparing Non-Absorbable Polypropylene (Prolene®) and Delayed Absorbable Polyglactin 910 (Vicryl®) Suture Material in Mass Closure of Vertical Laparotomy Wounds. Indian J Surg 2013; 75(4):306–310.
20. Albertsmeier M, Seiler CM, Fischer L, et al. Evaluation of the Safety and Efficacy of MonoMax® Suture Material for Abdominal Wall Closure after Primary Midline Laparotomy—a Controlled Prospective Multicentre Trial: ISSAAC [NCT005725079]. Langenbeck's Arch Surg 2012; 397(3):363–371.
21. Deerenberg EB, Harlaar JJ, Steyerberg EW, et al. Small Bites Versus Large Bites for Closure of Abdominal Midline Incisions (STITCH): a Double-Blind, Multicentre, Randomised Controlled Trial. Lancet 2015; 386(10000):1254–1260.
22. Wolf S, Arbona de Gracia L, Sommer F, et al. Continuous and interrupted abdominal-wall closure after primary emergency midline laparotomy (CONIAC-trial): study protocol for a randomised controlled single centre trial. BMJ Open 23; 12(11):e059709.
23. Mishra PR, Kumar S, Mishra S, et al. Interrupted X-Suture Prevents Burst Abdomen: Analysis of 5 Randomised Controlled Trials from India. Indian J Surg 2022; 85:233–240.
24. Lara FJ, Jiminez RZ, Donoso FJ, et al. A Novel Suturing Technique, Based on Physical Principles. World J Adv Res Rev 2020; 8(3):80–90.
25. Fischer JP, Basta MN, Wink JD, et al. Cost–utility analysis of the use of prophylactic mesh augmentation compared with primary fascial suture repair in patients at high risk for incisional hernia. Surgery 2015; 158:700–711.

26. Gutiérrez de la Peña C, Medina Achirica C, Domínguez-Adame E, et al. Primary closure of laparotomies with high risk of incisional hernia using prosthetic material: analysis of usefulness. Hernia 2003; 7:134–136.
27. Bhangu A, Nepogodiev D, Ives N, et al. Prophylactic Biological Mesh Reinforcement Versus Standard Closure of Stoma Site (ROCSS): a Multicentre, Randomised Controlled Trial. Lancet 2022; 395(10222):417–426.
28. Coccolini F, Tarasconi A, Petracca GL, et al. PROPHYlactic Implantation of BIOlogic Mesh in Peritonitis (PROPHYBIOM): a Prospective Multicentric Randomized Controlled Trial. Trials 2022: 23(1):198.
29. Jairam AP, Timmermans L, Eker HH, et al. PRIMA Trialist Group. Prevention of incisional hernia with prophylactic onlay and sublay mesh reinforcement versus primary suture only in midline laparotomies (PRIMA): 2-year follow-up of a multicentre, double-blind, randomised controlled trial. Lancet 2017; 390(10094):567–576.
30. Rawstorne E, Smart CJ, Fallis SA, et al. Component separation in abdominal trauma. J Surg Case Rep 2014; 2014(1):rjt133.
31. Poulakidas S, Kowal-Vern A. Component separation technique for abdominal wall reconstruction in burn patients with decompressive laparotomies. J Trauma 2009; 67(6):1435–1438.
32. Esmat M. A New Technique in Closure of Burst Abdomen: TI, TIE and TIES Incisions. World J Surg 2006; 30(6):1063–1073.
33. Iype S, Butler A, Jamieson N, et al. Delayed Dynamic Abdominal Wall Closure Following Multi-Visceral Transplantation. Int J Surg Case Rep 2014; 5(12):988–991.
34. Kamamoto F, Batista BN, Tokeshi F. New Technique for Dynamic Closure of the Abdominal Wall. Rev Col Bras Cir 2010; 37(5):376–378.
35. Fung S, Ashmawy H, Krieglstein C, et al. Vertical traction device prevents abdominal wall retraction and facilitates early primary fascial closure of septic and non-septic open abdomen. Langenbecks Arch Surg 2022; 407:2075–2083.

Section 3

Breast surgery

Chapter 6

Neoadjuvant endocrine therapy and agents for early breast cancer

Aglaia Skolariki, Simon Lord, Ramsey I Cutress

INTRODUCTION

Neoadjuvant therapy in breast cancer, also known as presurgical or induction therapy, is commonly used in locally advanced and inoperable disease to downstage tumours and improve surgical outcomes by minimising the extent of the procedure in the breast and axilla. Where mastectomy is indicated, neoadjuvant therapy can also be offered to achieve tumour shrinkage that will allow breast-conservation surgery (BCS) and optimise cosmetic results. More recently, the ability to determine whether a patient has residual disease following neoadjuvant treatment has facilitated personalisation of systemic therapy intensification with improved survival outcomes in poor responders in clinical trials [1] and practice.

Neoadjuvant therapies for breast cancer generally either include chemotherapy or endocrine therapy (ET). Neoadjuvant chemotherapy (NCT) is typically recommended in patients with stages II and III human epidermal growth factor receptor 2 positive (HER2+) and triple-negative breast cancer (TNBC) subtypes, as response to neoadjuvant treatment can provide prognostic and predictive value and guide treatment decisions following surgery in the adjuvant setting [2]. So far, NCT has also been considered the treatment of choice to downstage tumours, albeit advances in gene signatures and gene expression profiles (GEP) have allowed the incorporation of alternative and less toxic strategies for that scope, including endocrine and targeted treatments.

Neoadjuvant endocrine therapy (NET) has proven to be an attractive and better-tolerated option in patients with strongly oestrogen hormone receptor positive (HR+) cancers, and is rapidly gaining ground in clinical practice as more evidence accumulates showing comparable objective response (OR) and BCS rates with NCT [3–5]. ET is widely prescribed

---

Aglaia Skolariki MD MSc, designation Clinical Research Fellow, Centre for Immuno-Oncology, Department of Oncology, University of Oxford, Oxford, UK
E-mail: aglaia.skolariki@immonc.ox.ac.uk (for correspondence)

Simon Lord BM BS MRCP DPHIL, Department of Oncology, University of Oxford, Oxford, UK
E-mail: simon.lord@oncology.ox.ac.uk (for correspondence)

Ramsey I Cutress PhD FRCS, Professor of Breast Surgery, University of Southampton and University Hospital Southampton, Southampton, UK
E-mail: r.i.cutress@soton.ac.uk (for correspondence)

in the surgical setting and current guidelines recommend the use of NET in early-stage disease settings, in patients who are not suitable for NCT or primary hormone therapy (hormone therapy without surgery) in those who are considered unfit for surgery. A 2014 meta-analysis of seven trials comparing surgery with primary ET in elderly women concluded that there was no evidence of overall survival (OS) benefit in favour of either, hence, supporting the use of the latter as an alternative approach [6].

Neoadjuvant endocrine therapy has also been used as 'bridging' therapy when surgery is not immediately feasible for reasons other than the disease stage. This approach was widely adopted during the COVID-19 pandemic, as waiting times for surgical procedures had increased and a rationalised prioritisation of resources had to be implemented [7–9]. The B-MaP-C study gathered real-world evidence on the preoperative use of ET as a bridge to therapy demonstrating it to be both tolerable, and in the short term, safe [10].

Lastly, the perioperative window from breast cancer diagnosis to definitive surgery creates an excellent chance for window-of-opportunity trials to explore the effect of NET and its translational potential, and to investigate the pharmacological properties and anticancer activity of new investigational products and combinations [11,12].

TYPES OF ENDOCRINE THERAPY

There are three distinct classes of hormone therapy agents currently in use, each associated with a different mechanism of action and toxicity profile. These include the selective oestrogen receptor modulators (SORMs), the aromatase inhibitors (AIs) and the selective oestrogen receptor degraders or downgraders (SORDs), which work by inhibiting the effect, and/or reducing the levels of oestrogen receptor (OR). They have been extensively employed in the treatment of HR+ breast cancer, from the neoadjuvant to the metastatic setting, as well as in hormone-sensitive and OR-expressing malignancies, most commonly of gynaecologic origin [13,14].

Selective oestrogen receptor modulators

Selective oestrogen receptor modulators, previously known as anti-oestrogens, have been designed to inhibit the OR signalling pathway, by competitively binding to ORs, thus preventing their homodimerisation and subsequent activation of the OR transcriptional complex, as well as their downstream effects implicated in breast cancer cell proliferation [15–18]. The antagonistic effect of SORMs, as observed in mammary tissue, is nevertheless not ubiquitous; their selective binding ability allows them to have both oestrogenic and anti-oestrogenic properties, and varies according to the target tissue and OR isoform, therefore, exhibiting a wide spectrum of anticancer and tissue-specific effects according to their distinct molecular structure and individual pharmacodynamic profile [19–21].

Three agents have been primarily used in breast cancer treatment and these include tamoxifen, which had been the cornerstone of ET for decades, followed by raloxifene and toremifene [22]. Among the three, tamoxifen has been by far the most extensively studied SORM, currently utilised in all disease settings, as well as a preventative approach in women at high risk of breast cancer [23]. While its effect in breast tissue is antiproliferative, its oestrogenic activity in uterine tissue has been associated with endometrial hyperplasia, uterine fibroids and polyps, and secondary malignancies, predominantly endometrial cancers, and sarcomas [24,25]. Toremifene shares a very similar side effect profile, but, interestingly, raloxifene has a neutral effect on the uterus, therefore, not conferring increased risk of uterine cancers [26-28].

Side effects that have also been linked to tamoxifen and to a lesser extent to raloxifene include thromboembolic events. An increased risk of deep vein thrombosis, strokes and pulmonary embolisms has been demonstrated in large double-blind trials of tamoxifen compared to placebo [24,29-31]. These risks should particularly be noted if given in the perisurgical setting and a strategy for management of this is outlined in national guidance [32]. Evidence suggests that vascular events are more common during the first 2 years of treatment, and older age, hypertension, obesity and history of cardiovascular disease are considered independent factors [33,34]. On the other hand, SORMs have a lipid-lowering effect with evidence suggesting that they might modestly protect against coronary heart disease [35-37].

Gynaecological adverse events such as vaginal dryness and discharge, and menopausal symptoms including hot flushes and decreased libido, are among the most frequently observed in women treated with SORMs [24,29-31], with a profound and direct impact in the patient's quality of life [38]. A list of common side effects associated with the different types of ET can be found in **Table 6.1**.

Aromatase inhibitors

Instead of blocking the OR, AIs target its ligand, oestradiol, by inhibiting the enzyme aromatase which is responsible for the conversion of androgens to oestrogens in a process called aromatisation [39,40]. Aromatase expression is abundant in ovaries, but the enzyme is also active in peripheral tissues, including breast and adipose tissue [41].

Table 6.1 Adverse events of endocrine treatment agents and their respective frequencies [90-93]

Side effects	Aromatase inhibitors	Selective oestrogen receptor modulators	Selective oestrogen receptor degraders
Very common (≥1/10)		• Vasomotor symptoms • Fatigue • Nausea	
	• Joint/Musculoskeletal pain • Hypercholesterolaemia • Headache	• Vaginal discharge/bleeding • Peripheral oedema • Headache	• Joint/Musculoskeletal pain • Hepatic enzyme elevations • Hypersensitivity/Injection site reactions
Common (≥1/100 to <1/10)	• Osteoporosis • Bone fractures • Vaginal dryness/bleeding • Peripheral oedema • Hepatic enzyme elevations	• Thromboembolic events • Uterine fibroids • Cataract • Endometrial hyperplasia/polyps • Hepatic enzyme elevations	• Thromboembolic events • Headache • Vaginal bleeding • Injection site-related sciatica • Thrombocytopaenia
Uncommon (≥1/1,000 to <1/100)	• Cataract • Thromboembolic events • Cardiovascular events	• Endometrial cancer • Interstitial pneumonitis	• Anaphylactic reactions • Injection-site haematoma

As peripheral aromatisation is the main source of oestrogen in postmenopausal women, its inhibition results in oestrogen deprivation and abrogation of its detrimental effect in breast cancer growth [42–44]. In contrast, oestrogen production in premenopausal women is regulated by a negative feedback system involving the hypothalamus–pituitary–gonadal axis. Blocking aromatisation alone in women with intact ovarian function would lead to gonadotrophin secretion, ovarian stimulation and inefficient oestrogen synthesis inhibition [45]. Therefore, AIs are always combined with ovarian function suppression (OFS) when offered to premenopausal and perimenopausal women [46,47]. Pharmacological OFS is achieved with gonadotropin-releasing hormone agonists (GnRHa), but permanent methods such as oophorectomy can also be considered on an individual basis [48].

The three AIs currently approved for breast cancer treatment comprise the third-generation non-steroidal inhibitors anastrozole and letrozole, and the steroidal inactivator exemestane. The latter binds irreversibly and inactivates aromatase, while anastrozole and letrozole inhibit the enzyme in a reversible manner [49-53]. Although these agents have distinct pharmacological profiles, with letrozole being a more potent oestrogen suppressor than anastrozole, this has not translated into clinical relevance [54,55].

Unlike SORMs and their tissue-specific effects, toxicities secondary to oestrogen deprivation in peripheral tissues are common among all AIs [56-58]. Osteopenia and osteoporosis are among the main considerations when selecting the type of ET and women need to be carefully assessed and monitored for their individual fracture risk, which has been a secondary endpoint in most AI trials alongside bone mineral density measurement [59-62]. Patients who have abruptly transitioned to a menopausal status appear to be in increased risk of significant bone loss and associated skeletal events [63,64].

Menopausal, vasomotor and vaginal symptoms are frequently encountered, while signs of sexual dysfunction are more conspicuous compared to treatment with tamoxifen [65,66]. Notably, the intensity of adverse events related to oestrogen deprivation is usually magnified by the combined used of AIs and OFS in premenopausal patients [67].

The most common toxicity among AIs is known as AI-associated musculoskeletal syndrome (AIMSS) and presents with a wide range of symptoms including musculoskeletal aches, arthralgia and joint stiffness [68]. Finally, evidence from two meta-analyses comparing tamoxifen and AIs suggests that there is an increased incidence of cardiovascular events with the latter [62,69], although it is not clear whether this discrepancy is attributed to the cardioprotective effects of tamoxifen instead [70]. In contrast to tamoxifen AIs do not increase the risk of thromboembolic events making their use safe in the perisurgical setting.

Selective oestrogen receptor degraders or downgraders

Fulvestrant has been the main representative from a third category of ET, known as selective oestrogen receptor degraders or downgraders (SORDs), and is currently licensed for the first and second-line treatment of advanced HR+ breast cancer [71,72]. The efficacy of SORDs, considered to be complete antagonists of OR-α activity, stems from their ability to bind to the OR, forming a complex with impaired nuclear translocation and transcriptional activity, which elicits receptor turnover and protein degradation by activation of the ubiquitin-mediated proteasome [73-75]. These unique features of SORDs have the potential to overcome resistance mechanisms and are excellent candidates for use in patients with endocrine-resistant disease following treatment with other types of ET [76].

The ability to retain endocrine sensitivity is of particular importance in the neoadjuvant or primary ET setting, however, more evidence is needed to confirm superiority of SORDs over other classes of ET agents [77,78].

Fulvestrant shares a similar toxicity profile to AIs, with a global anti-oestrogenic behaviour and no known agonist effect [79,80]. However, its poor pharmacodynamic profile and limited bioavailability, allowing only intramuscular administration, have had a negative impact on both its potency and clinical utility [81,82]. Therefore, novel oral and more potent SORDs are currently in development [83–85], with elacestrant being the first of its class to receive Food and Drug Administration (FDA) approval for the treatment of endocrine-resistant, *ESR1*-mutated, advanced breast cancer patients [76].

Both AIs and fulvestrant have been successfully combined with targeted treatments such as cyclin-dependent kinase 4 and 6 inhibitors (CDK4/6i), and there is currently a plethora of novel ET agents under development [86]. New treatment strategies are under investigation with potent and orally available agents designed to disrupt the OR pathway in multiple points.

The new classes of complete oestrogen receptor antagonists (CORANs) and selective oestrogen receptor covalent antagonists (SORCAs) act by stimulating OR degradation and downregulating gene transcription [87]. Targeted protein degradation, the concept behind the development of another promising technology using proteolysis-targeting chimeras (PROTACs), is a particularly attractive approach, as treatment can now target previously out of range proteins [86]. Despite recent encouraging results from the first early phase trials [88,89], robust evidence is needed to identify the optimal sequence of ET in the era of multiple therapeutic options.

ENDOCRINE THERAPY IN THE ADJUVANT SETTING

Endocrine therapy is an effective treatment for HR+ breast cancer. It has been used effectively in both metastatic and adjuvant settings, as well as a prevention strategy in women at high risk of breast cancer [94]. Its versatility as a treatment option and the significant reduction in mortality rates following its use as adjuvant therapy has been one of oncology's greatest success stories [95].

For more than two decades, tamoxifen was the mainstay of adjuvant endocrine treatment [96,97]. Three randomised controlled trials were initiated between 1976 and 1978; the Christie Hospital trial investigating 1 year of adjuvant tamoxifen [98], the NATO trial which randomised patients to 2 years or no further therapy [99], and the Scottish trial which tested adjuvant tamoxifen for 5 years [100]. These trials enrolled patients irrespective of their nodal, menopausal or OR status, and they concluded that there was significant improvement in disease-free survival (DFS) in the tamoxifen arms, with a concurrent reduction in mortality rates.

The number of adjuvant trials increased exponentially in the following decade. A systematic review of the collective data of 28,896 women with early breast cancer was carried out by the Early Breast Cancer Trialists' Collaborative Group (EBCTCG) in 1988, establishing tamoxifen as a pillar of adjuvant therapy, especially in women over 50 years [96]. Evidence continued to accumulate and further EBCTCG reports and meta-analyses shed light on the predictive role of OR expression and prolonged survival benefit following 5 years of adjuvant tamoxifen [101,102].

Adjuvant ET saw a second breakthrough in the early 2000s, with the introduction of AIs in the clinic. Initial and mature results of the ATAC trial comparing the combination of anastrozole to either tamoxifen or anastrozole alone showed better outcomes with respect to DFS and contralateral breast cancers in the anastrozole arm [103,104]. Similarly, DFS and OS benefit was demonstrated for letrozole over tamoxifen in the phase 3 BIG 1-98 trial [105,106]. Finally, EBCTCG reported a meta-analysis of 9 trials that settled the argument, confirming that AIs were superior in reducing recurrence rates, breast cancer and all-cause mortality [107].

Subsequently, multiple trials were designed to assess superiority among the available AIs [65,108], to investigate sequential and extended strategies [109–111], as well as the optimal duration of ET [112–114]. Evidence from the aTTom and ATLAS trial of extended tamoxifen showed that tamoxifen for 10 instead of 5 years, significantly improved survival and reduced recurrence rates, a risk that remains substantial for decades, as shown in studies confirming recurrences up to 32 years post initial diagnosis [115–118].

The absolute benefit gained from different types of ET in premenopausal women has also been shown to favour AIs against tamoxifen, and adding OFS to either of the two significantly improves survival and reduces recurrences [119,120]. The pivotal SOFT and TEXT trials concluded that AIs are superior to tamoxifen in reducing risk of recurrence, while evidence on OS and mortality rates are still inconclusive, although less so in high-risk patients [121,122]. Finally, the phase 3 monarchE trial of the CDK4/6i abemaciclib in combination with ET versus ET alone, demonstrated benefit with regard to invasive DFS in node-positive, high-risk women [123].

Extended ET and treatment intensification with OFS and/or CDK4/6i have been associated with increased risk of toxicities, therefore, careful consideration is required to recognise the subgroup of patients who will benefit most from these strategies. Traditionally, decisions were made based on prognostic factors such as age, nodal status, tumour size, and Ki-67, a known proliferation and prognostic marker which has been underused due to poor analytical performance [124]. Today, gene signatures estimating recurrence risk have been developed as companion diagnostics to guide adjuvant chemotherapy decision [125], with the oncotype *DX 21*-gene assay used in the TAILORx and RxPONDER studies being the most popular [126,127]. Currently, predictive models combining genomic and clinical data are being validated in clinical trials.

ENDOCRINE THERAPY IN THE NEOADJUVANT SETTING

Successfully tailoring anticancer treatments to address the individual needs of the patients remains one of oncology's greatest challenges. Treatment escalation and de-escalation strategies in breast cancer are being implemented more widely and are facilitated by the development of accurate prognostic and prediction models to estimate disease course and response to different treatment modalities.

Several trials have compared the efficacy of NCT to adjuvant chemotherapy in early-stage breast cancer, suggesting that outcomes are comparable [128]. Conversely, HR+ breast cancers respond less dramatically to NCT, therefore, neoadjuvant systemic approaches integrating ET, which is associated with considerably less toxicities, have been utilised [129,130]. A meta-analysis of 20 trials published in 2016 solidified this argument and demonstrated the value of NET in achieving similar clinical, radiological and BCS rates to NCT [4]. However, the majority of these trials focussed on postmenopausal women and, therefore, caution is needed when generalising findings to premenopausal patients, as NET has been less extensively studied in this patient's population.

Trials in postmenopausal women

A pilot study in the 1980s was among the first to use tamoxifen as a surgery-sparing strategy in elderly women with early-stage disease, revealing a surprising 69% of responders [131]. A second trial prospectively randomised patients over the age of 70 years to upfront surgery or primary ET with tamoxifen, allowing crossover, and resulted in equivalent survival outcomes [132].

The integration of AIs for ER+ disease led to a number of studies assessing the efficacy of these agents in the neoadjuvant setting with main endpoints being the response rate, the reduction in tumour volumes and the conversion rate from mastectomy to BCS [133,134]. As in the case of adjuvant therapy, the superiority of AIs compared to tamoxifen was quickly recognised [135,136].

In a head-to-head comparison of neoadjuvant letrozole versus tamoxifen in 337 HR+ women, letrozole was associated with significantly better clinical and radiological objective response rates (ORR), and higher BCS rates [136]. Further supporting evidence was provided by three pivotal multicentre studies; the P024 trial which randomised women to letrozole versus tamoxifen, the PROACT trial which tested anastrozole against tamoxifen, and the IMPACT trial which investigated anastrozole and tamoxifen in combination versus each agent alone [137–139]. Apart from the latter, which failed to demonstrate statistical significance, both P024 and PROACT showed higher rates of responses and non-inferior or increased BCS rates in the AI arms. In each case, tolerability profiles were acceptable for both tamoxifen and AIs. The IMPACT trial was also the first to assess the prognostic value of the Preoperative Endocrine Prognostic Index (PEPI) model as a prognostic biomarker of recurrence [140].

Debates over superiority were put to rest after the publication of two meta-analyses of four and five studies respectively, which concluded that AIs were significantly more effective in achieving improved ORR and BCS rates compared to tamoxifen in postmenopausal women [141,142], evidence which were later validated in a third meta-analysis of 20 trials [4].

As a result, a phase II trial was designed to investigate differences among letrozole, anastrozole and exemestane with respect to clinical and biomarker outcomes [143,144]. The ACOSOG Z1031 trial enrolled 622 postmenopausal women with strongly ER+, stages II–III breast cancers to receive 16–18 weeks of NET with one of the three AIs. Arms were well-balanced, and clinical response rate was estimated at 62.9% for exemestane, 74.8% for letrozole and 69.1% for anastrozole. However, the treatment effect as assessed by the PEPI score and the Ki-67 changes led to the conclusion that the biological behaviour of the AIs was equivalent, a finding that was consistent with adjuvant trials of the time [65].

Fulvestrant's efficacy in the neoadjuvant setting has also been explored in phases II and III, multicentre trials with the hope of lowering the risk of endocrine resistance [145]. The NEWEST trial which evaluated different doses of neoadjuvant fulvestrant for 16 weeks concluded that the biological activity of the 500 mg dose was superior to the 250 mg one, by means of reduction in OR/progesterone (PR) expression and Ki-67 levels [146]. These biomarker changes were more pronounced in the 4-week compared to the 16-week assessment. Clinically, this was also translated into increased ORR.

The UNICANCER CARMINA 02 French trial randomised patients to either anastrozole or fulvestrant for 4–6 months according to clinical response [78]. Both treatments succeeded in producing satisfactory clinical response rates in 4 and 6 months, albeit anastrozole was associated with a higher number of responders, a finding which was consistent with the difference in pathological and BCS rates.

Finally, initial results of the ALTERNATE trial, which randomised patients to 6 months of fulvestrant, anastrozole or their combination, failed to show superiority of fulvestrant over anastrozole [145]. An overview of the NET trials in postmenopausal women can be found in **Table 6.2**.

Table 6.2 Randomised trials of neoadjuvant endocrine therapy (NET) in postmenopausal women. *Continues on pages 80–82*

Study	Phase	N	Treatment arms	NET duration	Primary endpoint*	Reference
Dixon et al., 2000	N/A	24	• Anastrozole 1 mg • Anastrozole 10 mg	3 months	ORR:§ 89.3% vs. 99.6%¥	[133]
Harper-Wynne et al, 2002	N/A	53	• Vorozole • Tamoxifen	12 weeks	• Ki-67 reduction at 2 weeks: 58% vs. 43%, $p = 0.13$ • Ki-67 reduction at 12 weeks: 27% vs. 51%, $p = 0.17$	[147]
Polychronis et al., 2005	II	56	• Gefitinib + anastrozole • Gefitinib + placebo	4–6 weeks	Ki-67 reduction at 2 weeks: 98% vs. 92.4%, $p = 0.0054$	[148]
Semiglazov et al., 2007	II	239	• Anastrozole or exemestane • Doxorubicin plus paclitaxel x 4 cycles	3 months	• ORR:§ 62–67% vs. 63%, $p = 0.5$ • BCS rate: 33% vs. 24%, $p = 0.058$	[3]
Smith et al., 2007	II	206	• Anastrozole + gefitinib • Anastrozole plus placebo for 2 weeks, then anastrozole plus gefitinib for 14 weeks • Anastrozole + placebo	16 weeks	Ki-67 reduction at 16 weeks: 77.4% vs. 83.6% (arm 1 and 2 vs. 3), $p = 0.26$	[149]
Mohammadianpanah et al., 2011	III	101	• 5-FU, doxorubicin, cyclophosphamide × 3–5 cycles + letrozole daily up to the time of surgery • 5-FU, doxorubicin, cyclophosphamide × 3–5 cycles	9–13 weeks	• ORR:§ 27.6% vs. 10.2%, $p = 0.028$ • pCR: 25.5% vs. 10.2%, $p = 0.049$	[150]
FemZone	II	168	• Letrozole plus zoledronic acid • Letrozole	6 months	ORR:† 69.2% vs. 54.5%, $p = 0.106$	[151]
NEOCENT	III	44	• 5-FU, epirubicin, cyclophosphamide ± docetaxel × 6 cycles • Letrozole	18–23 weeks	Recruitment feasibility and tissue collection‡	[152]
IMPACT	III	330	• Anastrozole plus placebo • Tamoxifen plus placebo • Tamoxifen plus anastrozole	12 weeks	ORR:§ 37% vs. 36% vs. 39%, $p = 0.61$	[139,153]
P024	III	337	• Letrozole • Tamoxifen	4 months	ORR:§ 55 × vs. 36%, $p < 0.001$	[137]
PROACT	III	451	• Anastrozole plus placebo • Tamoxifen plus placebo	3 months	ORR:† 39.5 × vs. 35.4%, $p = 0.29$	[138]

Study	Phase	N	Treatment arms	NET duration	Primary endpoint*	Reference

ACOSOG Z1031	II	622	1. Exemestane
			2. Letrozole
			3. Anastrozole
				16–18 weeks	• ORR:§
					  62.9% vs. 74.8% vs. 69.1%¥
					• BCS rate: 67.2%
					  5-year cumulative LRR: 1.53%; 95% CI 0.7–3.0%
						[143,144]

NEWEST	II	211	1. Fulvestrant 500 mg 2. Fulvestrant 250 mg	16 weeks	Ki-67 reduction at 4 weeks: 78.8% vs. 47.4%, $p < 0.0001$	[146]
CARMINA	II	116	1. Anastrozole 2. Fulvestrant	Up to 6 months	ORR:§ 52.6% vs. 36.8%¥ at 6 months	[78]
ALTERNATE	III	1299	1. Anastrozole 2. Fulvestrant 3. Anastrozole plus fulvestrant	6 months	ESDR: 18.6% vs. 22.7% (arm 1 vs. 2, $p = 0.15$) vs. 20.5% (arm 1 vs. 3, $p = 0.55$)	[77]
PTEX46	II	52	1. Exemestane for 4 months 2. Exemestane for 6 months	4 or 6 months	ORR:§ 42.3% vs. 48%, $p = 0.89$	[154]
CHERLOB	IIb	92	1. Letrozole plus lapatinib 2. Letrozole plus placebo	6 months	ORR:† 69.2% vs. 57.8%¥	[155]
CAAN	N/A	82	1. Exemestane and celecoxib twice daily 2. Exemestane daily 3. Letrozole daily	3 months	ORR:§ 58.6% vs. 54.5% vs 62%¥	[156]
NeoPAL	II	106	1. Letrozole and palbociclib 2. 5-FU, epirubicin, cyclophosphamide × 3 cycles, followed by docetaxel × 3 cycles	19 weeks	RCB 0–I rate: 7.7% vs. 15.7%¥	[157]
PALLET	II	307	1. Letrozole 1. Letrozole for 2 weeks, then palbociclib plus letrozole to 14 weeks 2. Palbociclib for 2 weeks, then palbociclib plus letrozole to 14 weeks 3. Palbociclib plus letrozole	14 weeks	• Ki-67 reduction at EOT: 88.5% vs. 97.4%, $p < 0.001$ • ORR:† 49.5% (arm 1) vs. 54.4% (arm 2 + 3 + 4), $p = 0.20$	[158]
SAFIA	III	159	1. Fulvestrant for 4 months followed by fulvestrant plus palbociclib for 4 additional months 2. Fulvestrant for 4 months followed by fulvestrant plus placebo for 4 additional months	Up to 8 months	pCR 2% vs. 7%, $p = 0.1464$ (post- and premenopausal patients combined)	[159]
neoMONARCH	II	173	• Abemaciclib plus anastrozole for 16 weeks • Abemaciclib for 2 weeks, then abemaciclib plus anastrozole for 14 weeks • Anastrozole for 2 weeks, then abemaciclib plus anastrozole for 14 weeks	16 weeks	Ki-67 reduction at 2 weeks: 93.5% vs. 93.1% vs. 71%, $p < 0.001$ (arm 1 vs. arm 3; arm 2 vs. arm 3)	[160]

Table 6.2 Continues on pages 80–82

Study	Phase	N	Treatment arms	NET duration	Primary endpoint*	Reference
Baselga et al., 2009	II	270	• Letrozole plus everolimus • Letrozole plus placebo	16 weeks	ORR:[§] 68.1% vs. 59.1%, $p = 0.0616$	[161]
NEO-ORB	II	257	• Letrozole plus alpelisib • Letrozole plus buparlisib • Letrozole plus placebo	24 weeks	ORR[†] (arm 1 vs. arm 3): • PIK3CAm: 43.3% vs. 44.8%[¥] • PIK3CAwt: 63.4 ¥ vs. 61%[¥] pCR (arm 1 vs. arm 3): • PIK3CAm: 1.7% vs. 3%[¥] • PIK3CAwt: 2.8% vs. 1.7%[¥]	[162]
LORELEI	II	334	• Letrozole plus taselisib • Letrozole plus placebo	16 weeks	• ORR:[†] 50% vs. 39%, $p = 0.049$ – PIK3CAm: 56% vs. 38%, $p = 0.033$ • pCR: 2% vs. 1%, $p = 0.37$	[163]
POETIC	III	4,480	• Letrozole or anastrozole • Control	14 days	• Local recurrence: 9% vs. 10%, $p = 0.40$ • 5-year RFS: 91% vs. 90.4%[¥]	[11]

(BCS, breast-conservation surgery; CI, confidence interval; EOT, end of treatment; ESDR, endocrine-sensitive disease rate; LRR, locoregional recurrence; N, number; NET, neoadjuvant endocrine therapy; ORR, objective response rate; pCR, pathologic complete response; RCB, residual cancer burden; PIK3Cam, PIK3CA mutant; PIK3CAwt, PIK3CA wild-type; RFS, recurrence-free survival; vs., versus)

*Arm 1 versus arm 2 versus arm 3, etc. respectively
[†]Assessed with MRI/MMG/US
[§]Assessed with caliper/palpation
[‡]Terminated early due to slow accrual
[¥]p value not provided

Trials in premenopausal women

Premenopausal women with HR+ early-stage breast cancer have been traditionally offered chemotherapy, with NCT reserved for those with locally advanced disease and inoperable tumours. Evidence from a small phase II study comparing the efficacy of exemestane plus goserelin to standard NCT with anthracyclines and taxanes in premenopausal patients, suggests that NET is inferior to NCT with less responses noted (75% vs. 44% with NCT and NET, respectively) [129].

Similar outcomes were observed in a phase III study of tamoxifen plus goserelin versus NCT, and resulted in inferior outcomes with respect to ORR and pCR rate for

NET, albeit the latter was overall low in both arms (3.4% vs. 1.2% in NCT and NET, respectively) [164]. In comparison, BCS rates and Ki-67 changes were not appreciably different between arms.

The results of these studies have led to the widespread acceptance of NCT as the superior treatment option for premenopausal women in this setting. However, if NET is to be offered, AIs with OFS are, again, the preferred choice of treatment compared to tamoxifen on account of better clinical outcomes. In STAGE trial, 197 premenopausal patients were randomised to either tamoxifen/goserelin or anastrozole/goserelin for a total of 24 weeks [165]. Overall, clinical, radiological, and pathological responses were superior for the anastrozole group, Ki-67 levels were significantly lower and BCS rates were higher compared to patients on tamoxifen. Of note, there was baseline imbalance between treatment arms, with more patients with Grade 3 tumours and PR-negative status randomised to tamoxifen, which might have introduced some bias. A synopsis of the NET trials in premenopausal women can be found in **Table 6.3**.

Treatment duration

The optimal length of NET is another grey area, and current ASCO guidelines recommend a personalised approach and close treatment monitoring to assess response [2]. At present,

Table 6.3 Randomised trials of neoadjuvant endocrine therapy (NET) in premenopausal women

Study	Phase	N	Treatment arms	ORR*	BCS rate*	Reference
GEICAM/2006-03	II	51	• Epirubicin plus cyclophosphamide × 4 cycles followed by docetaxel × 4 cycles • Exemestane daily plus goserelin for 24 weeks	75% vs. 44%,[†] $p = 0.027$	47% vs. 56%,[¥] $p = 0.2369$	[129]
TREND	II	51	• Degarelix plus letrozole × 6, 28-day cycles • Triptorelin plus letrozole × 6, 28-day cycles	44% vs. 46.2%[‡,§]	52.2% vs. 42.3%[‡]	[166]
NEST	III	187	• Adriamycin plus cyclophosphamide × 4 cycles followed by docetaxel × 4 cycles • Tamoxifen plus goserelin for 24 weeks	83.7% vs. 52.9%,[†] $p < 0.001$	13.8% vs. 11.5%, $p = 0.531$	[164]
STAGE	III	197	• Anastrozole plus goserelin for 24 weeks • Tamoxifen plus goserelin for 24 weeks	64.3 vs. 37.4%,[†] $p = 0.0002$	86% vs. 68%[‡]	[165]
SAFIA	III	195	• Fulvestrant/goserelin plus palbociclib • Fulvestrant/goserelin plus placebo	Major response:[†,¥] 62% vs. 66%, $p = 0.4963$	47% vs. 48%[‡,¥]	

*Arm 1 versus arm 2, respectively
[†] Assessed with MRI
[§] Assessment method not specified
[‡] p value not provided
[¥] Results include postmenopausal women
(BCS, breast-conservation surgery; N, number; ORR, objective response rate; vs., versus)

most evidence is provided by small phase II trials which have opted for a 3- to 6-month period [4].

Tamoxifen, which was more widely used in the first NET trials, was shown to achieve responses within the first 3 months of treatment, although larger lesions usually required longer periods of treatment to achieve their best response, sometimes up to 12 months [131,167]. However, the small proportion of ongoing responders compared to those who are likely to progress after 3 months does not justify prolonged treatment.

Also, on the other hand, these are known to achieve ongoing responses beyond the first 3–4 months of treatment [168], with most studies agreeing to a 4- to 6-month duration. A study of 182 women receiving neoadjuvant letrozole, assessed responses in different time intervals from 0 to 3, 3 to 6, 6 to 12, and 12 to 24 months [169]. ORR increased from 69.8% at 3 months to 83.5% with prolonged NET and BCS rates from 60 to 72%, respectively.

A phase II prospective NET study with optimal letrozole duration as its primary endpoint concluded that 4–6 months are sufficient to gain significant response benefit [170]. Evidence from two other trials suggested that extended treatment of up to 8 months is more suitable when aiming for maximum tumour volume reduction [171–173]. The TEAM IIA trial assessing ORR and tumour downstaging at 3 and 6 months of treatment with exemestane demonstrated that 6 months of NET allowed better downstaging and increased BCS eligibility, while a small proportion of patients might be at risk of progression [174]. Finally, the PTEX46 trial described similar response rates at 4 and 6 months with exemestane, and therefore argued in favour of a shorter duration [154].

In conclusion, although extended NET might result in better objective responses and surgical outcomes, its prospective benefit should be carefully balanced against the risk of developing endocrine resistance and ligand-independent activation of OR, a risk which has been shown to increase when NET exceeds 6 months [175].

Treatment combinations

As expected, combinations that have proven successful in the adjuvant setting are now proposed as neoadjuvant strategies.

One approach opts to employ the added benefit of CDK4/6i when combined with the already effective AIs. These combination trials have so far failed to demonstrate superiority compared to NCT, albeit being effective in improving response rates. The NeoPAL trial randomly allocated 106 patients to either letrozole/palbociclib combination or NCT, before being terminated early, as the threshold for its primary objective, residual cancer burden (RCB), was not reached for the combination [176]. However, recently published results of the secondary endpoints demonstrated comparable long-term survival outcomes with both approaches, suggesting a potentially useful and less toxic alternative to chemotherapy [177].

Furthermore, the significance of their added benefit when combined with AIs is debatable, and the lack of survival data in view of the extra toxicity risk does not justify any escalation of treatment. In PALLET, a trial of palbociclib plus letrozole versus letrozole alone this time, clinical responses were not improved, although the co-primary Ki-67 was significantly suppressed [158]. The latter was also evident in the NeoPalAna singe-arm study of palbociclib and anastrozole, which reported high complete cell cycle arrest rates [178]. The recently published results of SAFIA showed that the addition of Palbociclib to fulvestrant did not result in superior pCR rates [159]. Finally, the first results of the neoMONARCH trial proved that abemaciclib either alone or in combination with anastrozole performed better and achieved greater Ki-67 reductions compared to anastrozole alone, while maintaining a well-tolerated toxicity profile [160].

The *PI3K/AKT/mTOR* pathway has also been targeted and promising results have been observed in combination trials with AIs. The mTOR inhibitor everolimus was combined with letrozole in a phase II study of 270 postmenopausal women, showing higher rates of clinical responses and reductions in Ki-67 compared to letrozole monotherapy, both in the overall and in the *PIK3CA* mutant population [161]. Contradictory evidence regarding the efficacy of *PI3K* inhibitors and AI combinations has been produced by the NEO-ORB and LORELEI study, investigating combinations of letrozole with alpelisib and taselisib, respectively, versus letrozole monotherapy [162,163]. While LORELEI met its primary endpoint of objective responses in all subgroups including the *PIK3CA* mutant population, NEO-ORB failed to do so, and this was consistent across all cohorts.

PATIENT SELECTION

Appropriate candidate selection for NET and development of clinical prediction tools have been at the forefront of ongoing research ever since NET strategy started to be adopted and clinical practice guidelines provide evidence-based recommendations.

An important factor for NET consideration is the patient's menopausal status, and this was highlighted in the ASCO guidelines of 2021 [2]. NET is considered a valid strategy in postmenopausal women for tumour downstaging; however, as described earlier, its value is less well-established in premenopausal women, and therefore, NET should not be routinely offered to this population.

Oestrogen receptor expression has also been shown to directly impact the effectiveness of NET. The strong correlation between response to ET and OR expression was known from trials in the adjuvant setting, but further insight on the matter was provided by the OR and PR expression analyses that were conducted within the P024 trial [137]. Clinical responses to the study drugs, letrozole and tamoxifen, were shown to increase in a linear aspect to increasing OR Allred expression scores, with higher responses observed in women with OR Allred score 7 and 8. Following these findings, inclusion of women in ACOSOG Z1031 trial was restricted to those with OR Allred score of 6 and above [179].

Several predictive biomarkers to guide patient's selection have been proposed and investigated in trials, usually serving as secondary objectives. Gene signatures and GEP have been in the spotlight since the validation of the 21- and 70-gene assays as diagnostic companions for adjuvant chemotherapy decision making [125–127,180]. Their value in patient's stratification according to recurrence score (RS) has been both predictive and prognostic, and further established in the neoadjuvant setting, with high RS correlating to increased pCR rates and predictive of chemotherapy benefit [181–185]. Recent results from KARMA Dx study confirm their significance in selecting patients for systemic treatment de-escalation [186]. Reports from the adaptive I-SPY 2 trial integrating the 70-gene assay for patient's stratification according to their molecular classification are also highly anticipated [187].

With respect to their utilisation in patient's selection, the PAM50 classifier, using a 50-gene set to predict molecular subtypes has been evaluated in the ACOSOG Z1031 trial [143,188]. Its ability to identify tumours with aggressive biological behaviour and intrinsic resistance to ET suggested a possible role. Its predictive value of endocrine-sensitivity was also validated in a dataset with inputs from 103 postmenopausal patients who received NET [189]. Assigned values were 'chemotherapy-sensitive', 'endocrine-sensitive' and 'uncertain'. A chemo-endocrine score (CES) was then provided and shown to be significantly associated with clinical response ($p = 0.009$).

The 21-gene assay is also actively investigated for its role in patient's selection, and this strategy was implemented in the SAFIA trial, which recruited patients with a breast recurrence score (RS) < 31 [159]. This approach builds on previous evidence demonstrating the value of the RS in predicting response to NET [182,190,191], with the TransNEOS study offering validating data for its use in postmenopausal ER+, HER2- and clinically node-negative breast cancer patients [190]. In addition, this study demonstrated that post-NET RS was also predictive of BCS conversion and eligibility, with a better likelihood observed in patients with RS < 18.

Furthermore, a pooled analysis of 109 patients who received either NET or NCT according to their RS, suggested that omission of chemotherapy in patients with RS ≤ 25 was not detrimental with respect to pathological responses, although lack of data on premenopausal women, nodal status, and long-term follow-up limits their generalisability [193]. Finally, the positive results of the ADAPT trial further validated the use of the 21-gene assay in successfully selecting suitable NET candidates [194].

TREATMENT MONITORING

Treatment monitoring is equally important when NET strategies are considered. A fine balance needs to be established between gaining maximum treatment benefit and risk of developing treatment resistance which can adversely affect survival outcomes. It is speculated that intrinsic endocrine resistance can be as high as 20%, while acquired resistance after prolonged ET remains inevitable and is the focus of intensive research [195]. Of note, results of a recent genomic analysis of pre- and post-treatment samples of 35 patients treated with NET revealed a complicated landscape of genomic and transcriptomic variations, with *ESR1* variants more commonly associated with acquired resistance [195]. Therefore, different mitigation strategies have been implemented to prevent treatment resistance and progression, incorporating imaging, molecular and genomic biomarkers.

Radiological assessment of response is standard practice in the neoadjuvant setting and most trials have incorporated ultrasound (US), mammography (MMG) and/or magnetic resonance imaging (MRI) in a multimodal approach. In the CARMINA study, patients were primarily assessed by US and MRI, with positron emission tomography (PET) scans as optional, at 1, 4 and 6 months for those continuing on the extended treatment, or prior to surgery for the rest [78]. Reported ORR was similar for US and MRI, as were the estimated tumour volume reductions. The only timepoint in which either the US or MRI could predict clinical response was prior to surgery. In contrast, both the 1-month and the presurgical US showed statistically significant predictive value for pathological response assessment ($p = 0.006$ and $p = 0.03$ for 1-month and presurgical US, respectively).

At the same time, retrospective and prospective findings from further NCT and NET studies have shown that MRI is superior to US for pathological response assessment and pathological tumour size prediction [197,198], although it may not be as effective in successfully predicting pathological nodal status [199]. On balance, both US and MRI are acceptable methods for treatment monitoring, albeit additional evidence is needed to determine the optimal strategy depending on the specific type of neoadjuvant therapy being used.

Although monitoring imaging response is recommended, it is not sufficient to accurately predict non-responders. Furthermore, pCR is a rare finding in patients with HR+ disease receiving neoadjuvant treatment [200]. Therefore, other markers of response have been explored, with Ki-67 being the most promising and easy to integrate in a monitoring strategy [11,201].

The IMPACT trial was designed to assess changes in OR expression and Ki-67 staining for patients receiving NET and determine whether these changes related to outcome [202]. Although the level of Ki-67 suppression was not predictive of clinical response at the time, it was shown that it correlated positively with the biological activity of the treatment, and that the greatest reductions were achieved in ER-rich tumours. Further reports from the IMPACT group showed that Ki-67 reduction was more profound after 12 compared to 2 weeks of treatment for anastrozole, and suggested a possible association between levels of suppression and response prediction [153].

A separate multivariable analysis of 158 patients with paired biopsies showed that increase in the 2-week Ki-67 expression was independently and significantly associated with a higher chance of recurrences ($p = 0.004$), alongside the larger baseline tumour size and low OR status at 2 weeks [201].

Building on this evidence, the P024 trial developed the PEPI model and subsequently used a dataset of 203 women from IMPACT trial for validation. The PEPI score is generated by four factors comprising OR expression, Ki-67 index, pathological tumour size and nodal status [140]. Patients who had a PEPI score of 0 at surgery and a low pathological stage were considered good candidates for treatment de-escalation in the adjuvant setting.

Following this new development, PEPI scores were integrated in several trials and a positive correlation with pathological responses was noted [168,203]. In particular, the ACOSOG Z1031 trial was able to prove that a score of 0 was predictive of favourable recurrence free survival in patients who had induction treatment with an AI, compared to those who scored higher (hazard ratio for recurrence 0.27, $p = 0.014$) [203]. More importantly, they showed that a Ki-67 level > 10% after 2–4 weeks of NET, was significantly associated with higher PEPI scores, paving the way for Ki-67 to become a surrogate biomarker of response to guide treatment decisions and management.

The pivotal POETIC trial was designed to assess the prognostic role and the clinical relevance of the cut-off threshold of Ki-67 which was set at 10% [11]. Patients were allocated to either 2 weeks of AIs followed by surgery, or no NET, and adjuvant ET was given according to standard practice. Women with low Ki-67 at baseline and post-NET had the best prognosis with a low recurrence rate. On the other hand, women who started with a high Ki-67 status which was able to drop below 10% within 2 weeks of treatment had slightly worse outcomes than the previous group, but better prognosis compared to those whose Ki-67 remained over 10% after treatment. The latter was shown to represent a high-risk group that could benefit from treatment escalation.

This Ki-67 monitoring strategy was put to the test in two phase III NET trials with a biomarker-driven treatment design [77,194]. The ALTERNATE trial selected Ki-67 at 4 and 12 weeks and a modified PEPI scoring system at surgery to guide treatment decisions, while ADAPT was the first trial to use Ki-67 and the 21-gene assay at 3 weeks following NET to allocate non-responders to adjuvant chemotherapy. The recently published results of the latter showed no differences in survival outcomes in the different treatment groups, including premenopausal patients, and established the feasibility and validity of de-escalation strategies guided by GEP and molecular biomarkers [194].

IMPLICATIONS FOR SURGERY

Neoadjuvant systemic therapy is a key treatment modality in the management of early breast cancer and the preferred approach when BCS is considered. While there is some data to guide surgical strategies in the NET setting there is more information available from the NCT setting and techniques and pathways are often extrapolated. Cosmetic outcomes and impact on quality of life are important aspects in the selection of the surgical strategy, and careful consideration of the associated risks and benefits is warranted. EndoNET, a prospective phase III trial, is underway and aims to investigate quality of life outcomes and conversion rates of mastectomy to BCS in postmenopausal women treated with NET [204].

Survival benefit is another major consideration when selecting the therapeutic approach. NCT has repeatedly shown equivalent outcomes to adjuvant chemotherapy with respect to distant recurrences and long-term survival [128,205,206]. However, concerns were raised following conflicting evidence on locoregional disease control, as well as increased local recurrence rates in patients having NCT and BCS [207,208]. Similarly, the lack of validated predictive recurrence risk models and long-term survival data have led to the underutilisation of NET [4,208]. Only recently, results of the ACOSOG Z1031 trial were able to confirm the overall low 5-year locoregional recurrence rate (1.53% at 5 years), indicative of the safety of this approach, considering 50% of surgeries were de-escalated to BCS after NET [144]. Still, careful candidate selection followed by an extensive discussion of the associated risks and benefit is essential.

Surgery de-escalation and breast-conservation surgery rates

Despite the growing utilisation of neoadjuvant treatments that enables less extensive surgeries, a prospective study of women aged 40 years or younger, showed no significant increase in BCS rates over the years [209]. At the same time, significantly more women opted for radical surgery, and in particular bilateral mastectomies, probably mirroring the adoption of widespread genetic testing and cancer family history considerations in decision making.

Initial results of the NeST study, which collected data on stated practice from 39 UK-based breast multidisciplinary teams (MDTs), confirmed that tumour downstaging remains the predominant indication for neoadjuvant therapy, although NET was offered to a rather small subgroup of patients with primarily inoperable or locally advanced disease [210]. A 2016 meta-analysis of 20 randomised trials demonstrated non-significant differences in BCS rates for NET compared to NCT (OR 0.65; 95% CI 0.41–1.03; $p = 0.07$; $n = 334$), establishing the value of this less toxic approach in this setting [4]. Further data of a large cohort of 19,829 patients in the National Cancer Database (NCDB) study showed NET utilisation growing linearly with increasing T and N stage, and a steady change in practice along the years [211,212]. Conversely, T and N downstaging were achieved in significantly higher rates in patients receiving NCT compared to those on NET, especially in more advanced stages [212]. Notwithstanding, 40–50% of T3–4 lesions were also successfully downstaged to a level allowing BCS following NET.

Recently published surgical outcomes from the ACOSOG Z1031 study of 509 eligible for analysis women with clinical stage 2–3 HR+ breast cancer revealed a BCS rate of 67.2% [144]. While the first cohort of patients (Cohort A) was not required to have an interval biopsy, the protocol was later amended, and patients allocated to Cohort B would undergo a biopsy 2–4 weeks after initiation of NET. If Ki-67 was >10%, a decision was made to either proceed to surgery or switch to NCT. De-escalation from mastectomy to BCS was implemented in similar proportions (22.8% and 20% of patients in Cohort A and B, respectively). In contrast, treatment escalation was more pronounced in Cohort B (9.4% vs. 13.3% in Cohort A and B, respectively). This can be potentially explained by the additional evidence provided regarding Ki-67 trend and tumour response to NET, therefore shaping decisions towards a more radical surgical approach.

Strategies to improve tumour localisation and long-term local control following neoadjuvant therapy and BCS have also been implemented. These include clip-marking of the breast lesion and the biopsy-proven metastatic axillary lymph nodes with radio-opaque markers or other identifiers [213–216]. This facilitates appropriate excision of involved sites, and guides decisions on axilla management when Sentinel lymph node biopsy (SLNB) or targeted axillary dissection (TAD) are considered [217,218]. Although pCR is less frequent with either NET or NCT in luminal A cancers [200,219], marking suspicious nodes prior to systemic treatment has shown a considerable reduction in the false-negative rates observed when SLNB is performed [220]. Furthermore, accurate pathological staging, tumour regression grading and repeat evaluation of receptor expression in the surgical specimen of women receiving NET are vital to inform further treatment decisions such as adjuvant chemotherapy and radiotherapy to the tumour bed and axilla [218,221].

Axillary surgery considerations

Axillary management is less straightforward in the case of neoadjuvant therapy and data from most randomised trials regarding axillary surgery are scarce. Although choice of axillary surgery was not predefined in the ACOSOG Z1031 trial, evidence from the two cohorts reflects the gradual change in practice [222]. The protocol amendment in 2009 and the introduction of an interval biopsy led to a higher rate of SLNB without axillary lymph node dissection (ALND) in Cohort B patients (45.6% vs. 63.3% in Cohort A and B, respectively), which could have been driven by confidence gained from the Ki-67 trend results [144].

However, at present, there is no prospective evidence to support surgery de-escalation in the axilla. According to data collected from the NCDB between 2012 and 2015, patients receiving NET with clinical N0 and N1 disease underwent similar axillary management strategies compared to those having primary surgery [223]. This approach was justified as nodal pCR rates were typically low, therefore, decisions were based on factors other than expected response. Interestingly, patients treated with NET and pathological N1 disease following SLNB were less likely to have completion ALND compared to patients receiving primary surgery or NCT. Multivariate and interaction analyses followed to control for confounding factors such as age, with no significant findings. Nonetheless, the authors recognised the limitations in the interpretation of retrospective data.

In a separate analysis of NCDB, patients with clinical node-negative disease treated with NET had pathologically negative lymph nodes in 65% of the cases, while minimal residual nodal disease, characterised by the presence of isolated tumour cells and/or micrometastases, was evident in 8.7% [224]. A modest pathological response was seen in cN1 patients, with a modest pathological response was seen with only 10% of cN1 patients achieving pCR after NET and 4% of cN1 patients residual nodal burden. Subsequent survival analyses of patients with clinical T1-3N0-1 disease revealed no significant differences in the 5-year OS of those with nodal pCR compared to those with minimal residual nodal disease. Moreover, OS rates in patients stratified by their pathological nodal status were similar regardless of whether they were treated with NET or had upfront surgery. Optimal management in the case of the latter has been investigated in several randomised trials [225–227].

In an effort to identify a larger group of patients who could be candidates for de-escalating axillary approach, complementary data were extracted from the Dana-Farber/Brigham and Women's Cancer Center and the NCDB cohorts regarding post-NET axillary surgery and associated survival benefit [228]. Patients with less than three positive nodes after surgery were considered as having low-residual nodal disease burden, and these were estimated to represent >90% of the subgroup with clinically negative nodes. The strongest predictive factors for low-residual disease were the initial node-negative status, followed by clinical T1 tumours and absence of lymphovascular invasion.

These findings suggest that axillary de-escalation strategies similar to the ones implemented when primary surgery is considered, and are reasonable in patients with clinical node-negative disease after NET. Future prospective data will unravel differences in local recurrences and survival.

CONCLUSION

The more accurate our predictive markers of benefit become, the more likely it is for NET to become widely adopted. The widespread utilisation of genomic signatures in patient's stratification according to their recurrence risk and presumed chemotherapy benefit is expected to reduce further the use of chemotherapy in the pre- and postoperative setting and give way to NET approaches. As the clinical practice trends in favour of de-escalation in all treatment modalities, new ET combinations are currently investigated in the neoadjuvant setting and are likely to result in improved outcomes, with a view to less toxicity. Nonetheless, mature survival data from large prospective NET trials are still eagerly awaited.

> **Key points for clinical practice**
> - Endocrine therapy can be used as a neoadjuvant option particularly for post-menopausal women where chemotherapy is not recommended
> - Increased utilisation of tumour genomic testing is likely to further clarify where ET alone is sufficient as adjuvant therapy
> - NET appears to be effective and safe for surgical downstaging in appropriately selected patients
> - NET also provides an opportunity for bridging therapy, window of opportunity studies, potential responsive adapted therapies, as well as primary endocrine therapy in those unfit or unable to have surgery
> - Currently AI's are the agent of choice for NET however newer agents that selectively target the OR are increasingly being evaluated, as are combinations of endocrine and targeted therapies

REFERENCES

1. Radovich M, Jiang G, Hancock BA, et al. Association of Circulating Tumor DNA and Circulating Tumor Cells After Neoadjuvant Chemotherapy With Disease Recurrence in Patients With Triple-Negative Breast Cancer: Preplanned Secondary Analysis of the BRE12-158 Randomized Clinical Trial. JAMA Oncol [Internet] 2020; 6:1410–1415.

2. Korde LA, Somerfield MR, Carey LA, et al. Neoadjuvant Chemotherapy, Endocrine Therapy, and Targeted Therapy for Breast Cancer: ASCO Guideline. J Clin Oncol 2021; 39:1485–1505.
3. Semiglazov VF, Semiglazov VV, Dashyan GA, et al. Phase 2 randomized trial of primary endocrine therapy versus chemotherapy in postmenopausal patients with estrogen receptor-positive breast cancer. Cancer [Internet] 2007; 110:244–254.
4. Spring LM, Gupta A, Reynolds KL, et al. Neoadjuvant Endocrine Therapy for Estrogen Receptor-Positive Breast Cancer: A Systematic Review and Meta-analysis. JAMA Oncol [Internet] 2016; 2:1477–1486.
5. Brett B, Savva C, Mirshekar-Syahkal B, et al. Surgical outcomes of neoadjuvant endocrine treatment in early breast cancer: meta-analysis, BJS Open, 2024; 8:100.
6. Morgan J, Wyld L, Collins KA, Reed MW. Surgery versus primary endocrine therapy for operable primary breast cancer in elderly women (70 years plus). Cochrane Database Syst Rev [Internet] 2014; CD004272.
7. Huang J, Feinberg J, Dabiri B, et al. Neoadjuvant endocrine therapy (NET) as bridge therapy for early stage breast cancer during COVID-19: A single institution experience. Cancer Res [Internet] 2022; 82:P2-15-03-P2-15-03.
8. Feinberg J, Cen C, Schnabel F, et al. 'Bridge' Neoadjuvant Endocrine Therapy for Early Stage Breast Cancer Patients During COVID-19 at an Academic Hospital in NYC: Lessons Learned and Future Directions. Int J Clin Oncol Cancer Res 2021; 6:38.
9. Thompson CK, Lee MK, Baker JL, Attai DJ, DiNome ML. Taking a Second Look at Neoadjuvant Endocrine Therapy for the Treatment of Early Stage Estrogen Receptor Positive Breast Cancer During the COVID-19 Outbreak. Ann Surg [Internet] 2020; 272(2):e96.
10. Dave RV, Elsberger B, Taxiarchi VP, et al. Bridging pre-surgical endocrine therapy for breast cancer during the COVID-19 pandemic: outcomes from the B-MaP-C study. Breast Cancer Res Treat [Internet] 2023; 199:265–279.
11. Smith I, Robertson J, Kilburn L, et al. Long-term outcome and prognostic value of Ki67 after perioperative endocrine therapy in postmenopausal women with hormone-sensitive early breast cancer (POETIC): an open-label, multicentre, parallel-group, randomised, phase 3 trial. Lancet Oncol [Internet] 2020; 21:1443–1454.
12. Robertson JFR, Evans A, Henschen S, et al. A Randomized, Open-label, Presurgical, Window-of-Opportunity Study Comparing the Pharmacodynamic Effects of the Novel Oral SERD AZD9496 with Fulvestrant in Patients with Newly Diagnosed ER+ HER2- Primary Breast Cancer. Clin Cancer Res [Internet] 2020; 26:4242–4249.
13. George A, McLachlan J, Tunariu N, et al. The role of hormonal therapy in patients with relapsed high-grade ovarian carcinoma: A retrospective series of tamoxifen and letrozole. BMC Cancer [Internet] 2017; 17:1–8.
14. Lindemann K, Gibbs E, Åvall-Lundqvist E, et al. Chemotherapy vs tamoxifen in platinum-resistant ovarian cancer: a phase III, randomised, multicentre trial (Ovaresist). Br J Cancer [Internet] 2017; 116:455–463.
15. Kumar V, Chambon P. The estrogen receptor binds tightly to its responsive element as a ligand-induced homodimer. Cell 1988; 55:145–156.
16. Shiau AK, Barstad D, Loria PM, et al. The Structural Basis of Estrogen Receptor/Coactivator Recognition and the Antagonism of This Interaction by Tamoxifen. Cell 1998; 95:927–937.
17. Nicholson RI, Davies P, Griffiths K. Effects of oestradiol-17β and tamoxifen on nuclear oestradiol-17β receptors in DMBA-induced rat mammary tumours. Eur J Cancer 1977; 13:201–208.
18. Nicholson RI, Golder MP. The effect of synthetic anti-oestrogens on the growth and biochemistry of rat mammary tumours. Eur J Cancer 1975; 11:571–579.
19. Brzozowski AM, Pike ACW, Dauter Z, et al. Molecular basis of agonism and antagonism in the oestrogen receptor. Nature 1997; 3896652 [Internet]. 1997; 389:753–758.
20. Grese TA, Sluka JP, Bryant HU, et al. Molecular determinants of tissue selectivity in estrogen receptor modulators. Proc Natl Acad Sci U S A [Internet] 1997; 94:14105–14110.
21. Pasqualini JR, Sumida C, Giambiagi N. Pharmacodynamic and biological effects of anti-estrogens in different models. J Steroid Biochem 1988; 31:613–643.
22. Wood AJJ, Riggs BL, Hartmann LC. Selective Estrogen-Receptor Modulators — Mechanisms of Action and Application to Clinical Practice. N Engl J Med 2003; 348:618–629.
23. Visvanathan K, Fabian CJ, Bantug E, et al. Use of Endocrine Therapy for Breast Cancer Risk Reduction: ASCO Clinical Practice Guideline Update. J Clin Oncol [Internet] 2019; 37:3152–3165.

24. Fisher B, Costantino JP, Wickerham DL, et al. Tamoxifen for Prevention of Breast Cancer: Report of the National Surgical Adjuvant Breast and Bowel Project P-1 Study. JNCI J Natl Cancer Inst [Internet] 1998; 90:1371–1388.
25. Kedar RP, Bourne TH, Powles TJ, et al. Effects of tamoxifen on uterus and ovaries of postmenopausal women in a randomised breast cancer prevention trial. Lancet (London, England) [Internet] 1994; 343:1318–1321.
26. Buzdar AU, Hortobagyi GN. Tamoxifen and toremifene in breast cancer: comparison of safety and efficacy. J Clin Oncol 1998; 16:348–353.
27. Pyrhönen S, Valavaara R, Modig H, et al. Comparison of toremifene and tamoxifen in post-menopausal patients with advanced breast cancer: a randomized double-blind, the 'nordic' phase III study. Br J Cancer 1997; 76:270–277.
28. Delmas PD, Bjarnason NH, Mitlak BH, et al. Effects of raloxifene on bone mineral density, serum cholesterol concentrations, and uterine endometrium in postmenopausal women. N Engl J Med [Internet] 1997; 337:1641–1647.
29. Veronesi U, Maisonneuve P, Rotmensz N, et al. Tamoxifen for the prevention of breast cancer: late results of the Italian Randomized Tamoxifen Prevention Trial among women with hysterectomy. J Natl Cancer Inst [Internet] 2007; 99:727–737.
30. Powles TJ, Ashley S, Tidy A, Smith IE, Dowsett M. Twenty-year follow-up of the Royal Marsden randomized, double-blinded tamoxifen breast cancer prevention trial. J Natl Cancer Inst [Internet] 2007; 99:283–290.
31. Cuzick J, Sestak I, Cawthorn S, et al. Tamoxifen for prevention of breast cancer: extended long-term follow-up of the IBIS-I breast cancer prevention trial. Lancet Oncol [Internet] 2015; 16:67–75.
32. Gilmour A, Cutress R, Gandhi A, et al. Oncoplastic breast surgery: A guide to good practice. Eur J Surg Oncol 2021; 47:2272–2285.
33. Decensi A, Maisonneuve P, Rotmensz N, et al. Effect of tamoxifen on venous thromboembolic events in a breast cancer prevention trial. Circulation [Internet] 2005; 111:650–656.
34. Hernandez RK, Sørensen HT, Pedersen L, Jacobsen J, Lash TL. Tamoxifen treatment and risk of deep venous thrombosis and pulmonary embolism: a Danish population-based cohort study. Cancer [Internet] 2009; 115:4442–4449.
35. Grey AB, Stapleton JP, Evans MC, Reid IR. The effect of the anti-estrogen tamoxifen on cardiovascular risk factors in normal postmenopausal women. J Clin Endocrinol Metab [Internet] 1995; 80:3191–3195.
36. Early Breast Cancer Trialists' Collaborative Group (EBCTCG); Davies C, Godwin J, et al. Relevance of breast cancer hormone receptors and other factors to the efficacy of adjuvant tamoxifen: patient-level meta-analysis of randomised trials. Lancet [Internet] 2011; 378:771–784.
37. Ierre P, Elmas DD, Jarnason IHB, et al. Effects of Raloxifene on Bone Mineral Density, Serum Cholesterol Concentrations, and Uterine Endometrium in Postmenopausal Women. N Engl J Med 1997; 337:1641–1647.
38. Day R, Ganz PA, Costantino JP, et al. Health-related quality of life and tamoxifen in breast cancer prevention: a report from the National Surgical Adjuvant Breast and Bowel Project P-1 Study. J Clin Oncol [Internet]. 1999; 17:2659–2669.
39. Geisler J, Haynes B, Anker G, Dowsett M, Lønning PE. Influence of letrozole and anastrozole on total body aromatization and plasma estrogen levels in postmenopausal breast cancer patients evaluated in a randomized, cross-over study. J Clin Oncol [Internet] 2002; 20:751–757.
40. Hristian C, Ruber JG, Alter W, et al. Production and Actions of Estrogens. N Engl J Med 2002; 346:340–352.
41. Miller WR. Aromatase activity in breast tissue. J Steroid Biochem Mol Biol 1991; 39:783–790.
42. Geisler J, Detre S, Berntsen H, et al. Influence of neoadjuvant anastrozole (Arimidex) on intratumoral estrogen levels and proliferation markers in patients with locally advanced breast cancer. Clin Cancer Res 2001; 7:1230–1236.
43. Miller WR, Dixon JM. Local endocrine effects of aromatase inhibitors within the breast. J Steroid Biochem Mol Biol 2001; 79:93–102.
44. Geisler J, King N, Anker G, et al. In vivo inhibition of aromatization by exemestane, a novel irreversible aromatase inhibitor, in postmenopausal breast cancer patients. Clin Cancer Res 1998; 4:2089–2093.
45. Smith IE, Dowsett M. Aromatase Inhibitors in Breast Cancer. N Engl J Med 2003; 348:2431–2442.
46. Smith IE, Dowsett M, Yap YS, et al. Adjuvant aromatase inhibitors for early breast cancer after chemotherapy-induced amenorrhoea: Caution and suggested guidelines. J Clin Oncol 2006; 24:2444–2447.

47. Guerrero A, Gavilá P, Folkerd E, et al. Incidence and predictors of ovarian function recovery (OFR) in breast cancer (BC) patients with chemotherapy-induced amenorrhea (CIA) who switched from tamoxifen to exemestane. Ann Oncol [Internet] 2013; 24:674–679.
48. Bui KT, Willson ML, Goel S, Beith J, Goodwin A. Ovarian suppression for adjuvant treatment of hormone receptor-positive early breast cancer. Cochrane database Syst Rev [Internet] 2020; 3:CD013538.
49. Zaccheo T, Giudici D, Lombardi P, di Salle E. A new irreversible aromatase inhibitor, 6-methylenandrosta-1,4-diene-3,17-dione (FCE 24304): antitumor activity and endocrine effects in rats with DMBA-induced mammary tumors. Cancer Chemother Pharmacol [Internet] 1989; 23:47–50.
50. di Salle E, Ornati G, Giudici D, et al. Exemestane (FCE 24304), a new steroidal aromatase inhibitor. J Steroid Biochem Mol Biol [Internet] 1992; 43:137–143.
51. Buzdar A, Jonat W, Howell A, et al. Anastrozole, a potent and selective aromatase inhibitor, versus megestrol acetate in postmenopausal women with advanced breast cancer: results of overview analysis of two phase III trials. Arimidex Study Group. J Clin Oncol 1996; 14(7):2000–2011.
52. Lipton A, Demers LM, Harvey HA, et al. Letrozole (CGS 20267). A phase I study of a new potent oral aromatase inhibitor of breast cancer. Cancer [Internet] 1995; 75:2132–2138.
53. Bhatnagar AS, Häusler A, Schieweck K, Lang M, Bowman R. Highly selective inhibition of estrogen biosynthesis by CGS 20267, a new non-steroidal aromatase inhibitor. J Steroid Biochem Mol Biol [Internet] 1990; 37:1021–1027.
54. Geisler J, Helle H, Ekse D, et al. Letrozole is Superior to Anastrozole in Suppressing Breast Cancer Tissue and Plasma Estrogen Levels. Clin Cancer Res [Internet] 2008; 14:6330–6335.
55. Dixon JM, Renshaw L, Young O, et al. Letrozole suppresses plasma estradiol and estrone sulphate more completely than anastrozole in postmenopausal women with breast cancer. J Clin Oncol [Internet] 2008; 26:1671–1676.
56. Coombes R, Kilburn L, Snowdon C, et al. Survival and safety of exemestane versus tamoxifen after 2-3 years' tamoxifen treatment (Intergroup Exemestane Study): a randomised controlled trial. Lancet (London, England) [Internet] 2007; 369:559–570.
57. Coates AS, Keshaviah A, Thürlimann B, et al. Five years of letrozole compared with tamoxifen as initial adjuvant therapy for postmenopausal women with endocrine-responsive early breast cancer: update of study BIG 1-98. J Clin Oncol [Internet] 2007; 25:486–492.
58. Arimidex, Tamoxifen, Alone or in Combination Trialists' Group; Buzdar A, Howell A, et al. Comprehensive side-effect profile of anastrozole and tamoxifen as adjuvant treatment for early-stage breast cancer: long-term safety analysis of the ATAC trial. Lancet Oncol [Internet] 2006; 7:633–643.
59. Coleman RE, Banks LM, Girgis SI, et al. Skeletal effects of exemestane on bone-mineral density, bone biomarkers, and fracture incidence in postmenopausal women with early breast cancer participating in the Intergroup Exemestane Study (IES): a randomised controlled study. Lancet Oncol [Internet] 2007; 8:119–127.
60. Rabaglio M, Sun Z, Price KN, et al. Bone fractures among postmenopausal patients with endocrine-responsive early breast cancer treated with 5 years of letrozole or tamoxifen in the BIG 1-98 trial. Ann Oncol Off J Eur Soc Med Oncol [Internet] 2009; 20:1489–1498.
61. Eastell R, Adams JE, Coleman RE, et al. Effect of anastrozole on bone mineral density: 5-year results from the anastrozole, tamoxifen, alone or in combination trial 18233230. J Clin Oncol [Internet] 2008; 26:1051–1058.
62. Amir E, Seruga B, Niraula S, Carlsson L, Ocaña A. Toxicity of adjuvant endocrine therapy in postmenopausal breast cancer patients: a systematic review and meta-analysis. J Natl Cancer Inst [Internet] 2011; 103:1299–1309.
63. Shapiro CL, Manola J, Leboff M. Ovarian failure after adjuvant chemotherapy is associated with rapid bone loss in women with early-stage breast cancer. J Clin Oncol [Internet] 2001; 19:3306–3311.
64. Saarto T, Blomqvist C, Välimäki M, et al. Chemical castration induced by adjuvant cyclophosphamide, methotrexate, and fluorouracil chemotherapy causes rapid bone loss that is reduced by clodronate: a randomized study in premenopausal breast cancer patients. J Clin Oncol [Internet] 1997; 15:1341–1347.
65. Goss PE, Ingle JN, Pritchard KI, et al. Exemestane versus anastrozole in postmenopausal women with early breast cancer: NCIC CTG MA.27--a randomized controlled phase III trial. J Clin Oncol [Internet] 2013; 31:1398–1404.
66. Derzko C, Elliott S, Lam W. Management of sexual dysfunction in postmenopausal breast cancer patients taking adjuvant aromatase inhibitor therapy. Curr Oncol [Internet] 2007; 14:S20–S40.

67. Bernhard J, Luo W, Ribi K, et al. Patient-reported outcomes with adjuvant exemestane versus tamoxifen in premenopausal women with early breast cancer undergoing ovarian suppression (TEXT and SOFT): a combined analysis of two phase 3 randomised trials. Lancet Oncol [Internet] 2015; 16:848–858.
68. Henry NL, Giles JT, Ang D, et al. Prospective characterization of musculoskeletal symptoms in early stage breast cancer patients treated with aromatase inhibitors. Breast Cancer Res Treat [Internet] 2008; 111:365–372.
69. Cuppone F, Bria E, Verma S, et al. Do adjuvant aromatase inhibitors increase the cardiovascular risk in postmenopausal women with early breast cancer? Meta-analysis of randomized trials. Cancer [Internet] 2008; 112:260–267.
70. Khosrow-Khavar F, Filion KB, Al-Qurashi S, et al. Cardiotoxicity of aromatase inhibitors and tamoxifen in postmenopausal women with breast cancer: a systematic review and meta-analysis of randomized controlled trials. Ann Oncol Off J Eur Soc Med Oncol [Internet] 2017; 28:487–496.
71. Di Leo A, Jerusalem G, Petruzelka L, et al. Results of the CONFIRM phase III trial comparing fulvestrant 250 mg with fulvestrant 500 mg in postmenopausal women with estrogen receptor positive advanced breast cancer. J Clin Oncol [Internet] 2010; 28:4594–4600.
72. Robertson JFR, Bondarenko IM, Trishkina E, et al. Fulvestrant 500 mg versus anastrozole 1 mg for hormone receptor-positive advanced breast cancer (FALCON): an international, randomised, double-blind, phase 3 trial. Lancet [Internet] 2016;388:2997–3005.
73. Long X, Nephew KP. Fulvestrant (ICI 182,780)-dependent Interacting Proteins Mediate Immobilization and Degradation of Estrogen Receptor-α. J Biol Chem 2006; 281:9607–9615.
74. Guan J, Zhou W, Hafner M, et al. Therapeutic Ligands Antagonize Estrogen Receptor Function by Impairing Its Mobility. Cell [Internet] 2019; 178:949–963.e18.
75. Wittmann BM, Sherk A, McDonnell DP. Definition of Functionally Important Mechanistic Differences among Selective Estrogen Receptor Down-regulators. Cancer Res [Internet] 2007; 67:9549–9560.
76. Bidard FC, Kaklamani VG, Neven P, et al. Elacestrant (oral selective estrogen receptor degrader) Versus Standard Endocrine Therapy for Estrogen Receptor-Positive, Human Epidermal Growth Factor Receptor 2-Negative Advanced Breast Cancer: Results From the Randomized Phase III EMERALD Trial. J Clin Oncol [Internet] 2022; 40:3246–3256.
77. Ma CX, Suman VJ, Leitch AM, et al. ALTERNATE: Neoadjuvant endocrine treatment (NET) approaches for clinical stage II or III estrogen receptor-positive HER2-negative breast cancer (ER+ HER2- BC) in postmenopausal (PM) women: Alliance A011106. J Clin Oncol 2020; 38:504.
78. Lerebours F, Rivera S, Mouret-Reynier MA, et al. Randomized phase 2 neoadjuvant trial evaluating anastrozole and fulvestrant efficacy for postmenopausal, estrogen receptor-positive, human epidermal growth factor receptor 2-negative breast cancer patients: Results of the UNICANCER CARMINA 02 French trial (UCBG 0609). Cancer [Internet] 2016; 122:3032–3040.
79. Howell A, DeFriend DJ, Blamey RW, Robertson JF, Walton P. Response to a specific antioestrogen (ICI 182780) in tamoxifen-resistant breast cancer. Lancet (London, England) [Internet] 1995; 345:29–30.
80. Robertson JFR, Llombart-Cussac A, Rolski J, et al. Activity of fulvestrant 500 mg versus anastrozole 1 mg as first-line treatment for advanced breast cancer: results from the FIRST study. J Clin Oncol [Internet] 2009; 27:4530–4535.
81. Robertson JFR, Odling-Smee W, Holcombe C, Kohlhardt SR, Harrison MP. Pharmacokinetics of a single dose of fulvestrant prolonged-release intramuscular injection in postmenopausal women awaiting surgery for primary breast cancer. Clin Ther 2003; 25:1440–1452.
82. Kuter I, Sapunar F, McCormack P. Pharmacokinetic profile of fulvestrant 500 mg vs 250 mg: Results from the NEWEST study. J Clin Oncol 2008; 26:579.
83. Jhaveri KL, Boni V, Sohn J, et al. Safety and activity of single-agent giredestrant (GDC-9545) from a phase Ia/b study in patients (pts) with estrogen receptor-positive (ER+), HER2-negative locally advanced/metastatic breast cancer (LA/mBC). J Clin Oncol 2021; 39:1017.
84. Baird R, Oliveira M, Gil EMC, et al. Abstract PS11-05: Updated data from SERENA-1: A Phase 1 dose escalation and expansion study of the next generation oral SERD AZD9833 as a monotherapy and in combination with palbociclib, in women with ER-positive, HER2-negative advanced breast cancer. Cancer Res [Internet] 2021; 81:PS11-05.
85. Linden HM, Campone M, Bardia A, et al. Abstract PD8-08: A phase 1/2 study of SAR439859, an oral selective estrogen receptor (ER) degrader (SERD), as monotherapy and in combination with other anti-cancer therapies in postmenopausal women with ER-positive (ER+)/human epidermal growth factor receptor 2-negative (HER2-) metastatic breast cancer (mBC): AMEERA-1. Cancer Res [Internet] 2021; 81:PD8-08.

86. Jhaveri K. Abstract TF1-2: ER+ word salad decoded: SERD, SERM, SERCA, CERAN, PROTAC. Cancer Res [Internet] 2022; 82:TF1-2.
87. Lloyd MR, Wander SA, Hamilton E, Razavi P, Bardia A. Next-generation selective estrogen receptor degraders and other novel endocrine therapies for management of metastatic hormone receptor-positive breast cancer: current and emerging role. Ther Adv Med Oncol [Internet] 2022; 14:17588359221113694.
88. Hamilton EP, Wang JS, Pluard TJ, et al. Phase I/II study of H3B-6545, a novel selective estrogen receptor covalent antagonist (SERCA), in estrogen receptor positive (ER plus), human epidermal growth factor receptor 2 negative (HER2-) advanced breast cancer. J Clin Oncol [Internet] 2021; 39:1018.
89. Hamilton E, Vahdat L, Han HS, et al. Abstract PD13-08: First-in-human safety and activity of ARV-471, a novel PROTAC® estrogen receptor degrader, in ER+/HER2- locally advanced or metastatic breast cancer. Cancer Res 2022; 82:PD13-08-PD13-08.
90. emc. Fulvestrant 250 mg solution for injection in pre-filled syringe — Summary of Product Characteristics (SmPC) - (emc) [Internet]. (2023). Available from: https://www.medicines.org.uk/emc/product/12018/smpc#gref [Last accessed 29th July 2025].
91. emc. Anastrozole 1 mg film-coated tablets — Summary of Product Characteristics (SmPC) - (emc) [Internet]. (2023). Available from: https://www.medicines.org.uk/emc/product/5950/smpc#gref [Last accessed 29th July 2025].
92. emc. Exemestane 25 mg film-coated tablets — Patient Information Leaflet (PIL) - (emc) [Internet]. (2023). Available from: https://www.medicines.org.uk/emc/product/4664/pil#gref [Last accessed 29th July 2025].
93. emc. Tamoxifen 20 mg Film-Coated Tablets — Summary of Product Characteristics (SmPC) - (emc) [Internet]. (2023). Available from: https://www.medicines.org.uk/emc/product/2248/smpc#gref [Last accessed 29th July 2025].
94. Nelson HD, Fu R, Zakher B, Pappas M, McDonagh M. Medication Use for the Risk Reduction of Primary Breast Cancer in Women: Updated Evidence Report and Systematic Review for the US Preventive Services Task Force. JAMA [Internet] 2019; 322:868–886.
95. Daly B, Olopade OI, Hou N, et al. Evaluation of the Quality of Adjuvant Endocrine Therapy Delivery for Breast Cancer Care in the United States. JAMA Oncol [Internet] 2017; 3:928–935.
96. Group EBCTC. Effects of Adjuvant Tamoxifen and of Cytotoxic Therapy on Mortality in Early Breast Cancer. N Engl J Med 2010; 319:1681–1692.
97. Abe O, Abe R, Enomoto K, et al. Tamoxifen for early breast cancer: an overview of the randomised trials. Lancet 1998; 351(9114):1451–1467.
98. The National Institutes of Health (NIH) Consensus Development Program: Adjuvant Chemotherapy for Breast Cancer [Internet]. (2023). Available from: https://consensus.nih.gov/1985/1985AdjuvantChemoBreastCancer052html.htm [Last accessed 29th July 2025].
99. Controlled trial of tamoxifen as single adjuvant agent in management of early breast cancer: Analysis at Six Years by Nolvadex Adjuvant Trial Organisation. Lancet 1985; 325:836–840.
100. Legault-Poisson S. Adjuvant tamoxifen in the management of operable breast cancer: The Scottish Trial: Report from the Breast Cancer Trials Committee, Scottish Cancer Trials Office (MRC), Edinburgh. Lancet 1987; 330:171–175.
101. Abe O, Abe R, Enomoto K, et al. Relevance of breast cancer hormone receptors and other factors to the efficacy of adjuvant tamoxifen: patient-level meta-analysis of randomised trials. Lancet 2011; 378:771–784.
102. Abe O, Abe R, Enomoto K, et al. Tamoxifen for early breast cancer: An overview of the randomised trials. Lancet [Internet] 1998; 351:1451–1467.
103. Results of the ATAC (Arimidex, Tamoxifen, Alone or in Combination) trial after completion of 5 years' adjuvant treatment for breast cancer. Lancet [Internet] 2005; 365:60–62.
104. Baum M, Buzdar AU, Cuzick J, et al. Anastrozole alone or in combination with tamoxifen versus tamoxifen alone for adjuvant treatment of postmenopausal women with early breast cancer: First results of the ATAC randomised trial. Lancet [Internet] 2002; 359:2131–2139.
105. Regan MM, Neven P, Giobbie-Hurder A, et al. Assessment of letrozole and tamoxifen alone and in sequence for postmenopausal women with steroid hormone receptor-positive breast cancer: the BIG 1-98 randomised clinical trial at 8·1 years median follow-up. Lancet Oncol [Internet] 2011; 12:1101–1108.
106. Ruhstaller T, Giobbie-Hurder A, Colleoni M, et al. Adjuvant Letrozole and Tamoxifen Alone or Sequentially for Postmenopausal Women With Hormone Receptor-Positive Breast Cancer: Long-Term Follow-Up of the BIG 1-98 Trial. J Clin Oncol [Internet] 2019; 37:105–114.
107. Bradley R, Burrett J, Clarke M, et al. Aromatase inhibitors versus tamoxifen in early breast cancer: patient-level meta-analysis of the randomised trials. Lancet 2015; 386:1341–1352.

108. De Placido S, Gallo C, De Laurentiis M, et al. Adjuvant anastrozole versus exemestane versus letrozole, upfront or after 2 years of tamoxifen, in endocrine-sensitive breast cancer (FATA-GIM3): a randomised, phase 3 trial. Lancet Oncol [Internet] 2018; 19:474–485.
109. Jin H, Tu D, Zhao N, Shepherd LE, Goss PE. Longer-term outcomes of letrozole versus placebo after 5 years of tamoxifen in the NCIC CTG MA.17 trial: analyses adjusting for treatment crossover. J Clin Oncol [Internet] 2012; 30:718–721.
110. Tjan-Heijnen VCG, van Hellemond IEG, Peer PGM, et al. Extended adjuvant aromatase inhibition after sequential endocrine therapy (DATA): a randomised, phase 3 trial. Lancet Oncol [Internet] 2017; 18:1502–1511.
111. Mamounas EP, Bandos H, Lembersky BC, et al. Use of letrozole after aromatase inhibitor-based therapy in postmenopausal breast cancer (NRG Oncology/NSABP B-42): a randomised, double-blind, placebo-controlled, phase 3 trial. Lancet Oncol [Internet] 2019; 20:88–99.
112. Blok EJ, Kroep JR, Kranenbarg EMK, et al. Optimal Duration of Extended Adjuvant Endocrine Therapy for Early Breast Cancer; Results of the IDEAL Trial (BOOG 2006-05). J Natl Cancer Inst [Internet] 2018; 110:40–48.
113. Gnant M, Fitzal F, Rinnerthaler G, et al. Duration of Adjuvant Aromatase-Inhibitor Therapy in Postmenopausal Breast Cancer. N Engl J Med [Internet] 2021; 385:395–405.
114. Goss PE, Ingle JN, Pritchard KI, et al. Extending Aromatase-Inhibitor Adjuvant Therapy to 10 Years. N Engl J Med [Internet] 2016; 375:209–219.
115. Gray RG, Rea D, Handley K, et al. aTTom: Long-term effects of continuing adjuvant tamoxifen to 10 years versus stopping at 5 years in 6,953 women with early breast cancer. J Clin Oncol 2013; 31:5.
116. Davies C, Pan H, Godwin J, et al. Long-term effects of continuing adjuvant tamoxifen to 10 years versus stopping at 5 years after diagnosis of oestrogen receptor-positive breast cancer: ATLAS, a randomised trial. Lancet [Internet] 2013; 381:805–816.
117. Pan H, Gray R, Braybrooke J, et al. 20-Year Risks of Breast-Cancer Recurrence after Stopping Endocrine Therapy at 5 Years. N Engl J Med [Internet] 2017; 377:1836–1846.
118. Pedersen RN, Esen BÖ, Mellemkjær L, et al. The Incidence of Breast Cancer Recurrence 10-32 Years After Primary Diagnosis. J Natl Cancer Inst [Internet] 2022; 114:391–399.
119. LHRH-agonists in Early Breast Cancer Overview group; Cuzick J, Ambroisine L, et al. Use of luteinising-hormone-releasing hormone agonists as adjuvant treatment in premenopausal patients with hormone-receptor-positive breast cancer: a meta-analysis of individual patient data from randomised adjuvant trials. Lancet (London, England) [Internet] 2007; 369:1711–1723.
120. Francis PA, Pagani O, Fleming GF, et al. Tailoring Adjuvant Endocrine Therapy for Premenopausal Breast Cancer. N Engl J Med [Internet] 2018; 379:122–137.
121. Bradley R, Braybrooke J, Gray R, et al. Aromatase inhibitors versus tamoxifen in premenopausal women with oestrogen receptor-positive early-stage breast cancer treated with ovarian suppression: a patient-level meta-analysis of 7030 women from four randomised trials. Lancet Oncol [Internet] 2022; 23:382–392.
122. Pagani O, Walley BA, Fleming GF, et al. Adjuvant Exemestane With Ovarian Suppression in Premenopausal Breast Cancer: Long-Term Follow-Up of the Combined TEXT and SOFT Trials. J Clin Oncol [Internet] 2023; 41:1376–1382.
123. Harbeck N, Rastogi P, Martin M, et al. Adjuvant abemaciclib combined with endocrine therapy for high-risk early breast cancer: updated efficacy and Ki-67 analysis from the monarchE study. Ann Oncol Off J Eur Soc Med Oncol [Internet] 2021; 32:1571–1581.
124. Nielsen TO, Leung SCY, Rimm DL, et al. Assessment of Ki67 in Breast Cancer: Updated Recommendations From the International Ki67 in Breast Cancer Working Group. J Natl Cancer Inst [Internet] 2021; 113(7):808–819.
125. Cardoso F, van't Veer LJ, Bogaerts J, et al. 70-Gene Signature as an Aid to Treatment Decisions in Early-Stage Breast Cancer. N Engl J Med [Internet] 2016; 375:717–729.
126. Sparano JA, Gray RJ, Makower DF, et al. Adjuvant Chemotherapy Guided by a 21-Gene Expression Assay in Breast Cancer. N Engl J Med [Internet] 2018; 379:111–121.
127. Kalinsky K, Barlow WE, Gralow JR, et al. 21-Gene Assay to Inform Chemotherapy Benefit in Node-Positive Breast Cancer. N Engl J Med [Internet] 2021; 385:2336–2347.
128. Rastogi P, Anderson SJ, Bear HD, et al. Preoperative chemotherapy: Updates of national surgical adjuvant breast and bowel project protocols B-18 and B-27. J Clin Oncol 2008; 26:778–785.
129. Alba E, Calvo L, Albanell J, et al. Chemotherapy (CT) and hormonotherapy (HT) as neoadjuvant treatment in luminal breast cancer patients: results from the GEICAM/2006-03, a multicenter, randomized, phase-II study. Ann Oncol Off J Eur Soc Med Oncol [Internet] 2012; 23:3069–3074.

130. Rouzier R, Perou CM, Symmans WF, et al. Breast cancer molecular subtypes respond differently to preoperative chemotherapy. Clin Cancer Res [Internet] 2005; 11:5678–5685.
131. Preece PE, Wood RAB, Mackie CR, Cuschieri A. Tamoxifen as initial sole treatment of localised breast cancer in elderly women: a pilot study. Br Med J (Clin Res Ed) [Internet] 1982; 284:869.
132. Gazet JC, Ford HT, Bland JM, et al. Prospective randomised trial of tamoxifen versus surgery in elderly patients with breast cancer. Lancet 1988; 331:679–681.
133. Dixon JM, Renshaw L, Bellamy C, et al. The effects of neoadjuvant anastrozole (Arimidex) on tumor volume in postmenopausal women with breast cancer: a randomized, double-blind, single-center study. Clin cancer Res an Off J Am Assoc Cancer Res 2000; 6:2229–2235.
134. Dixon JM, Love CDB, Bellamy COC, et al. Letrozole as primary medical therapy for locally advanced and large operable breast cancer. Breast Cancer Res Treat [Internet] 2001; 66:191–199.
135. Ellis MJ, Coop A, Singh B, et al. Letrozole is more effective neoadjuvant endocrine therapy than tamoxifen for ErbB-1- and/or ErbB-2-positive, estrogen receptor-positive primary breast cancer: evidence from a phase III randomized trial. J Clin Oncol [Internet] 2001; 19:3808–3816.
136. Eiermann W, Paepke S, Appfelstaedt J, et al. Preoperative treatment of postmenopausal breast cancer patients with letrozole: A randomized double-blind multicenter study. Ann Oncol Off J Eur Soc Med Oncol [Internet] 2001; 12:1527–1532.
137. Ellis MJ, Ma C. Letrozole in the neoadjuvant setting: the P024 trial. Breast Cancer Res Treat [Internet] 2007; 105:33–43.
138. Cataliotti L, Buzdar AU, Noguchi S, et al. Comparison of anastrozole versus tamoxifen as preoperative therapy in postmenopausal women with hormone receptor-positive breast cancer: the Pre-Operative 'Arimidex' Compared to Tamoxifen (PROACT) trial. Cancer [Internet] 2006; 106:2095–2103.
139. Smith IE, Dowsett M, Ebbs SR, et al. Neoadjuvant treatment of postmenopausal breast cancer with anastrozole, tamoxifen, or both in combination: the Immediate Preoperative Anastrozole, Tamoxifen, or Combined with Tamoxifen (IMPACT) multicenter double-blind randomized trial. J Clin Oncol [Internet] 2005; 23:5108–5116.
140. Ellis MJ, Tao Y, Luo J, et al. Outcome prediction for estrogen receptor-positive breast cancer based on postneoadjuvant endocrine therapy tumor characteristics. J Natl Cancer Inst [Internet] 2008; 100:1380–1388.
141. Leal F, Liutti VT, Antunes dos Santos VC, et al. Neoadjuvant endocrine therapy for resectable breast cancer: A systematic review and meta-analysis. Breast [Internet] 2015;24:406–412.
142. Seo JH, Kim YH, Kim JS. Meta-analysis of pre-operative aromatase inhibitor versus tamoxifen in postmenopausal woman with hormone receptor-positive breast cancer. Cancer Chemother Pharmacol [Internet] 2009; 63:261–266.
143. Ellis MJ, Suman VJ, Hoog J, et al. Randomized phase II neoadjuvant comparison between letrozole, anastrozole, and exemestane for postmenopausal women with estrogen receptor-rich stage 2 to 3 breast cancer: Clinical and biomarker outcomes and predictive value of the baseline PAM50-based intrinsic subtype - ACOSOG Z1031. J Clin Oncol 2011; 29:2342–2349.
144. Hunt KK, Suman VJ, Wingate HF, et al. Local-Regional Recurrence After Neoadjuvant Endocrine Therapy: Data from ACOSOG Z1031 (Alliance), a Randomized Phase 2 Neoadjuvant Comparison Between Letrozole, Anastrozole, and Exemestane for Postmenopausal Women with Estrogen Receptor-Positive Clinical Stage 2 or 3 Breast Cancer. Ann Surg Oncol [Internet] 2023; 30:2111–2118.
145. Suman VJ, Ellis MJ, Ma CX. The ALTERNATE trial: assessing a biomarker driven strategy for the treatment of post-menopausal women with ER+/Her2− invasive breast cancer. Chinese Clin Oncol [Internet] 2015; 4:34.
146. Kuter I, Gee JMW, Hegg R, et al. Dose-dependent change in biomarkers during neoadjuvant endocrine therapy with fulvestrant: results from NEWEST, a randomized Phase II study. Breast Cancer Res Treat 2012; 133:237–246.
147. Harper-Wynne CL, Sacks NPM, Shenton K, et al. Comparison of the systemic and intratumoral effects of tamoxifen and the aromatase inhibitor vorozole in postmenopausal patients with primary breast cancer. J Clin Oncol Off J Am Soc Clin Oncol 2002; 20:1026–1035.
148. Polychronis A, Sinnett HD, Hadjiminas D, et al. Preoperative gefitinib versus gefitinib and anastrozole in postmenopausal patients with oestrogen-receptor positive and epidermal-growth-factor-receptor-positive primary breast cancer: a double-blind placebo-controlled phase II randomised trial. Lancet Oncol 2005; 6:383–391.
149. Smith IE, Walsh G, Skene A, et al. A phase II placebo-controlled trial of neoadjuvant anastrozole alone or with gefitinib in early breast cancer. J Clin Oncol 2007; 25:3816–3822.

150. Mohammadianpanah M, Ashouri Y, Hoseini S, et al. The efficacy and safety of neoadjuvant chemotherapy +/2 letrozole in postmenopausal women with locally advanced breast cancer: A randomized phase III clinical trial. Breast Cancer Res Treat [Internet] 2012; 132:853–861.
151. Fasching PA, Jud SM, Hauschild M, et al. FemZone trial: a randomized phase II trial comparing neoadjuvant letrozole and zoledronic acid with letrozole in primary breast cancer patients. BMC Cancer [Internet] 2014; 14:66.
152. Palmieri C, Cleator S, Kilburn LS, et al. NEOCENT: a randomised feasibility and translational study comparing neoadjuvant endocrine therapy with chemotherapy in ER-rich postmenopausal primary breast cancer. Breast Cancer Res Treat 2014; 148:581–590.
153. Dowsett M, Smith IE, Ebbs SR, et al. Short-Term Changes in Ki-67 during Neoadjuvant Treatment of Primary Breast Cancer with Anastrozole or Tamoxifen Alone or Combined Correlate with Recurrence-Free Survival. Clin Cancer Res [Internet] 2005; 11:951s–958s.
154. Hojo T, Kinoshita T, Imoto S, et al. Use of the neo-adjuvant exemestane in post-menopausal estrogen receptor-positive breast cancer: a randomized phase II trial (PTEX46) to investigate the optimal duration of preoperative endocrine therapy. Breast [Internet] 2013; 22:263–267.
155. Guarneri V, Generali DG, Frassoldati A, et al. Double-blind, placebo-controlled, multicenter, randomized, phase IIb neoadjuvant study of letrozole-lapatinib in postmenopausal hormone receptor-positive, human epidermal growth factor receptor 2-negative, operable breast cancer. J Clin Oncol Off J Am Soc Clin Oncol 2014; 32:1050–1057.
156. Chow LWC, Yip AYS, Loo WTY, Lam CK, Toi M. Celecoxib anti-aromatase neoadjuvant (CAAN) trial for locally advanced breast cancer. J Steroid Biochem Mol Biol 2008; 111:13–17.
157. Cottu P, D'Hondt V, Dureau S, et al. Letrozole and palbociclib versus chemotherapy as neoadjuvant therapy of high-risk luminal breast cancer. Ann Oncol Off J Eur Soc Med Oncol [Internet] 2018; 29:2334–2340.
158. Johnston S, Puhalla S, Wheatley D, et al. Randomized Phase II Study Evaluating Palbociclib in Addition to Letrozole as Neoadjuvant Therapy in Estrogen Receptor-Positive Early Breast Cancer: PALLET Trial. J Clin Oncol [Internet] 2019; 37:178–189.
159. Alsaleh K, Al Zahwahry H, Bounedjar A, et al. Neoadjuvant endocrine therapy with or without palbociclib in low-risk patients: a phase III randomized double-blind SAFIA trial. J Cancer Res Clin Oncol [Internet] 2023; 149:6171–6179.
160. Hurvitz S, Abad MF, Rostorfer R, et al. Breast cancer, early stage Interim results from neoMONARCH: A neoadjuvant phase II study of abemaciclib in postmenopausal women with HR + /HER2- breast cancer (BC). Ann Oncol [Internet] 2016; 27:vi552.
161. Baselga J, Semiglazov V, Van Dam P, et al. Phase II randomized study of neoadjuvant everolimus plus letrozole compared with placebo plus letrozole in patients with estrogen receptor-positive breast cancer. J Clin Oncol [Internet] 2009; 27:2630–2637.
162. Mayer IA, Prat A, Egle D, et al. A Phase II Randomized Study of Neoadjuvant Letrozole Plus Alpelisib for Hormone Receptor-Positive, Human Epidermal Growth Factor Receptor 2-Negative Breast Cancer (NEO-ORB). Clin Cancer Res [Internet] 2019; 25:2975–2987.
163. Saura C, Hlauschek D, Oliveira M, et al. Neoadjuvant letrozole plus taselisib versus letrozole plus placebo in postmenopausal women with oestrogen receptor-positive, HER2-negative, early-stage breast cancer (LORELEI): a multicentre, randomised, double-blind, placebo-controlled, phase 2 trial. Lancet Oncol [Internet] 2019; 20:1226–1238.
164. Kim HJ, Noh WC, Lee ES, et al. Efficacy of neoadjuvant endocrine therapy compared with neoadjuvant chemotherapy in pre-menopausal patients with oestrogen receptor-positive and HER2-negative, lymph node-positive breast cancer. Breast Cancer Res [Internet] 2020; 22:54.
165. Masuda N, Sagara Y, Kinoshita T, et al. Neoadjuvant anastrozole versus tamoxifen in patients receiving goserelin for premenopausal breast cancer (STAGE): a double-blind, randomised phase 3 trial. Lancet Oncol 2012;13:345–352.
166. Dellapasqua S, Gray KP, Munzone E, et al. Neoadjuvant Degarelix Versus Triptorelin in Premenopausal Patients Who Receive Letrozole for Locally Advanced Endocrine-Responsive Breast Cancer: A Randomized Phase II Trial. J Clin Oncol [Internet] 2019; 37:386–395.
167. Dixon JM, Anderson TJ, Miller WR. Neoadjuvant endocrine therapy of breast cancer: a surgical perspective. Eur J Cancer 2002; 38:2214–2221.
168. Toi M, Saji S, Masuda N, et al. Ki67 index changes, pathological response and clinical benefits in primary breast cancer patients treated with 24 weeks of aromatase inhibition. Cancer Sci [Internet] 2011; 102:858–865.
169. O-115. Is there an optimal duration of neoadjuvant letrozole therapy? Eur J Cancer Suppl 2005; 3:36–37.

170. Llombart-Cussac A, Guerrero Á, Galán A, et al. Phase II trial with letrozole to maximum response as primary systemic therapy in postmenopausal patients with ER/PgR[+] operable breast cancer. Clin Transl Oncol [Internet] 2012; 14:125–131.
171. Carpenter R, Doughty JC, Cordiner C, et al. Optimum duration of neoadjuvant letrozole to permit breast conserving surgery. Breast Cancer Res Treat [Internet] 2014; 144:569–576.
172. Dixon JM, Renshaw L, Macaskill EJ, et al. Increase in response rate by prolonged treatment with neoadjuvant letrozole. Breast Cancer Res Treat [Internet] 2009; 113:145–151.
173. Krainick-Strobel UE, Lichtenegger W, Wallwiener D, et al. Neoadjuvant letrozole in postmenopausal estrogen and/or progesterone receptor positive breast cancer: a phase IIb/III trial to investigate optimal duration of preoperative endocrine therapy. BMC Cancer [Internet] 2008; 8:62.
174. Fontein DBY, Charehbili A, Nortier JWR, et al. Efficacy of six month neoadjuvant endocrine therapy in postmenopausal, hormone receptor-positive breast cancer patients – A phase II trial. Eur J Cancer 2014; 50:2190–2200.
175. Leal MF, Haynes BP, Schuster E, et al. Early Enrichment of ESR1 Mutations and the Impact on Gene Expression in Presurgical Primary Breast Cancer Treated with Aromatase Inhibitors. Clin cancer Res an Off J Am Assoc Cancer Res 2019; 25:7485–7496.
176. Cottu P, D'Hondt V, Dureau S, et al. Letrozole and palbociclib versus chemotherapy as neoadjuvant therapy of high-risk luminal breast cancer. Ann Oncol [Internet] 2018; 29:2334–2340.
177. Delaloge S, Dureau S, D'Hondt V, et al. Survival outcomes after neoadjuvant letrozole and palbociclib versus third generation chemotherapy for patients with high-risk oestrogen receptor-positive HER2-negative breast cancer. Eur J Cancer 2022; 166:300–308.
178. Ma CX, Gao F, Luo J, et al. NeoPalAna: Neoadjuvant Palbociclib, a Cyclin-Dependent Kinase 4/6 Inhibitor, and Anastrozole for Clinical Stage 2 or 3 Estrogen Receptor-Positive Breast Cancer. Clin Cancer Res [Internet] 2017; 23:4055–4065.
179. Ellis MJ, Babiera G, Unzeitig GW, et al. ACOSOG Z1031: A randomized phase II trial comparing exemestane, letrozole, and anastrozole in postmenopausal women with clinical stage II/III estrogen receptor-positive breast cancer. J Clin Oncol 2010; 28:LBA513–LBA513.
180. Dubsky PC, Singer CF, Egle D, et al. The EndoPredict score predicts response to neoadjuvant chemotherapy and neoendocrine therapy in hormone receptor-positive, human epidermal growth factor receptor 2-negative breast cancer patients from the ABCSG-34 trial. Eur J Cancer [Internet] 2020; 134:99–106.
181. Whitworth P, Beitsch P, Mislowsky A, et al. Chemosensitivity and Endocrine Sensitivity in Clinical Luminal Breast Cancer Patients in the Prospective Neoadjuvant Breast Registry Symphony Trial (NBRST) Predicted by Molecular Subtyping. Ann Surg Oncol 2017; 24:669–675.
182. Bear HD, Wan W, Robidoux A, et al. Using the 21 Gene Assay from Core Needle Biopsies to Choose Neoadjuvant Therapy for Breast Cancer: A Multicenter Trial. J Surg Oncol [Internet] 2017; 115:917.
183. Pease AM, Riba LA, Gruner RA, Tung NM, James TA. Oncotype DX® Recurrence Score as a Predictor of Response to Neoadjuvant Chemotherapy. Ann Surg Oncol [Internet] 2019; 26:366–371.
184. Boland MR, Al-Maksoud A, Ryan EJ, et al. Value of a 21-gene expression assay on core biopsy to predict neoadjuvant chemotherapy response in breast cancer: systematic review and meta-analysis. Br J Surg [Internet] 2021; 108:24–31.
185. Gianni L, Zambetti M, Clark K, et al. Gene expression profiles in paraffin-embedded core biopsy tissue predict response to chemotherapy in women with locally advanced breast cancer. J Clin Oncol [Internet] 2005; 23:7265–7277.
186. Llombart-Cussac A, Anton-Torres A, Rojas B, et al. Impact of the 21-Gene Assay in Patients with High-Clinical Risk ER-Positive and HER2-Negative Early Breast Cancer: Results of the KARMA Dx Study. Cancers (Basel) [Internet] 2023; 15:1529.
187. Wang H, Yee D. I-SPY 2: a Neoadjuvant Adaptive Clinical Trial Designed to Improve Outcomes in High-Risk Breast Cancer. Curr Breast Cancer Rep [Internet] 2019; 11:303–310.
188. Bernard PS, Parker JS, Mullins M, et al. Supervised Risk Predictor of Breast Cancer Based on Intrinsic Subtypes. J Clin Oncol [Internet] 2009; 27:1160–1167.
189. Prat A, Lluch A, Turnbull AK, et al. A PAM50-based Chemo-Endocrine Score for Hormone Receptor-Positive Breast Cancer with an Intermediate Risk of Relapse. Clin Cancer Res [Internet] 2017; 23:3035–3044.
190. Akashi-Tanaka S, Shimizu C, Ando M, et al. 21-Gene expression profile assay on core needle biopsies predicts responses to neoadjuvant endocrine therapy in breast cancer patients. Breast [Internet] 2009; 18:171–174.

191. Ueno T, Masuda N, Yamanaka T, et al. Evaluating the 21-gene assay Recurrence Score® as a predictor of clinical response to 24 weeks of neoadjuvant exemestane in estrogen receptor-positive breast cancer. Int J Clin Oncol [Internet] 2014; 19:607–613.
192. Iwata H, Masuda N, Yamamoto Y, et al. Validation of the 21-gene test as a predictor of clinical response to neoadjuvant hormonal therapy for ER+, HER2-negative breast cancer: the TransNEOS study. Breast Cancer Res Treat [Internet] 2019; 173:123–133.
193. Taylor C, Meisel J, Foreman AJ, et al. Using Oncotype DX breast recurrence score® assay to define the role of neoadjuvant endocrine therapy in early-stage hormone receptor-positive breast cancer. Breast Cancer Res Treat [Internet] 2023; 199:91–98.
194. Nitz UA, Gluz O, Kümmel S, et al. Endocrine Therapy Response and 21-Gene Expression Assay for Therapy Guidance in HR+/HER2- Early Breast Cancer. J Clin Oncol [Internet] 2022; 40:2557–2567.
195. Anurag M, Ellis MJ, Haricharan S. DNA damage repair defects as a new class of endocrine treatment resistance driver. Oncotarget 2018; 9:36252–36253.
196. Xia Y, He X, Renshaw L, et al. Integrated DNA and RNA Sequencing Reveals Drivers of Endocrine Resistance in Estrogen Receptor–Positive Breast Cancer. Clin Cancer Res [Internet] 2022; 28:3618–3629.
197. Yeh E, Slanetz P, Kopans DB, et al. Prospective comparison of mammography, sonography, and MRI in patients undergoing neoadjuvant chemotherapy for palpable breast cancer. AJR Am J Roentgenol [Internet] 2005; 184:868–877.
198. Zhang C, Kosiorek HE, Patel BK, et al. Accuracy of Posttreatment Imaging for Evaluation of Residual in Breast Disease After Neoadjuvant Endocrine Therapy. Ann Surg Oncol [Internet] 2022; 29:6207–6212.
199. Reis J, Boavida J, Tran HT, et al. Assessment of preoperative axillary nodal disease burden: breast MRI in locally advanced breast cancer before, during and after neoadjuvant endocrine therapy. BMC Cancer [Internet] 2022; 22:702.
200. Haque W, Verma V, Hatch S, et al. Response rates and pathologic complete response by breast cancer molecular subtype following neoadjuvant chemotherapy. Breast Cancer Res Treat [Internet] 2018; 170:559–567.
201. Dowsett M, Group O behalf of the IT, Smith IE, et al. Prognostic Value of Ki67 Expression After Short-Term Presurgical Endocrine Therapy for Primary Breast Cancer. J Natl Cancer Inst [Internet] 2007; 99:167–170.
202. Dowsett M, Ebbs SR, Dixon JM, et al. Biomarker changes during neoadjuvant anastrozole, tamoxifen, or the combination: influence of hormonal status and HER-2 in breast cancer--a study from the IMPACT trialists. J Clin Oncol Off J Am Soc Clin Oncol 2005; 23:2477–2492.
203. Ellis MJ, Suman VJ, Hoog J, et al. Ki67 Proliferation Index as a Tool for Chemotherapy Decisions During and After Neoadjuvant Aromatase Inhibitor Treatment of Breast Cancer: Results From the American College of Surgeons Oncology Group Z1031 Trial (Alliance). J Clin Oncol [Internet] 2017; 35:1061.
204. ISRCTN - ISRCTN11896599: Does the timing and order of breast surgery and hormone treatment affect the quality of life and the amount of surgery required in post-menopausal women with breast cancer? The EndoNET study [Internet]. (2023). Available from: https://www.isrctn.com/ISRCTN11896599 [Last accessed 29th July 2025].
205. Mieog JSD, Van Der Hage JA, Van De Velde CJH. Neoadjuvant chemotherapy for operable breast cancer. Br J Surg [Internet] 2007; 94:1189–1200.
206. Mauri D, Pavlidis N, Ioannidis JPA. Neoadjuvant versus adjuvant systemic treatment in breast cancer: a meta-analysis. J Natl Cancer Inst [Internet] 2005; 97:188–194.
207. Valachis A, Mamounas EP, Mittendorf EA, et al. Risk factors for locoregional disease recurrence after breast-conserving therapy in patients with breast cancer treated with neoadjuvant chemotherapy: An international collaboration and individual patient meta-analysis. Cancer 2018; 124:2923–2930.
208. Pariser AC, Sedghi T, Soulos PR, et al. Utilization, duration, and outcomes of neoadjuvant endocrine therapy in the United States. Breast Cancer Res Treat 2019; 178:419–426.
209. Kim HJ, Dominici L, Rosenberg SM, et al. Surgical Treatment After Neoadjuvant Systemic Therapy in Young Women With Breast Cancer: Results From a Prospective Cohort Study. Ann Surg [Internet] 2022; 276:173–179.
210. Whitehead I, Irwin GW, Bannon F, et al. The NeST (Neoadjuvant systemic therapy in breast cancer) study: National Practice Questionnaire of United Kingdom multi-disciplinary decision making. BMC Cancer [Internet] 2021; 21:1–9.
211. Chiba A, Hoskin TL, Heins CN, et al. Trends in Neoadjuvant Endocrine Therapy Use and Impact on Rates of Breast Conservation in Hormone Receptor Positive Breast Cancer: A National Cancer Data Base Study. Ann Surg Oncol [Internet] 2017; 24:418–424.

212. Cao L, Sugumar K, Keller E, et al. Neoadjuvant Endocrine Therapy as an Alternative to Neoadjuvant Chemotherapy Among Hormone Receptor-Positive Breast Cancer Patients: Pathologic and Surgical Outcomes. Ann Surg Oncol [Internet] 2021; 28:5730–5741.
213. Donker M, Straver ME, Wesseling J, et al. Marking axillary lymph nodes with radioactive iodine seeds for axillary staging after neoadjuvant systemic treatment in breast cancer patients the mari procedure. Ann Surg [Internet] 2015; 261:378–382.
214. Dash N, Chafin SH, Johnson RR, Contractor FM. Usefulness of tissue marker clips in patients undergoing neoadjuvant chemotherapy for breast cancer. AJR Am J Roentgenol [Internet] 1999; 173:911–917.
215. Minella C, Villasco A, D'alonzo M, et al. Surgery after Neoadjuvant Chemotherapy: A Clip-Based Technique to Improve Surgical Outcomes, a Single-Center Experience. Cancers (Basel) [Internet] 2022;14:2229.
216. Espinosa-Bravo M, Sao Avilés A, Esgueva A, et al. Breast conservative surgery after neoadjuvant chemotherapy in breast cancer patients: comparison of two tumor localization methods. Eur J Surg Oncol [Internet] 2011; 37:1038–1043.
217. Caudle AS, Yang WT, Krishnamurthy S, et al. Improved axillary evaluation following neoadjuvant therapy for patientswith node-positive breast cancer using selective evaluation of clipped nodes: Implementation of targeted axillary dissection. J Clin Oncol 2016; 34:1072–1078.
218. Thomssen C, Balic M, Harbeck N, Gnant M. St. Gallen/Vienna 2021: A Brief Summary of the Consensus Discussion on Customizing Therapies for Women with Early Breast Cancer. Breast Care (Basel) [Internet] 2021; 16:135–143.
219. Semiglazov VF, Semiglazov VV, Dashyan GA, et al. Phase 2 randomized trial of primary endocrine therapy versus chemotherapy in postmenopausal patients with estrogen receptor-positive breast cancer. Cancer [Internet] 2007; 110:244–254.
220. Boughey JC, Ballman KV, Le-Petross HT, et al. Identification and resection of the clipped node decreases the false negative rate of sentinel lymph node surgery in patients presenting with node positive breast cancer (T0-T4, N1-2) who receive neoadjuvant chemotherapy – results from ACOSOG Z1071 (Alliance). Ann Surg [Internet] 2016; 263:802.
221. Kindts I, Laenen A, Depuydt T, Weltens C. Tumour bed boost radiotherapy for women after breast-conserving surgery. Cochrane database Syst Rev [Internet] 2017; 11:CD011987.
222. Ellis M, Luo J, Tao Y, et al. Tumor Ki67 Proliferation Index within 4 Weeks of Initiating Neoadjuvant Endocrine Therapy for Early Identification of Non-Responders. Cancer Res [Internet] 2009; 69:78.
223. Weiss A, Wong S, Golshan M, et al. Patterns of Axillary Management in Stages 2 and 3 Hormone Receptor-Positive Breast Cancer by Initial Treatment Approach. Ann Surg Oncol [Internet] 2019; 26:4326–4336.
224. Kantor O, Wong S, Weiss A, et al. Prognostic significance of residual nodal disease after neoadjuvant endocrine therapy for hormone receptor-positive breast cancer. npj Breast Cancer 2020 61 [Internet] 2020; 6:1–6.
225. Sávolt Á, Péley G, Polgár C, et al. Eight-year follow up result of the OTOASOR trial: The Optimal Treatment Of the Axilla – Surgery Or Radiotherapy after positive sentinel lymph node biopsy in early-stage breast cancer: A randomized, single centre, phase III, non-inferiority trial. Eur J Surg Oncol [Internet] 2017; 43:672–679.
226. Donker M, van Tienhoven G, Straver ME, et al. Radiotherapy or surgery of the axilla after a positive sentinel node in breast cancer (EORTC 10981-22023 AMAROS): A randomised, multicentre, open-label, phase 3 non-inferiority trial. Lancet Oncol [Internet] 2014; 15:1303–1310.
227. Giuliano AE, Ballman KV, McCall L, Beitsch PD, et al. Effect of Axillary Dissection vs No Axillary Dissection on 10-Year Overall Survival Among Women With Invasive Breast Cancer and Sentinel Node Metastasis: The ACOSOG Z0011 (Alliance) Randomized Clinical Trial. JAMA [Internet] 2017; 318:918–926.
228. Kantor O, Wakeman M, Weiss A, et al. Axillary Management After Neoadjuvant Endocrine Therapy for Hormone Receptor-Positive Breast Cancer. Ann Surg Oncol [Internet] 2021; 28:1358–1367.

Chapter 7

Percutaneous treatment for breast cancer

Jenny Yijian Wang, Francesca Holt, Gloria Petralia, Gurdeep S Mannu

ABSTRWACT

Breast cancer is the most common cancer in women in the UK and with mammographic screening, many breast cancers are diagnosed at an early stage. There has been a general trend towards de-escalation of local therapy for early breast cancer. Innovative advances in technology have yielded a new generation of percutaneous treatment options for breast cancer and these can be divided into methods of tumour ablation using ionising radiation (radiotherapy using photons, protons, or carbon ions), using thermal techniques [microwaves, radio waves, laser, high-intensity frequency ultrasound (US), or cryoablation] and vacuum-assisted excision. This chapter discusses the literature on these options and their potential in future breast cancer treatment.

INTRODUCTION

Breast cancer is the most common type of cancer among women in the UK [1]. With the introduction of breast screening, breast cancers are now detected earlier than in previous years. Early breast cancer is defined as when all detected invasive cancer cells in the breast or regional lymph nodes and can be removed surgically and there is no evidence of distant spread of the disease.

Routine management of early breast cancer involves surgery to remove the whole or part of the breast containing the cancer. Women who receive breast-conserving surgery are recommended adjuvant radiotherapy to the whole breast to treat any potential residual microscopic disease. Adjuvant radiotherapy for early breast cancer using high-energy X-rays (photons) has been shown in randomised trials to reduce the risk of local recurrence

---

Jenny Yijian Wang BA, Medical Student, University of Oxford, UK
E-mail: jenny.wang@gtc.ox.ac.uk (for correspondence)

Francesca Holt MRCP, Clinical Research Fellow, University of Oxford, UK
E-mail: francesca.holt@ndph.ox.ac.uk (for correspondence)

Gloria Petralia FRCS, Consultant Breast Surgeon, Oxford University Hospitals, UK
E-mail: Gloria.Petralia@ouh.nhs.uk (for correspondence)

Gurdeep S Mannu FRCS, Clinical Research Fellow, University of Oxford, UK
E-mail: gurdeep.mannu@nds.ox.ac.uk (for correspondence)

and improve survival from breast cancer [2,3]. In addition to surgery and radiotherapy, many women receive some form of adjuvant systemic anticancer therapy, such as endocrine therapy, chemotherapy, targeted biological therapy and/or bisphosphates to further reduce the risk of cancer recurrence and improve survival [4].

Over time surgical techniques for early breast cancer treatment have both de-escalated in intensity and optimised in terms of oncological outcomes. Through incremental advances, Halstead's radical mastectomy has eventually been replaced by the sophisticated oncoplastic techniques for breast conserving surgery used today that maintain the oncological benefit but also achieve excellent cosmetic outcomes [5]. However, no matter how far surgical techniques evolve, surgery by its very nature involves a scar and the potential for bleeding and haematoma, infection, cosmetic defect, seroma formation and the potential for further surgery in the event of involved margins. This is in addition to the risks and side effects of general anaesthesia. Compared with the standard surgical procedure, the main advantages of minimally invasive percutaneous methods include the absence of general anaesthesia (and the associated side effects, risks and monitoring), no cut in the skin or a small incision for needle/probe insertion compared with incisions used for conventional surgical excision, and, therefore, less scarring, better cosmetic outcome, less pain, shorter recovery time and the corresponding health economic benefits [6–8].

Non-surgical systemic treatments for breast cancer in the form of endocrine therapies have been used in older women who may be unsuitable for surgery due to frailty and/or multiple comorbidities. Outside this particular group, treatment of early breast cancer without surgery is not recommended as part of standard care. However, therapies under investigation include: (1) ionising radiation (radiotherapy using photons, protons, or carbon ions), (2) thermal ablation [using microwaves, radio waves, laser, high-intensity frequency ultrasound (US) or cryoablation], (3) image-guided vacuum needle excision. Each of these therapies aims to achieve either precisely targeted lethal damage to cancer cells within the unresected breast, termed 'ablation', or vacuum excision of a small area of low-grade disease and may offer an alternative to surgery in select cases in the future. In this chapter, we describe these percutaneous treatments, highlight their benefits and risks, and discuss how they may fit into future clinical practice in breast cancer treatment.

ABLATIVE RADIOTHERAPY

Radiotherapy uses ionising radiation to cause cancer cell death. Normal healthy cells can also be damaged by radiation which results in adverse effects, but unlike cancer cells, normal cells are better at repair. Nowadays, most women being treated for early breast cancer receive adjuvant photon radiotherapy after their surgery to treat any potential residual microscopic disease. Randomised trials have shown that external beam radiotherapy using photons (± electrons) reduces the risk of local recurrence and improves survival from breast cancer when targeted at the whole breast after breast conserving surgery, or the chest wall after mastectomy in lymph node positive cancer [2,3]. Adjuvant radiotherapies using other types of ionising radiation, such as protons and carbon ions, are under investigation because for some women, they may better minimise doses to normal cells and, therefore, carry fewer adverse effects [9]. Radiotherapy for unresected breast cancer is not currently recommended as part of routine breast cancer management in the UK.

The majority of studies reporting outcomes after ablative radiotherapy for early breast cancer were published before the 1990s [10–20]. These studies mainly reported retrospectively upon non-randomised cohorts of patients treated in France, Belgium, Canada and the USA between the 1950s and 1990s. The characteristics of patients eligible for inclusion in these studies were wide-ranging. Some patients were offered ablative radiotherapy as their small operable breast cancers were considered potentially curable with radiation. Others were offered ablative radiation because they were considered inoperable.

The techniques used to deliver the course of radiotherapy in these studies varied but most commonly involved two phases of treatment. First, approximately 40–60 Gy was delivered in 2–3 Gy fractions to the affected whole breast using external photon beams (e.g. Cobalt-60, 4 MV). Second, a boost of between 10 and 40 Gy was delivered in 2–3 Gy fractions to the breast cancer using either external beams of photons, electrons, or interstitial implantation of Iridium-192, Cesium-137 or Radium-226.

Later publications from centres in France reported on the use of hypofractionated ablative external beam photon radiotherapy for patients with breast cancer over the age of 70 years considered unsuitable for surgery for reasons of a locally advanced breast cancer, significant medical co-morbidities, or declining surgery [14,21]. Doses of 32.5 Gy in 6.5 Gy fractions were given once weekly to the whole breast. This was followed by a boost to the breast cancer of between one and three 6.5 Gy fractions, using external beam photons or electrons. Such high doses per fraction were considered acceptable because the study population was elderly and, therefore, the slight increased risk of late adverse effects tolerated.

Many of these early publications demonstrated the relationship between radiation dose and the probability of local breast cancer control, and its variation with breast cancer size [15,22]. Many studies also reported that the higher doses of radiation used to achieve local control of breast cancer resulted in considerable adverse cosmetic effects on normal breast tissue [13,17]. In comparison, adjuvant radiotherapy directed at microscopic disease required lower doses of radiation to achieve local breast cancer control and, therefore, could achieve better cosmetic outcomes. The focus of clinical research shifted away from ablative radiotherapy towards comparing outcomes from mastectomy with breast conserving surgery and adjuvant radiotherapy [2]. The radiotherapy technology and techniques used in these early studies of ablative radiotherapy are now considered outdated.

There are few published outcomes from ablative radiotherapy for early breast cancer delivered after the year 2000, but those available report on the use advanced radiotherapy technologies such as stereotactic radiotherapy, proton beam therapy, and carbon ion therapy. These technologies can theoretically improve doses to the cancer and better spare surrounding normal tissues and organs. For example, one pilot study from Japan treated 11 patients with breast cancer using stereotactic ablative photon radiotherapy. A dose of 50 Gy in 25 fractions was delivered to the whole breast followed by a boost of 21 Gy in three fractions of stereotactic radiotherapy to the tumour [23,24]. Stereotactic radiotherapy accounts for tumour motion and is delivered using intensity-modulated radiotherapy techniques which result in dose distributions that tightly cover the cancer with steep dose gradients away from neighbouring normal tissues and organs. All patients had a complete or partial response on computed tomography (CT) or magnetic resonance imaging (MRI) scans. However, two patients developed locoregional recurrence, and one distant metastasis.

There are no randomised comparisons between ablative radiotherapy and standard of care. However, there are non-randomised clinical trials of ablative radiotherapy for early breast cancer underway, e.g. NCT03585621 and NCT02316561, and new applications of ablative radiotherapy for early breast cancer are emerging in the literature [25,26]. For example, there are some case reports describing the experimental use of stereotactic ablative radiotherapy for early breast cancer in place of surgery without adjuvant whole breast radiotherapy [21,27,28]. Similarly, one centre in Japan has published outcomes after using passive delivery of 60 Gy carbon ions given in once weekly fractions of 15 Gy for early breast cancer [29]. 14 patients considered unsuitable for surgical management of their ≥2 cm invasive ductal carcinomas (IDC) were included. A complete response as assessed on US and MRI was seen in 13 patients and one patient had a partial response. After a median follow-up of 61 months (range 51–87), there had been one local recurrence. The maximum grade toxicity was grade 1 acute skin reaction seen in 10 patients.

With so few data available, it is not yet possible to evaluate whether modern ablative radiotherapy techniques can replace surgery in the management of early breast cancer in specific cases, but the increasing availability of advanced radiotherapy technologies are likely to drive further research in this area.

THERMAL ABLATION

Techniques for thermal ablation involve non-surgical percutaneous treatment to induce necrosis in tumour cells and with a shorter recovery time and better cosmetic result than surgical excision. Currently, thermal ablation techniques include cryoablation, radiofrequency ablation (RFA), laser ablation (LA), microwave ablation (MWA) and high-intensity focused ultrasound (HIFU) ablation. Each of these is described below.

Cryoablation

Cryoablation is the use of localised extreme cooling to induce necrotic tumour cell death. The cryoablation probe is inserted into the centre of the tumour guided by US and cooled to below −30°C. A spinal needle parallel to the cryoablation probe is used to inject sterile saline to maintain at least 2 mm separation between probe and skin. Cryoablation devices can either use liquid nitrogen or argon gas. The cooling occurs through a freeze-thaw-freeze pattern to maximise the area of necrosis within the tumour, as previously damaged tissue is a better conductor of cold temperatures.

The majority of recent trials of cryoablation have included patients with unifocal IDC or ductal carcinoma in situ (DCIS) ≤ 1.5 cm [30–32]. Some trials specified an inclusion criterion of breast cancers with low risk of recurrence, such as those with a favourable receptor profile and no extensive intraductal component. Invasive lobular carcinomas tended to be excluded because of the difficulty visualising their indiscrete margins on US. A minority of trials included patients with unresectable breast cancers or patients considered unsuitable for surgery.

Recent studies reported success rates of around 76–97% [30–34]. Success was usually defined as complete ablation and lack of recurrence after 5 years as measured on MRI and/or histologically. One of the largest trials in the field was ACOSOG Z1072, a phase II trial of cryoablation for unifocal IDC or DCIS of ≤2 cm, which reported successful cryoablation in 75.9% of cancers [35]. Reported adverse events in cryoablation trials include mild effects such as bruising, localised oedema, pain and bleeding. Moderate adverse effects included freeze burns, inflammation, infection and skin retraction. Fat necrosis, a serious adverse effect, was rare [30,32–35].

Cryoablation has previously been approved by the Food and Drug Administration (FDA) for kidney and liver cancers and benign breast tumours but has not yet been approved in the UK or USA for breast cancers. Ongoing non-randomised trials of cryoablation for breast cancer include ICE3 (Cryoablation Without Excision for Low-Risk Early-Stage Breast Cancer) and FROST (Freezing Instead of Removal Of Small Tumours) [30,32]. The interim results of ICE3 estimate the ipsilateral breast tumour recurrence rate to be 2.06% after a median follow-up of 5 years, for early-stage breast cancer ≤1.5 cm HR+ and HER2- in 194 women [32]. There is an ongoing randomised trial, COOL-IT (NCT05505643), which plans to randomise 256 participants with ≤2 cm breast cancer to either cryoablation or lumpectomy [36]. Planned primary outcomes are safety and ipsilateral breast cancer recurrence [36].

Radiofrequency ablation

For RFA, an electrode is inserted into the tumour, where radiofrequency alternating currents cause resistive heating leading to localised coagulative necrosis of the surrounding tumour cells. The heating procedure takes approximately 30 minutes. The power is initially set to 12–15 W and increased stepwise till a maximum of 60 W until the maximum resistance and a temperature of 68–100°C is reached.

One of the first reports of the use of RFA for breast cancer was in 1999. Jeffrey and colleagues reported the use of RFA in five patients with locally advanced invasive breast cancers measuring >5 cm. The procedure was performed under general anaesthesia [37]. More recent studies perform RFA under local anaesthesia and aim to treat smaller breast cancers (≤2 cm).

Most patients included in studies of RFA underwent surgical excision, radiotherapy and systemic adjuvant therapy after the intervention in alignment with standard care. Therefore, the success of RFA was mostly defined as complete resection, determined through histological staining of biopsy tissue. Response on MRI was also reported in some studies. Reported success rates ranged from around 80–100%. As with other thermal ablation techniques, the probability of successful ablation was greatest for tumours of ≤2 cm. For example, a study by Ito and colleagues reported an ipsilateral breast tumour recurrence-free rate of 94% after 5 years in tumours ≤2 cm compared with 84% in tumours >2 cm [38].

A recent randomised control phase II trial found that RFA was effective for local tumour control [39]. However, recruitment was terminated due to higher rates of breast inflammation and infection in the RFA compared to the lumpectomy group [39]. In general, recorded side effects of RFA include pain, burns, nipple retraction and calcified lump formation [27,28]. RFA has previously been approved in the UK for hepatocellular carcinoma, but not currently for early breast cancer [40].

Laser ablation

Laser ablation uses an image-guided laser optical fibre inserted percutaneously into the target tumour to heat the tumour to a specified temperature, resulting in the tumour cell death. Cell damage can be induced by prolonged exposure of 45–55°C or short exposure of over 60°C, where the laser can be delivered on high or low power and pulsed or continuous [41]. Two incisions are made in the tumour, one in the centre for the laser probe and a peripheral one for a thermal probe to measure ablation progress.

Laser ablation was first used for small breast cancers in 1994 [42]. Trials of LA since this time have included patients with breast cancers of varying stages, for example, those with unifocal IDCs of ≤2 cm, as well as those with stages 2-3 multifocal breast cancer or unresectable breast cancer. Recent trials have reported success rates of around 84-100%, validated using MRI, biopsy histology, mammogram, or positron emission tomography (PET). Pain was a commonly reported adverse effect, with others including lump formation, haematoma and erythema. Fat necrosis was rare. The Novilase Br-002 phase II trial showed 84% complete tumour ablation after one LA procedure [43]. Novilase Br-003 is currently underway in a larger cohort of patients [44].

Microwave ablation

Microwave ablation uses electromagnetic microwaves (≥900 MHz) to generate heat from a probe which induces tumour cell death by coagulative necrosis. Microwaves heat up tumour cells preferentially to adipose tissue, minimising damage to the surrounding breast. The procedure is normally US-guided, where the probe is inserted into the tumour for 2-3 minutes. Multiple probes may be used for larger lesions.

Recent studies of MWA for early breast cancer have usually included patients with unifocal IDC ≤ 5 cm. One study was indicated in locally advanced unresectable breast cancer. These preliminary studies have shown a complete ablation rate of around 91-95%, with side effects including mild burns and pain.

A larger scale non-randomised trial (NCT04626986) of 300 patients with IDC of ≤5 cm is currently ongoing comparing MWA to breast conserving surgery [45]. Primary outcome measures are overall survival and cosmetic satisfaction. Another ongoing randomised trial (NCT04805736) is investigating the safety and complete ablation rate of MWA with or without the addition of Camrelizumab, an immunotherapy agent to determine whether there may be a synergistic effect [46]. MWA for breast cancer is currently not approved for use in the UK or USA.

High-intensity focussed ultrasound

High-intensity focussed ultrasound is amongst the most advanced of the thermal ablative approaches for breast cancer treatment. It works by passing US waves through the skin that are then focussed onto the cancer [47]. Once targeted, these US waves increase the temperature at the site of the cancer and within a few millimetres of it, destroying the cancer cells by thermal ablation without damaging surrounding normal tissue [48]. On a microscopic level, the tissue undergoes a process of protein denaturation, epithelial necrosis and coagulation [48].

Building on the promising body of preclinical research showing HIFU ablation to be non-toxic and effective for the treatment of implanted breast malignancies, phases I and II clinical trials from China and Europe have since provided further evidence in favour of using HIFU for early breast cancer [49]. However, there has been a wide variation in the reported efficacy from HIFU, with successful ablation rates ranging from 20 to 100% [50]. The reason for this discrepancy is likely multifactorial and due to a combination of use of different HIFU devices amongst the studies, each with varying specifications, lack of 'real-time' imaging efficacy feedback and lack of long-term experience in its use.

Kim and colleagues undertook a systematic review of the effectiveness of HIFU in breast cancer and noted that in order to examine HIFU ablation as an alternative treatment option for breast cancer, further long-term follow-up studies on safety, technical effectiveness and survival rate are required [50]. In a recent systematic review of the published literature, Peek and colleagues concluded that large scale prospective clinical trials were required to confirm the utility of HIFU for breast cancer [7]. However, prior to undertaking such trials, evidence of consistent tumour and margin necrosis is required.

TRANSCUTANEOUS VACUUM-ASSISTED NEEDLE EXCISION

Vacuum-assisted needle excision is used as standard of care in the treatment of various lesions of uncertain malignant potential, termed 'B3' lesions. These lesions include: atypical intraductal epithelial proliferation (AIDEP), classical (not pleomorphic) lobular neoplasia, flat epithelial atypia, radial scar with or without epithelial atypia and mucocoele-like lesion with or without epithelial atypia. Amongst B3 lesions, surgical excision is reserved for papillary lesions with epithelial atypia, cellular fibroepithelial lesions and for certain other lesions [51]. The use of VAE in the context of invasive breast cancer is currently being investigated by the ongoing SMALL trial [52].

The SMALL trial is a phase III, randomised controlled trial that includes women aged ≥47 years old with small (≤15 mm), screen-detected, grade 1 breast cancers that are strongly oestrogen and progesterone receptor positive and HER2 negative. It is randomising between conventional surgical excision versus VAE for these lesions and will examine both re-excision following initial procedure at 3 months after the end of the recruitment period and local recurrence-free survival time as primary outcome measures. The results of this trial will help to identify whether clinical practice should move away from conventional surgical excision for small, prognostically favourable invasive breast cancer.

DISCUSSION

Patient's selection

Percutaneous ablative approaches have mainly been studied in patients with small breast cancers considered to carry a low risk of recurrence, and/or those considered unsuitable for surgery. For both ablative radiotherapy and thermal ablation, the effectiveness of the interventions varies according to tumour size [53]. The potential future role of these percutaneous approaches is, therefore, likely to be in carefully selected patient groups, such as those with prognostically very favourable tumours or potentially those not fit for general anaesthesia and, therefore, breast surgery. Mechanical needle excision, already used in the treatment of B3 lesions, could also be used in the same setting.

Advantages compared with surgery

Many of the advantages from avoiding the risks of general anaesthesia and complications associated with a larger cut in the skin from surgery have been listed above. However, a potential advantage of certain minimally invasive percutaneous techniques is that ablating breast cancer cells in situ may provide antigens to train the immune system to eradicate residual cancer cells elsewhere in the body [25,54].

An association between ablative therapies and the immune system has been recognised since the 1960s. For example, there has been evidence to suggest that HIFU in itself activates a systemic antitumour immunity, thereby priming the body's immune system to detect and thereby attack circulating or in situ cancer cells [55]. Although this research is at too early a stage to provide concrete conclusions, it does suggest some possible advantages from HIFU treatment over surgery which have the potential to translate into longer terms benefits of reduced breast cancer recurrence and improved survival.

Preclinical evidence has shown immunostimulatory effects of ablation. Tumour cell necrosis induced by ablation releases damage associated with molecular patterns, which is detected by dendritic cells, which, in turn, co-stimulates T-cells to produce a systemic immune response [56]. A clinical study suggests that as well as directly inducing tumour necrosis, MWA also primes the T-helper 1 pathway which results in a secondary antitumour effect [42].

Disadvantages compared with surgery

One of the main disadvantages of ablative approaches in comparison with standard surgical techniques is that as the ablated tumour is not resected, it would not be available for histopathological assessment. Postoperative pathological assessment of the resected tumour provides information about whether the cancer has been completely removed with a clear margin and pathological information that guides prognostication and adjuvant treatment decisions. It may be possible to obtain some of this information from imaging and biopsy tissue. While lack of pathology information is not an issue with percutaneous vacuum needle excision, margin assessment remains a constraint.

In the case of ablative radiotherapy, treatment is delivered in divided doses over a period of days or weeks, and, therefore, takes longer than surgery. It also carries risks of acute and late adverse effects on surrounding normal tissues and organs, the extent of which likely varies according to the type of ionising radiation and delivery technique used.

CONCLUSION

Percutaneous ablative and vacuum excision approaches offer the potential to avoid primary surgery and the associated complications in carefully selected patient groups, for example, those with small breast cancers considered to carry a low risk of recurrence, and/or those considered unsuitable for surgery. However, there are technical challenges to resolve before percutaneous ablative methods that can be used in routine care. Advancements in preoperative imaging and technological developments in prognostication for adjuvant treatment decision-making will address some of these current limitations. At present, there is insufficient evidence gathered to support the use of percutaneous treatments for breast cancer outside of clinical trials, but there may be a role for these minimally invasive techniques in future following further research.

Key points for clinical practice

- Routine management of early breast cancer usually involves surgery. This is often followed by adjuvant radiotherapy. In many cases, one or more systemic adjuvant therapies (endocrine therapy, chemotherapy, targeted biological therapy and bisphosphonates) are also recommended

- Percutaneous ablative techniques cause targeted lethal damage to cancer cells, and some healthy cells within a very short distance of the target
- Percutaneous methods are often performed with the patient awake or under light sedation, and, therefore, have advantages over surgery, such as avoiding the risks of general anaesthesia, avoiding surgical complications, and minimising any cosmetic defect
- There are technical challenges to resolve before percutaneous ablative methods can be used in routine care, such as ascertainment of margins, identification of the optimal post-treatment surveillance of ablated tumours, and while not as relevant for needle excision approaches, ablative methods may also lack tissue availability to guide adjuvant treatment if pretreatment biopsies are insufficient
- Percutaneous methods have shown the most promise in early stage and small tumours but also have shown benefit in patients unsuitable for resection
- Ablative approaches are currently only used in clinical trials but may have a role in selected cases of breast cancer in future

REFERENCES

1. Mannu GS, Darby S. Cancer Epidemiology. In: Poston G, Wyld L, Audisio RA (Eds). Textbook of Surgical Oncology, Second Edition, CRC publishing; 2016. pp. 3–16.
2. Early Breast Cancer Trialists' Collaborative Group (EBCTCG); Darby S, McGale P, et al. Effect of radiotherapy after breast-conserving surgery on 10-year recurrence and 15-year breast cancer death: meta-analysis of individual patient data for 10,801 women in 17 randomised trials. Lancet 2011; 378:1707–1716.
3. EBCTCG (Early Breast Cancer Trialists' Collaborative Group); McGale P, Taylor C, et al. Effect of radiotherapy after mastectomy and axillary surgery on 10-year recurrence and 20-year breast cancer mortality: meta-analysis of individual patient data for 8135 women in 22 randomised trials. Lancet 2014; 383:2127–2135.
4. Kerr AJ, Dodwell D, McGale P, et al. Adjuvant and neoadjuvant breast cancer treatments: A systematic review of their effects on mortality. Cancer Treat Rev 2022; 105:102375.
5. Mannu GS, Bhalerao A. A century of breast surgery: from radical to minimal. Can J Surg. 2014; 57:E147–E148.
6. Zhao Z, Wu F. Minimally-invasive thermal ablation of early-stage breast cancer: A systemic review. Eur J Surg Oncol 2010; 36:1149–1155.
7. Peek MC, Ahmed M, Napoli A, et al. Systematic review of high-intensity focused ultrasound ablation in the treatment of breast cancer. Br J Surg 2015; 102:873–882.
8. van de Voort EMF, Struik GM, Birnie E, et al. Thermal Ablation as an Alternative for Surgical Resection of Small (≤ 2 cm) Breast Cancers: A Meta-Analysis. Clin Breast Cancer 2021; 21:e715–e730.
9. Malouff TD, Mahajan A, Mutter RW, et al. Carbon ion radiation therapy in breast cancer: a new frontier. Breast Cancer Res Treat 2020; 181:291–296.
10. Amalric R, Santamaria F, Robert F, et al. Radiation therapy with or without primary limited surgery for operable breast cancer: A 20-year experience at the Marseilles Cancer Institute. Cancer 1982; 49:30–34.
11. Calle R, Pilleron JP, Schlienger P, Vilcoq JR. Conservative management of operable breast cancer. Ten years experience at the Foundation Curie. Cancer 1978; 42:2045–2053.
12. Bataini JP, Picco C, Martin M, Calle R. Relation between time-dose and local control of operable breast cancer treated by tumorectomy and radiotherapy or by radical radiotherapy alone. Cancer 1978; 42:2059–2065.
13. Beadle GF, Silver B, Botnick L, Hellman S, Harris JR. Cosmetic results following primary radiation therapy for early breast cancer. Cancer 1984; 54:2911–2918.
14. Pierquin B, Owen R, Maylin C, et al. Radical radiation therapy of breast cancer. Int J Radiat Oncol Biol Phys 1980; 6:17–24.
15. De Lena M, Varini M, Zucali R, et al. Multimodal treatment for locally advanced breast cancer. Result of chemotherapy-radiotherapy versus chemotherapy-surgery. Cancer Clin Trials 1981; 4:229–236.

16. Spitalier J, Brandone H, Ayme Y, et al. Cesiumtherapy of breast cancer. A five-year report on 400 consecutive patients. Int J Radiat Oncol Biol Phys 1977; 2:231–235.
17. Dubois JB, Salomon A, Gary-Bobo J, Pourquier H, Pujol H. Exclusive radical radiation therapy in breast carcinoma. Radiother Oncol 1991; 20:24–29.
18. Thomas F, Arriagada R, Mouriesse H, et al. Radical radiotherapy alone in non-operable breast cancer: The major impact of tumor size and histological grade on prognosis. Radiother Oncol 1988; 13:267–276.
19. Van Limbergen E, Rijnders A, van der Schueren E, Lerut T, Christiaens R. Cosmetic evaluation of breast conserving treatment for mammary cancer. 2. A quantitative analysis of the influence of radiation dose, fractionation schedules and surgical treatment techniques on cosmetic results. Radiother Oncol 1989; 16:253–267.
20. Fourquet A, Vilcoq JR, Zafrani B, Schlienger P, Jullien D. Medullary breast carcinoma: The role of radiotherapy as primary treatment. Radiother Oncol 1987; 10:1–6.
21. Chargari C, Kirova YM, Laki F, et al. The impact of the loco-regional treatment in elderly breast cancer patients: Hypo-fractionated exclusive radiotherapy, single institution long-term results. Breast (Edinburgh) 2010; 19:413–416.
22. Arriagada R, Mouriesse H, Sarrazin D, Clark RM, Deboer G. Radiotherapy alone in breast cancer. I. Analysis of tumor parameters, tumor dose and local control: the experience of the gustave-roussy institute and the princess margaret hospital. Int J Radiat Oncol Biol Phys (United States) 1985; 11:1751–1757.
23. Shibamoto Y, Takano S, Iida M, et al. Definitive radiotherapy with stereotactic or IMRT boost with or without radiosensitization strategy for operable breast cancer patients who refuse surgery. J Radiat Res 2022; 63:849–855.
24. Shibamoto Y, Murai T, Suzuki K, et al. Definitive Radiotherapy With SBRT or IMRT Boost for Breast Cancer: Excellent Local Control and Cosmetic Outcome. Technol Cancer Res Treat 2018; 17:1533033818799355.
25. Washington University School of Medicine. Cryoablation vs Lumpectomy in T1 Breast Cancers (COOL-IT). United States: Washington University School of Medicine, 2023. Available from https://clinicaltrials.gov/ct2/show/NCT05505643 [Last accessed 22 July 2025].
26. Charaghvandi KR, Van't Westeinde T, Yoo S, et al. Single dose partial breast irradiation using an MRI linear accelerator in the supine and prone treatment position. Clin Transl Radiat Oncol 2009; 14:1–7.
27. Vaidya JS, Hall-Craggs M, Baum M, et al. Percutaneous minimally invasive stereotactic primary radiotherapy for breast cancer. Lancet Oncol 2002; 3:252–253.
28. Veluvolu M, Patel M, Narayanasamy G, Kim T. Definitive single fraction stereotactic ablative radiotherapy for inoperable early-stage breast cancer: A case report. Rep Pract Oncol Radiother 2020; 25(5):760–764.
29. Karasawa K, Omatsu T, Shiba S, et al. A clinical study of curative partial breast irradiation for stage I breast cancer using carbon ion radiotherapy. Radiation oncology (London, England) 2020; 15:1–265.
30. Coronado G, Ho E, Holmes DR. Abstract OT2-01-04: Freezing instead of resection of small breast tumors (FROST): A study of cryoablation in the management of early stage breast cancer. Cancer Res (Chicago, Ill). 2018; 78:OT2-01-04-OT2-01-04.
31. Vesprini D. Stereotactic Body Radiation Therapy for Breast Cancer. 2022. Available from https://clinicaltrials.gov/ct2/show/NCT03585621 [Last accessed 22 July 2025].
32. Fine RE, Gilmore RC, Dietz JR, et al. Cryoablation Without Excision for Low-Risk Early-Stage Breast Cancer: 3-Year Interim Analysis of Ipsilateral Breast Tumor Recurrence in the ICE3 Trial. Ann Surg Oncol 2021; 28:5525–5534.
33. Cazzato RL, de Lara CT, Buy X, et al. Single-Centre Experience with Percutaneous Cryoablation of Breast Cancer in 23 Consecutive Non-surgical Patients. Cardiovasc Intervent Radiol 2015; 38:1237–1243.
34. Manenti G, Scarano AL, Pistolese CA, et al. Subclinical Breast Cancer: Minimally Invasive Approaches. Our Experience with Percutaneous Radiofrequency Ablation vs. Cryotherapy. Breast Care (Basel, Switzerland) 2013; 8:356–360.
35. Simmons RM, Ballman KV, Cox C, et al. A Phase II Trial Exploring the Success of Cryoablation Therapy in the Treatment of Invasive Breast Carcinoma: Results from ACOSOG (Alliance) Z1072. Ann Surg Oncol 2016; 23:2438–2445.
36. Washington University School of Medicine. Cryoablation vs Lumpectomy in T1 Breast Cancers (COOL-IT). United States: Washington University School of Medicine; 2023.
37. Jeffrey SS, Birdwell RL, Ikeda DM, et al. Radiofrequency Ablation of Breast Cancer: First Report of an Emerging Technology. Arch Surg 1999; 134:1064–1068.
38. Ito T, Oura S, Nagamine S, et al. Radiofrequency Ablation of Breast Cancer: A Retrospective Study. Clin Breast Cancer 2018; 18:e495–e500.

39. García-Tejedor A, Guma A, Soler T, et al. Radiofrequency Ablation Followed by Surgical Excision versus Lumpectomy for Early Stage Breast Cancer: A Randomized Phase II Clinical Trial. Radiology 2018; 289:317–324.
40. NICE. Radiofrequency ablation of hepatocellular carcinoma. London: NICE, 2003. Available from https://www.nice.org.uk/guidance/ipg2/chapter/1-Recommendations [Last accessed 22 July 2025].
41. Schena E, Saccomandi P, Fong Y. Laser Ablation for Cancer: Past, Present and Future. J Funct Biomater 2017; 8:19.
42. Harries SA, Amin Z, Smith ME, et al. Interstitial laser photocoagulation as a treatment for breast cancer. Br J Surg 1994; 81:1617–1619.
43. Schwartzberg B, Lewin J, Abdelatif O, et al. Phase 2 Open-Label Trial Investigating Percutaneous Laser Ablation for Treatment of Early-Stage Breast Cancer: MRI, Pathology, and Outcome Correlations. Ann Surg Oncol 2018; 25:2958–2964.
44. Novian Health Inc. Confirmatory Clinical Evaluation of Novilase® Laser Therapy for Focal Destruction of Malignant Breast Tumors.2021. Available from https://clinicaltrials.gov/study/NCT03463954?cond=Breast%20Cancer&aggFilters=status:rec&lastUpdPost=2021-06-07_&viewType=Table&rank=8 [Last accessed 22 July 2025].
45. Liang P. Chinese PLA General Hospital. Comparison of Microwave Ablation With Breast Conserving Surgery for Breast Tumor. 2021. Available from https://clinicaltrials.gov/ct2/show/NCT04626986 [Last accessed 22 July 2025].
46. Wang S, The First Affiliated Hospital with Nanjing Medical University. Microwave Ablation Combined With Camrelizumab in the Treatment of Early Breast Cancer. 2022. Available from https://clinicaltrials.gov/study/NCT04805736 [Last accessed 22 July 2025].
47. Wu F, Wang ZB, Chen WZ, et al. Extracorporeal high intensity focused ultrasound ablation in the treatment of 1038 patients with solid carcinomas in China: an overview. Ultrason Sonochem 2004; 11:149–154.
48. Kim SH, Jung SE, Kim HL, et al. The potential role of dynamic MRI in assessing the effectiveness of high-intensity focused ultrasound ablation of breast cancer. Int J Hyperthermia 2010; 26:594–603.
49. Wu F, ter Haar G, Chen WR. High-intensity focused ultrasound ablation of breast cancer. Expert Rev Anticancer Ther 2007; 7:823–831.
50. Peek MCL, Wu F. High-intensity focused ultrasound in the treatment of breast tumours. Ecancermedicalscience 2018; 12:794.
51. Public Health England. NHS Breast Screening Programme Clinical guidance for breast cancer screening assessment. London: Public Health England, 2016. Available from https://assets.publishing.service.gov.uk/media/5a808356e5274a2e8ab50931/Clinical_guidance_for_breast__cancer_screening__assessment_Nov_2016.pdf [Last accessed 22 July 2025].
52. Foster J. A study for women who have small breast cancers found by screening, comparing removal of the cancer by standard surgery with a smaller procedure, which is more like a biopsy. ISRCTNregistry 2022.
53. Dai Y, Liang P, Yu J. Percutaneous Management of Breast Cancer: a Systematic Review. Curr Oncol Rep 2022; 24:1443–1459.
54. Iyer SP, Hunt CR, Pandita TK. Cross Talk between Radiation and Immunotherapy: The Twain Shall Meet. Radiat Res 2018; 189:219–224.
55. Yantorno C, Soanes WA, Gonder MJ, Shulman S. Studies in cryo-immunology. I. The production of antibodies to urogenital tissue in consequence of freezing treatment. Immunology 1967; 12:395–410.
56. Slovak R, Ludwig JM, Gettinger SN, Herbst RS, Kim HS. Immuno-thermal ablations – boosting the anticancer immune response. J Immunother Cancer 2017; 5:78.

Section 4

Hepatobiliary surgery

Chapter 8

Contemporary management of incidentally detected gallstones

Chiranjiva Khandelwal, Utpal Anand, Kislay Kant

ABSTRACT

Asymptomatic gallstones are common incidental findings during abdominal imaging. While most remain silent, a minority will develop biliary colic, acute cholecystitis, gallstone pancreatitis, or—rarely—gallbladder carcinoma [1-4]. Management options include expectant observation or prophylactic laparoscopic cholecystectomy. Although surgery is curative, it carries measurable operative risks, making routine intervention unnecessary in most cases [5-7]. Current evidence recommends observation for the majority and prophylactic surgery only in well-defined high-risk situations, especially in gallbladder cancer–endemic populations [8-11]. Routine cholecystectomy for cancer prevention is not recommended.

INTRODUCTION

Asymptomatic cholelithiasis refers to the presence of gallstones discovered incidentally through imaging in asymptomatic individuals. The growing use of ultrasonography in antenatal care, non-specific abdominal evaluations, and occupational health screening has resulted in more frequent incidental detection in otherwise healthy people [1-3]. Management differs worldwide based on factors like incidence of local gallbladder cancer, patient risk profile, and healthcare resources.

PREVALENCE

Gallstone disease affects 10–20% of adults in many populations, with over 80% of cases remaining asymptomatic [1-3]. Among those with silent gallstones, only 1–2% per year

---

Chiranjiva Khandelwal MS DNB FRCS (England), Head, Surgical Oncology, Mahavir Cancer Sansthan, Patna, Former Professor, Department of Surgical Gastroenterology, Indira Gandhi Institute of Medical Sciences, Patna, Bihar, India
E-mail: khandelwal3250@gmail.com (for correspondence)

Utpal Anand MS MCh, Additional Professor, Surgical Gastroenterology, All India Institute of Medical Sciences, Patna, Bihar, India
E-mail: drutpalanad@aiimspatna.org (for correspondence)

Kislay Kant MS DNB-SS, Assistant Professor, Surgical Gastroenterology, All India Institute of Medical Sciences, Patna, Bihar, India
E-mail: kislay.kant@gmail.com (for correspondence)

develop symptomatic disease requiring intervention. Prevalence is high (10–15%) in the US, Mexico and Sweden, moderate in India (5–10%) and lower (3–6%) in Bangladesh, Japan and Thailand [8–11]. These regional differences are influenced by multiple factors such as diet, genetics, body mass index, age distribution, sex ratio, and access to imaging.

NATURAL HISTORY

Long-term observational studies demonstrate that the majority of individuals with asymptomatic gallstones never develop symptoms [4,12–14]. The University of Michigan longitudinal data showed symptoms in 10% at 5 years, 15% at 10 years, and 18% at 15 years, respectively. Nearly all symptomatic cases are preceded by episodes of biliary colic. Annual rate of symptom onset remains low (1–2%) and severe complications (cholecystitis and pancreatitis) rarely occur without warning pain. These findings support conservative management for the most asymptomatic cases, with the understanding that biliary pain typically provides adequate warning before serious complications develop.

ASYMPTOMATIC GALLSTONES AND GALLBLADDER CANCER

Although gallstones are present in most gallbladder carcinoma (GBC) patients, only 0.3–3% of gallstone carriers develop GBC over 20 years [15–19].

High-risk factors for gallbladder carcinoma development

Stone characteristics
Geographic risk:
- Stones >3 cm
- High stone volume
- Long-standing gallstone disease
- Cholesterol-predominant stones (common in endemic areas)
- *High-incidence regions:* Northern India, Chile, and parts of Japan [8,20–27]

Additional risk factors:
- Environmental exposures (arsenic and pesticides)
- Genetic predisposition
- Chronic *Salmonella typhi* carriage
- Congenital pancreaticobiliary mal-junction [26,28–31]

Clinical implications
- In low-risk areas, prophylactic cholecystectomy is not routinely recommended for silent gallstones due to the minimal cancer risk.
- In endemic areas like Chile, selective surgical prevention may be justified based on individual risk profiles.

This risk stratification helps to guide personalised management of asymptomatic gallstones carrier worldwide.

MANAGEMENT

Management of this condition balances its typically benign course in most patients against the rare but serious risks of future symptoms, complications, or malignancy. Three key strategies are employed:
1. *Expectant (conservative) management:* Monitoring without intervention
2. *Routine prophylactic cholecystectomy:* Preventive gallbladder removal in all cases
3. *Selective prophylactic cholecystectomy:* Surgery reserved for high-risk patients

Expectant management is appropriate for approximately 80% of carriers, given the slow annual progression rate of just 1–2%. It avoids operative risks such as bile duct injury (0.1–0.5%), major bleeding, visceral injury, and post-cholecystectomy syndromes, while remaining cost-effective [1–7].

Successful implementation requires:
- Patient education on warning signs (biliary colic, jaundice, fever, and pancreatitis)
- Regular follow-up to monitor for complications
- Lifestyle modifications (healthy weight, diet, exercise, and smoking cessation) mitigates risk

Routine prophylactic laparoscopic cholecystectomy prevents all gallstone-related complications and may reduce GBC incidence in endemic areas [6,7,32–34]. It is technically easier in asymptomatic patients but is not cost-effective in low-risk populations, exposes many to unnecessary surgery with inherent operative risks [5–7,31,32].

Current guidelines recommend this approach only for:
- Patients in endemic areas with a long-life expectancy
- Those with a strong family history of GBC

Selective prophylactic cholecystectomy focusses on patients with the greatest likelihood of future symptoms, complications, or malignant transformation, aiming to prevent these outcomes while avoiding unnecessary surgery in low-risk individuals.

High-risk stone features include:
- Stone diameter > 3 cm
- Clusters of tiny stones under (<3 mm) with a patent cystic duct predisposing to pancreatitis
- Floating calculi or multiple stones
- Large total stone volume

Key patient risk factors:
- Age <55 years with a life expectancy exceeding >20 years
- Female sex, obesity, and smoking
- Strong family history of gallbladder cancer
- Residence in high-incidence geographic regions

In these cases—particularly in endemic areas—prophylactic laparoscopic cholecystectomy is a reasonable, evidence-based intervention to mitigate elevated GBC risk.

Special consideration for prophylactic cholecystectomy

Certain high-risk patient subgroups may benefit from prophylactic cholecystectomy irrespective of standard risk stratification [15,22–24,26].

- *Chronic hemolytic disorders (e.g. thalassemia and sickle-cell disease):*
  - High complication rates and poorer outcomes with emergency surgery, supporting elective cholecystectomy.
- *Solid organ transplant recipients:*
  - Cardiac transplant patients: Benefit from routine post-transplant cholecystectomy
  - Renal recipients can usually be observed unless symptoms develop.
- *Bariatric surgery candidates:*
  - Rapid weight loss increases gallstone risk, making concurrent cholecystectomy advisable.
- *Long-term parenteral nutrition:*
  - High gallstone incidence and complication risk supports prophylactic removal.
- *Incidental gallstones during abdominal surgery:*
  - Elevated postoperative biliary event risk, often justifying removal during the index procedure.
- *Cirrhotic patients:*
  - Higher surgical risk can undergo laparoscopic cholecystectomy safely in selected symptomatic cases, though most asymptomatic cases are observed.
- *Diabetic patients:*
  - Higher gallstone prevalence, but similar complication rates to non-diabetics and thus are generally managed conservatively unless symptomatic.

Clinical decision-making in gallstone management

Decision-making should be individualised, integrating evidence, patient-specific risk factors, surgical fitness, and personal preferences [8,19–21].

Risk stratification

Factors favouring prophylactic cholecystectomy

Stone-related:
- Large stones (>3 cm)
- Multiple stones/high total stone volume
- Small stones (<3 mm) (↑ pancreatitis risk)

Patient-related:
- Younger age + long life expectancy
- Residence in endemic regions (↑ gallbladder cancer risk)
- High-risk conditions (e.g. chronic hemolytic anemia, post-cardiac transplant, and bariatric surgery candidates)

Factors favouring conservative management
- Elderly patients with significant comorbidities
- Low-risk stone features in asymptomatic patients
- Limited life expectancy

Shared decision-making

Clinicians should discuss:
- Absolute versus relative risks of complications (e.g. biliary colic, pancreatitis and malignancy)

- *Surgical risks:* Bile duct injury (0.1–0.5%) [5-7], bleeding, infection, post-cholecystectomy syndromes
- *Conservative management risks:* ~1-2% annual symptom/complication risk

Monitoring and lifestyle measures

- *Patient education:* Recognise red flags (biliary pain, jaundice, and fever).
- *Lifestyle optimisation:* Weight management, diet, and smoking cessation.
- *Structured surveillance:* Periodic ultrasound + clinical review for early intervention if risk evolves.

Health system considerations

- Cost-effectiveness and resource availability guide policies.
- Most settings prioritise observation + rapid referral pathway; surgery is reserved for high-risk cases.

> **Key points for clinical practice**
> - High-risk patients benefit from early surgery; low-risk groups often do well with monitoring
> - Transparent risk communication is critical for informed choices
> - Dynamic follow-up ensures timely intervention if risks change

REFERENCES

1. Attili AF, Carulli N, Roda E, et al. Epidemiology of gallstone disease in Italy: prevalence data of the Multicenter Italian Study on Cholelithiasis (M.I.COL.). Am J Epidemiol 1995; 141:158–165.
2. Barbara L, Sama C, Morselli Labate AM, et al. A population study on the prevalence of gallstone disease: the Sirmione Study. Hepatology 1987; 7:913–917.
3. Sakorafas GH, Milingos D, Peros G. Asymptomatic cholelithiasis: is cholecystectomy really needed? A critical reappraisal 15 years after the introduction of laparoscopic cholecystectomy. Dig Dis Sci 2007; 52:1313–1325.
4. Morris-Stiff G, Sarvepalli S, Hu B, et al. The Natural History of Asymptomatic Gallstones: A Longitudinal Study and Prediction Model. Clin Gastroenterol Hepatol 2023; 21:319–327.e4.
5. Flum DR, Cheadle A, Prela C, et al. Bile duct injury during cholecystectomy and survival in medicare beneficiaries. JAMA 2003; 290:2168–2173.
6. Waage A, Nilsson M. Iatrogenic bile duct injury: a population-based study of 152 776 cholecystectomies in the Swedish Inpatient Registry. Arch Surg 2006; 141:1207–1213.
7. Fletcher DR, Hobbs MST, Tan P, et al. Complications of cholecystectomy: risks of the laparoscopic approach and protective effects of operative cholangiography: a population-based study. Ann Surg 1999; 229:449–457.
8. Unisa S, Jagannath P, Dhir V, et al. Population-based study to estimate prevalence and determine risk factors of gallbladder diseases in the rural Gangetic basin of North India. HPBOxford) 2011; 13:117–125.
9. Gracie WA, Ransohoff DF. The natural history of silent gallstones: the innocent gallstone is not a myth. N Engl J Med 1982; 307:798–800.
10. Friedman GD, Raviola CA, Fireman B. Prognosis of gallstones with mild or no symptoms: 25 years of follow-up in a health maintenance organization. J Clin Epidemiol 1989; 42:127–136.
11. European Association for the Study of the Liver. EASL Clinical Practice Guidelines on the prevention, diagnosis and treatment of gallstones. J Hepatol 2016; 65:146–181.
12. Festi D, Reggiani MLB, Attili AF, et al. Natural history of gallstone disease: Expectant management or active treatment? Results from a population-based cohort study. J Gastroenterol Hepatol 2010; 25:719–724.

13. Henley SJ, Weir HK, Jim MA, et al. Gallbladder Cancer Incidence and Mortality, United States 1999-2011. Cancer Epidemiol Biomarkers Prev 2015; 24:1319–1326.
14. Torre LA, Siegel RL, Islami F, et al. Worldwide Burden of and Trends in Mortality From Gallbladder and Other Biliary Tract Cancers. Clin Gastroenterol Hepatol 2018; 16:427–437.
15. Supe A. Asymptomatic gall stones—revisited. Trop Gastroenterol 2011; 32:196–203.
16. Diehl AK. Gallstone size and the risk of gallbladder cancer. JAMA 1983; 250:2323–2326.
17. Lowenfels AB, Walker AM, Althaus DP, et al. Gallstone growth, size, and risk of gallbladder cancer: an interracial study. Int J Epidemiol 1989; 18:50–54.
18. Roa I, Ibacache G, Roa J, et al. Gallstones and gallbladder cancer-volume and weight of gallstones are associated with gallbladder cancer: a case-control study. J Surg Oncol 2006; 93:624–628.
19. Serra I, Yamamoto M, Calvo A, et al. Association of chili pepper consumption, low socioeconomic status and longstanding gallstones with gallbladder cancer in a Chilean population. Int J Cancer 2002; 102:407–411.
20. Kumar A, Ali M, Raj V, et al. Arsenic causing gallbladder cancer disease in Bihar. Sci Rep 2023; 13:4259.
21. Koshiol J, Wozniak A, Cook P, et al. Salmonella enterica serovar Typhi and gallbladder cancer: a case-control study and meta-analysis. Cancer Med 2016; 5:3310–3335.
22. El-Menoufy MAM, El-Barbary HM, Raslan SM. The Egyptian Journal of Haematology. 2019; 44:28–33.
23. Kao LS, Flowers C, Flum DR. Prophylactic cholecystectomy in transplant patients: a decision analysis. J Gastrointest Surg 2005; 9:965–972.
24. Plecka Östlund M, Wenger U, Mattsson F, et al. Population-based study of the need for cholecystectomy after obesity surgery. Br J Surg 2012; 99:864–869.
25. Gao X, Zhang L, Wang S, et al. Prevalence, Risk Factors, and Complications of Cholelithiasis in Adults With Short Bowel Syndrome: A Longitudinal Cohort Study. Front Nutr 2021; 8:762240.
26. Bragg LE, Thompson JS. Concomitant cholecystectomy for asymptomatic cholelithiasis. Arch Surg 1989; 124:460–462.
27. Shirah BH, Shirah HA, Zafar SH, et al. Clinical patterns of postcholecystectomy syndrome. Ann Hepatobiliary Pancreat Surg 2018; 22:52–57.
28. Zhang Y, Liu H, Li L, et al. Cholecystectomy can increase the risk of colorectal cancer: A meta-analysis of 10 cohort studies. PLoS One 2017; 12:e0181852.
29. de Goede B, Klitsie PJ, Hagen SM, et al. Meta-analysis of laparoscopic versus open cholecystectomy for patients with liver cirrhosis and symptomatic cholecystolithiasis. Br J Surg. 2013; 100:209–216.
30. Lee BJH, Yap QV, Low JK, et al. Cholecystectomy for asymptomatic gallstones: Markov decision tree analysis. World J Clin Cases 2022; 10:10399–10412.
31. Booij KAC, de Reuver PR, van Dieren S, et al. Long-term Impact of Bile Duct Injury on Morbidity, Mortality, Quality of Life, and Work Related Limitations. Ann Surg 2018; 268:143–150.
32. Shaffer EA. Epidemiology and risk factors for gallstone disease: has the paradigm changed in the 21st century? Curr Gastroenterol Rep 2005; 7:132–140.
33. Sianesi M, Capocasale E, Ferreri G, et al. The role of cholecystectomy in renal transplantation. Transplant Proc 2005; 37:2129–2130.
34. Sicklick JK, Camp MS, Lillemoe KD, et al. Surgical Management of Bile Duct Injuries Sustained During Laparoscopic Cholecystectomy. Ann Surg. 2005; 241:786–795.

Chapter 9

Recent advances in management of acute cholecystitis

Christian Macutkiewicz

ABSTRACT

Biliary disease accounts for up to 40% of the emergency general surgery workload and the management of acute cholecystitis has changed, from intravenous antibiotics and delayed elective cholecystectomy to emergency cholecystectomy and management at first presentation. The COVID-19 pandemic brought a halt to elective cholecystectomy worldwide and patients remained on waiting lists with worsening disease. This has brought different challenges with increasingly difficult gallbladders. This chapter highlights the latest Tokyo guidelines, strategies to diagnose and manage the difficult gallbladder, techniques in performing safe cholecystectomy and new technologies to help the surgeon.

INTRODUCTION

Around 10–15% of adults in the UK suffer from gallstones. This, in turn, reflects on the emergency general surgery workload, with symptomatic gallstone disease patients making up to 30–40% of admissions from the emergency department. Most require definitive operative management in the form of a laparoscopic cholecystectomy. Patients are often discharged home with analgesia to be placed on an elective waiting list, with a risk of a further episode of biliary colic in 50% of patients per year and the risk of developing complications is 1–2% per year [1].

WHAT IS ACUTE CALCULOUS CHOLECYSTITIS?

Acute cholecystitis is characterised by abrupt and painful gallbladder inflammation. Its main cause is blockage of the cystic duct, usually by a stone, which causes a build-up of pressure in the gallbladder and then colonisation by bacteria. Most patients arrive with pain in the right upper quadrant, a fever and raised blood inflammatory markers.

Christian Macutkiewicz MBChB MD FRCS, Consultant General and HPB Surgeon, Manchester University NHS Foundation Trust, Manchester, UK
E-mail: christian.macutkiewicz@mft.nhs.uk (for correspondence)

Imaging is frequently used to confirm the diagnosis, with ultrasonography being the first imaging of choice. Antibiotics are used for the treatment of the causative organism. In addition, pain management should be considered, and definitive therapy, which includes cholecystectomy, if the patient is fit, or cholecystostomy if unfit, should be planned.

Complications should be in mind when admitting patients with acute cholecystitis to avoid morbidity and mortality [2].

ACUTE ACALCULOUS CHOLECYSTITIS

Acute acalculous cholecystitis is an acute inflammation of the gallbladder without stones. It is mainly due to hypokinesia of the gallbladder and delayed emptying of bile. Acalculous cholecystitis is usually present with severe inflammation, which in some cases can be life-threatening, with a higher risk of perforation when compared to the traditional calculous acute cholecystitis. It is usually seen in severely ill patients [3]. The risk factors for developing acute acalculous cholecystitis include sudden severe weight loss, use of total parenteral nutrition and long periods of fasting. The mechanism includes bile stasis and concentration of bile which in turn leads to bile salt concentration and pressure building. This is typically followed by ischaemia and necrosis of the wall and perforation.

Diagnosis of acute cholecystitis

Diagnosis of acute cholecystitis requires the combination of symptoms, clinical signs and blood and imaging investigations. The updated Tokyo guidelines (**Box 9.1**) (2018) provide an approach for diagnosing acute cholecystitis [4].

Imaging modalities

Ultrasound

Ultrasound scan is the initial imaging modality for diagnosing acute cholecystitis. This is due to ultrasound being readily available, easy to use and non-invasive. It is worth mentioning

---

Box 9.1 Tokyo updated guidelines for the diagnosis of acute cholecystectomy [4]

- *Signs of local inflammation:*
  - Murphy's sign
  - Right hypochondrial mass, pain or tenderness
- *Signs of systemic inflammation:*
  - Elevated white cell count
  - Elevated CRP
  - Fever
- *Imaging:* Imaging findings characteristic of acute cholecystitis

Suspected diagnosis: One item in 1 + one item in 2
Definite diagnosis: one item in 1 + one item in 2 + 3

(CRP, C-reactive protein)

that ultrasound has a high rate of false-negative results in diagnosing acute cholecystitis with 18% specificity and 81% positive predictive value. Accurate diagnosis requires a combination of clinical assessment, blood investigation and imaging modalities [5].

Computed tomography scan

Despite the inability to spot all the gallstones due to radiolucency, computed tomography (CT) scans can help in diagnosing acute cholecystitis and might predict the difficulty of the operation that will be performed [6]. In addition, CT scan is the most useful investigation for diagnosing gangrenous and emphysematous cholecystitis. The finding of acute cholecystitis should include either wall thickening of >4 mm, or enlargement of the gallbladder of >8 cm on the long axis and >4 cm on the transverse axis. Pericholecystic fluid, gallstones or fat stranding around the gallbladder might also be seen.

Magnetic resonance cholangiopancreatography/magnetic resonance imaging

Magnetic resonance cholangiopancreatography (MRCP) has a high specificity and sensitivity for diagnosing acute cholecystitis, especially if the ultrasound was inconclusive for the diagnosis. In addition, it provides extra value in delineating the anatomy of the biliary tree to help diagnose complications if any are present, e.g. common bile duct stones and any common hepatic duct narrowing from an inflammatory mass. Additionally, it avoids exposing the patient to radiation and being suitable in pregnancy makes it superior to CT scans in diagnosing acute cholecystitis.

Grading the severity of acute cholecystitis is challenging as there are several classifications. The 2018 Tokyo guidelines are the most widely adopted and comprehensive.

Grades of acute cholecystitis [4]

Grade I (mild) acute cholecystitis

Neither 'Grade III' nor 'Grade II' acute cholecystitis requirements are met. It can also be described as acute cholecystitis in a healthy patient without organ failure and minimal inflammatory changes in the gallbladder.

Grade II (moderate) acute cholecystitis

It is associated with any one of the following conditions:
- Elevated WBC count (>18,000/mm^3)
- palpable and tender mass in the right upper abdominal quadrant
- Symptoms >72 hours
- Imaging evidence of gangrenous cholecystitis, pericholecystic abscess, hepatic abscess, biliary peritonitis or emphysematous cholecystitis

Grade III (severe) acute cholecystitis associated with organ/system failure

- Hypotension requiring vasopressor support
- Impaired level of consciousness
- *Renal impairment:* Oliguria, creatinine >176 µmol/L

- *Respiratory impairment:* Partial pressure of oxygen in arterial blood (PaO_2)/fraction of inspired oxygen (FiO_2) ratio <300
- *Hepatic impairment:* Prothrombin time/international normalised ratio (PT-INR) >1.5
- *Haematological impairment:* Platelet count <1,00,000/mm^3

Management of acute cholecystitis

Treatment of acute cholecystitis should be considered after assessment of the general patient condition and assessing the severity grade. National Institute for Health and Care Excellence (NICE) guidelines published in 2014 recommended that patients with acute cholecystitis should have their cholecystectomy within 7 days of their diagnosis [7].

Grade I (mild): Laparoscopic cholecystectomy should be performed if the patient can tolerate surgery. If the patient cannot tolerate surgery, general supportive care with antibiotics should be administrated until the patient's condition improves to allow safe surgery.

Grade II (moderate): General supportive care with antibiotics should be considered in the first instance. If there is improvement in the patient's condition, then laparoscopic cholecystectomy should be performed if the patient can tolerate surgery and the surgeon is experienced in dealing with acute cholecystectomies. An option for delayed cholecystectomy is still present if the patient's condition improves on the initial supportive measures but not enough to allow a cholecystectomy within 7 days. However, if the initial supportive measures fail to improve the patient's condition, then urgent biliary drainage in the form of a percutaneous cholecystostomy should be performed to provide sepsis source control.

Grade III (severe): Organ support together with antibiotics must be started first to normalise the physiological status of the patient. Following that, if the patient can tolerate surgery, early laparoscopic cholecystectomy can be performed, provided that an experienced surgeon and intensive care support are available on site. If the patient is not able to tolerate surgery or the organ support cannot establish the normal physiological status in a timely manner, biliary drainage should be considered to control the inflammation.

Antibiotic therapy

Acute cholecystitis can vary from a mild attack requiring only a course of oral antibiotics, to a severe attack which can lead to significant morbidity and mortality if not treated properly. If applicable, cultures of bile which can be collected during surgery or percutaneous interventions will help to identify the causative organism and will allow for more direct therapy. Until culture results are available, broad-spectrum antibiotics according to the local hospital protocols should be used. This should be ideally switched to a narrow-spectrum antibiotic when the causative organism is identified. The main purpose of antibiotic therapy in acute cholecystitis is to limit the inflammation locally and inhibit the septic response. Antibiotic therapy will also inhibit wound infection if surgery is planned and will prevent the progression of the disease to form a liver abscess [8]. Trials have shown that ampicillin, piperacillin and aminoglycosides are superior in the treatment of acute cholecystitis [8]. In general, antibiotics for acute cholecystitis should be selected according to the severity of the case.

Grade I (mild acute cholecystitis): Escherichia coli (E. coli) is usually the causative organism; therefore, treatment with antibiotics targeting *E. coli* is recommended. These include oral fluoroquinolones, oral cephalosporins, and penicillin/β-lactamase inhibitor combination.

Grade II (moderate acute cholecystitis): Grade 2 acute cholecystitis requires more potent antibiotic therapy that includes second-generation cephalosporins and broad-spectrum penicillin.

Grade III (severe acute cholecystitis): Grade 3 acute cholecystitis is usually caused by multiple and resistant bacteria. Third- and fourth-generation cephalosporins are recommended first-line antibiotics followed by fluoroquinolones and carbapenems [9].

Biliary drainage (cholecystostomy)

If the patient cannot tolerate surgery due to comorbidities, frailty or severe sepsis, biliary drainage (cholecystostomy) should be performed urgently to drain the biliary system and provide source control for sepsis. This will be ideally followed by laparoscopic cholecystectomy when the patient's condition permits. There is no strong evidence suggesting the optimal timing of laparoscopic cholecystectomy after biliary drainage (cholecystostomy). However, the evidence suggests that performing laparoscopic cholecystectomy early after cholecystostomy is associated with more bleeding, conversion to open surgery and more complications [10].

Laparoscopic cholecystectomy

Previously, laparoscopic cholecystectomy for acute cholecystitis was performed only when the acute attack had subsided. Acute cholecystitis was even considered a relative contraindication for laparoscopic cholecystectomy based on the SAGES guidelines published in 1993 [11]. This was mainly due to the consideration of technical difficulties during surgery, injury to bile ducts and conversion to open surgery. Therefore, most surgeons adopted a more conservative approach by starting the patients on antibiotics and performing the surgery after 6–8 weeks.

Recently, strong evidence from the literature showed that, although performing laparoscopic cholecystectomy early might be more technically challenging, there is no difference in the incidence rate of serious complications. In addition, early laparoscopic cholecystectomy involved shorter hospital stays than delayed laparoscopic cholecystectomy. It also prevents readmission and provides a better patient experience [12].

The definition of early laparoscopic cholecystectomy has changed over time. At first, the evidence from the literature suggested laparoscopic cholecystectomy be performed within 7 days of the onset of the symptoms. However, newer evidence shows that performing laparoscopic cholecystectomy within 72 hours has better outcomes in the form of hospital stay and overall cost with no significant change in the occurrence of serious complications such as bile duct injury. It is worth noting that there is no significant difference in performing laparoscopic cholecystectomy earlier than 72 hours [13].

The Chole-QuIC project [14]

The Royal College of Surgeons of England initiated a quality improvement project in October 2016. The aim of the project was to perform laparoscopic cholecystectomy within 8 days of admission in nearly 80% of eligible patients with gallstone disease. 13 hospitals around the UK shared in this project, which resulted in a significant improvement in the quality of service provided by the participating trusts and better patient outcomes.

This continued until the COVID-19 pandemic, which affected the ability to provide enough operating theatre space to treat benign conditions including cholecystectomies and hernia repairs. This has led to an expansion of the numbers of patients on the waiting list, and subsequent deterioration in their condition. Patients have had more attacks of biliary colic, pancreatitis, cholangitis and acute cholecystitis during this time and, therefore, their cholecystectomies have become more difficult. Further editions of Chole-QuIC projects have been released including CholeQuIC-ER, Chole-QuIC3 and lastly Chole-QuIC4. The aim of these projects is to reduce the waiting time for cholecystectomy for patients with gallstone disease and improve the patient experience.

DIFFICULT CHOLECYSTECTOMY

There is no consensus definition for difficult cholecystectomy, but it can be described as an increased risk and incidence of complication compared to an elective cholecystectomy. This is mainly due to repeated inflammatory attacks and distortion of the anatomy.

Factors predicting difficult cholecystectomy

Factors predicting difficult cholecystectomy are listed in **Box 9.2**.

Box 9.2 Factors predicting difficult cholecystectomy [15]

Factors predicting prolonged operation:
- Thick-walled gallbladder
- Impacted stone in the neck
- High BMI
- Abscess formation
- Absence of wall enhancement

Factors predicting conversion to open surgery:
- Gallbladder wall thickness >5 mm on ultrasound
- Age >60 years
- Male sex
- Contracted gallbladder
- High BMI
- High ASA score

(ASA, American Society of Anaesthesiologists; BMI, body mass index)

> **Box 9.3 Intraoperative difficulty scoring for cholecystectomy [16]**
>
> *Gallbladder appearance:*
> - Adhesions around the gallbladder <50%   1
> - Adhesions burying the gallbladder   3
>
> *Contraction/Distention:*
> - Distended gallbladder   1
> - Inability to grasp the gallbladder   1
> - Stone >1 cm impacted in the neck/Hartman's pouch   1
>
> *Access:*
> - BMI >30 kg/m^2 1
> - Previous intraperitoneal adhesions   1
>
> *Sepsis:* Pus or bile outside the gallbladder   1
>
> Time to identify cystic artery >90 minutes   1
>
> (BMI, body mass index)

Intraoperative difficulty scoring for cholecystectomy (Box 9.3)

Points above are added, and a final score is calculated. The final score can predict the degree of difficulty. Scores <2 are considered mild. Scores from 2 to 4 are considered moderate. Scores from 5 to 7 are considered severe and scores from 8 to 10 are considered extreme [16].

How to manage a difficult cholecystectomy?

The main aim to manage a difficult cholecystectomy is to perform it safely, avoiding any collateral damage to surrounding structures or bile duct injury. There is often distorted anatomy due to acute or prolonged severe chronic inflammation where the common bile duct can be mistaken for the cystic duct, leading to its transection. This will result in significant morbidity, commit the patient to further procedures and will affect the patient's quality of life. Other biliary tree and vascular injuries can occur including cystic stump leaks, iatrogenic or thermal injury to the bile ducts and clipping of the right hepatic artery. An acute laparoscopic cholecystectomy can range from being a straightforward procedure to one of the most difficult and challenging operations the surgeon has ever performed. There are, therefore, some important considerations when prepared for a difficult cholecystectomy:

Patient's selection

Safe cholecystectomy starts with preoperative planning and the selection of the patients. Specific factors have been found to be associated with an increased difficulty of cholecystectomy (**Box 9.2**). Impacted stones in the neck, thick-walled gallbladders, high BMI and absence of wall enhancement on imaging are associated with prolonged operation. Male sex, thickened wall of the gallbladder >5 mm, advanced age, high BMI and a contracted gallbladder are associated with a more difficult operation and a higher rate of open conversion. These patients with preoperative predictors of difficult cholecystectomy are better managed by a surgeon with experience of difficult cholecystectomy or in a specialised centre.

Access to the peritoneal cavity

The standard camera port placement in most patients is either supra- or infraumbilical. This will need to be tailored for obese patients as the umbilicus usually is shifted downwards. The camera port should be ideally located 15 cm from the xiphoid process. The triangulation rule should be used for the placement of other ports to allow for proper manipulation and safe dissection. Following access, positioning of the patient is vital to expose the gallbladder. Typically reversed Trendelenburg and a tilt to the left will help to visualise the gallbladder. However, in obese patients, the normal positioning might not be enough for proper visualisation of the gallbladder, as the omentum will be bulky and will obscure the view. In these cases, an extra 5-mm port might be needed, to allow the assistant to retract the omentum caudally or to place a liver retractor.

The critical view of safety

The concept of the 'critical view of safety' was first introduced in 1995 by Strasberg et al. [17]. It is a method to ensure normal anatomy is identified before any ligation or clipping of ductal structures and vessels is performed. It includes dissection of the cystic plate to expose at least the lower third of the gallbladder off the liver. This should be followed by careful dissection of the hepatocystic triangle to expose only two structures entering the gallbladder [18]. Stay close to the gallbladder.

Dissection should be in close proximity to the gallbladder, particularly in the hepatocystic triangle. This dissection should be done anterior to a plane that passes through Rouviere's sulcus in the liver, which is the landmark of the right posterior sectoral duct.

Avoidance of error traps

The infundibular or fundus-first technique has been described and used as a technique for difficult cholecystectomies. Surgeons should be careful when using this technique, as the cystic duct and right hepatic duct may become fused, with severe inflammation such that it can be easy to drift the dissection more proximally and very close to the major vessels and ducts of the liver, causing injuries.

Use of cholangiography/indocyanine green

Several modalities can be used to help identify the anatomy of the biliary system. Intraoperative cholangiography is useful to delineate the anatomy and can aid identification of aberrant ducts and cystic duct insertions. In cases of possible intraoperative bile duct injury, cholangiography or ICG may help to manage a difficult situation [19–21].

Indocyanine green (ICG) can also be used to perform intraoperative near-infrared fluorescence of the biliary structures. This is because ICG is selectively absorbed by the liver after intravenous administration and then secreted into the bile. The surgeon can then visualise the common hepatic duct and bile duct with the cystic duct insertion, using near-infrared fluorescence technology. Limiting factors include obesity and dense inflammation, and the fact that a specialised camera stack with a white light source and a near-infrared light source and a camera device recognising both sources is required.

Minimising the use of energy devices

It is a common practice to use diathermy to dissect the hepatocystic triangle and to fulgurate the gallbladder liver bed in case of bleeding. Although this is low risk for superficial bleeding, there is a risk of injury to superficial bile ducts which may only secrete bile once the eschar falls off the liver bed, which can happen a week later. Collateral diathermy heat can also spread burn the common bile duct. This can cause a delayed bile leak 5-7 days postoperatively. Using suction-irrigation instead of energy devices is particularly useful with severe inflammation, oedema and tissue fibrosis; this can help to delineate structures and reduces risk of collateral damage.

Team working and assistance

Having an external independent opinion from a colleague is always helpful. They will not be affected by stress and so be able to assist with clearer judgement. They may provide suggestions to help the progression of the operation and can scrub for assistance, especially if there is a decision to covert to an open operation.

Conversion to open procedure

Conversion to open surgery is favourable to provide proper access and tissue manipulation. However, the operation itself will still be difficult and challenging, as difficult laparoscopic cholecystectomies will still be difficult with the open approach. It is useful to ask for a second opinion before conversion, especially if the operating surgeon has no advanced experience in laparoscopic skills [22].

How to manage bleeding?

Bleeding is always stressful for surgeons. However, it is vital to stay calm when bleeding happens during cholecystectomy. The bleeding itself will eventually be controlled, but it is the collateral damage that may happen when a surgeon is trying to control the bleeding that can be irreversible, if proper care and techniques are not followed. Bleeding can be classified into four main categories—vessel injury, clip slippage from the cystic artery or other clipped vessels, liver bed bleeding and miscellaneous bleeding from anywhere else during the surgery.

Vessel injury

Pneumoperitoneum establishment is considered the risky step of the operation. Injury to major vessels, including the aorta, vena cava and iliac vessels, has been reported during port or Veress needle insertion, with an incidence of up to 0.18%. This becomes riskier in thin individuals where the distance between the aorta and the abdominal wall can be as low as 1 cm. Major vessel injury has also been reported following scalpel skin incisions for port placement [23]. The open Hasson technique for port insertion is considered the safest option for the initial umbilical port insertion. However, vessel injuries with the open Hasson technique are still reported [24]. Usually, the major vessels are retroperitoneal and, in some cases, there is no apparent bleeding in the intraperitoneal space. Exploratory laparoscopy should be performed always and any haematoma or expanding swelling in the area of insertion should raise suspicions of vascular injury. The insertion of other ports can be less risky if it happens under vision, with the tip of the trocar seen through the scope. Bleeding from the anterior abdominal wall due to injury to the epigastric vessel can also happen. Injury to the right hepatic artery or portal vein can happen during dissection of the Calot's triangle, particularly with distorted anatomy and sharp dissection [25].

If injury to one of the major vessels occurs, immediate identification and rapid response are required to save the patient. This includes immediate conversion to laparotomy and proper control of the situation, while seeking help and advice from a colleague with the correct level of expertise in managing the situation, usually a vascular surgeon. Injury to the right hepatic or portal vein will also require a prompt decision for open conversion, as trials to control this laparoscopically will lead to more morbidity and mortality. Injury to the vessels of the anterior abdominal wall can be prevented by proper illumination of the abdominal wall during the port insertion and by avoiding any visible epigastric vessels.

Slipped clips

Bleeding due to slipped clips can happen during cholecystectomy; this might obscure the field and will require the surgeon to be calm and act wisely. Clipping randomly without direct vision and overuse of diathermy should be avoided as it may not control the situation and can result in irreversible damage. The use of the suction device or swabs to dry the area, followed by application of direct pressure and reassessment of the situation, is recommended. After direct pressure, dissection of the bleeding vessel can usually be performed. If the surgeon thinks that clips can be applied safely under vision, to control the bleeding vessel, this should be tried. However, if this cannot be achieved, then conversion to open procedure to control the situation is the most appropriate next step.

Bleeding from liver venous sinusoids/venous bleeding

Most venous bleeding will stop by direct pressure. However, bleeding from liver sinusoids is sometimes refractory to pressure. Tributaries of the middle hepatic vein lie in close proximity to the gallbladder fossa and can cause torrential bleeding if entered. Again, random use of diathermy and clipping randomly should be avoided, as it may cause damage to the superficial bile ducts in the liver and cause further bleeding from another sinusoid. High-intensity diathermy to severe bleeding in the gallbladder fossa risks major haemorrhage developing from tributaries of the middle hepatic vein. This should also be avoided due to the added risk of injury to the deeper bile ducts causing significant bile leaks. Pressure should be used as the first step to control and the surgeon might continue the dissection elsewhere. This should then be followed by a reassessment of the situation and the use of topical haemostats to help achieve control. Products, such as Surgicel, Fibrillar and FloSeal, are useful adjuncts to haemostasis and avoid collateral damage to bile ducts [26].

Miscellaneous bleeding

This can be any bleeding encountered during the operation. Omental adhesions to the liver may cause liver capsule tears and bleeding during retraction of the gallbladder. Liver injury and bleeding can happen during manipulation and dissection. Minor and superficial bleeding from the liver capsule tear can be managed by diathermy or by applying absorbable haemostats or clips to visible vessels.

Difficult cholecystectomy

When to stop and how to bail out?

One of the most difficult decisions to take during laparoscopic cholecystectomy is to bail out before any irreversible vascular or bile injury could happen. Indicators which will help this decision include unclear anatomy, failure of progression and inability to obtain the critical view of safety in a safe manner. Once a decision has been taken that the operation is failing to progress, there are several bail-out options.

Abandoning the procedure

Simply stopping and abandoning the procedure is considered very safe and wise if the dissection planes and anatomy are not clear. Patient safety is paramount and abandoning the operation is better than causing serious bile duct injury, which will cause significant morbidity and have implications on the patient's quality of life. Interval cholecystectomy can be reattempted after 3 months, or it may be preferable to refer the patient to a specialist centre.

Biliary drainage (cholecystostomy)

This can be achieved by opening the gallbladder fundus and suctioning the contents. This is followed by placing a Foley catheter or drain into the gallbladder fundus with a purse-string suture to secure it. Interval cholecystectomy can be reattempted after 3 months or, referral to a specialist centre may be considered.

Subtotal cholecystectomy [27]

Two types of subtotal cholecystectomy (**Figure 9.1**) can be identified in the literature:
1. Subtotal reconstituting cholecystectomy – when the gallbladder wall is sutured to the top of the cystic duct/Hartmann's pouch and the stump closed. A small remnant gallbladder is created from the remaining portions of the gallbladder.
2. Subtotal fenestrating cholecystectomy – when the remaining part of the gallbladder is left open and the internal opening of the cystic duct either sutured with a purse-string or left open and drained.

Both are considered safe; however, the fenestrating subtotal cholecystectomy is more widely used as there are fewer risks of stone formation. The technique for both starts by

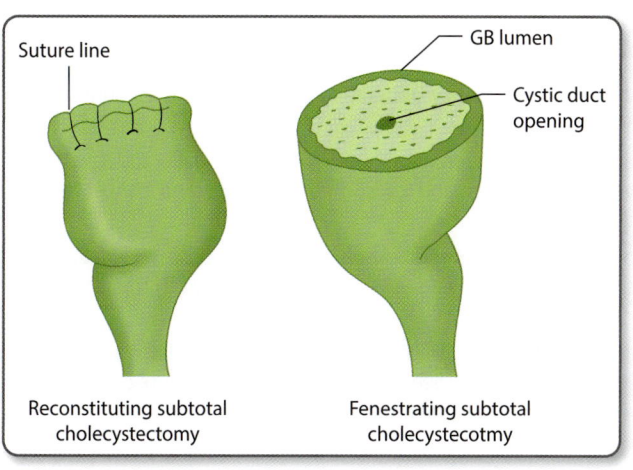

Figure 9.1 Two types of subtotal cholecystectomy. GB, gallbladder.

incision of the anterior wall of the gallbladder and extraction of stones and suction of any bile. The incision should be extended to remove most of the anterior wall of the gallbladder. The inside of the gallbladder then should be examined and if the cystic duct opening is draining bile, it should be closed by suturing. Finally, a drain should be left near the gallbladder fossa to drain any bile that may leak.

RECENT ADVANCES IN LAPAROSCOPIC CHOLECYSTECTOMY

Laparoscopic cholecystectomy is one of the most frequently performed surgeries worldwide. The traditional cholecystectomy is performed by insertion of 3 or 4 ports, with two 10-mm ports and two 5-mm ports. Technology has advanced to include mini laparoscopic cholecystectomy using 3-mm ports [28] and single-incision laparoscopic surgery (SILS) cholecystectomy [29,30]. Natural orifice cholecystectomy has been described but not widely adopted [31]. Robotic cholecystectomy is an emerging technique that may be useful in the treatment of acute cholecystitis [31–34].

CONCLUSION

Biliary disease accounts for up to 40% of the emergency general surgery workload and acute cholecystitis is a common presentation. The management of acute cholecystitis depends on the severity and patient's fitness for surgery, and cholecystectomy is safe and effective if performed within 7 days as advised by the NICE guidelines. Safe dissection techniques, management of complications such as bleeding and calling for help if there are doubts on the anatomy are important aspects of managing the 'hot gallbladder'. Techniques such as intraoperative cholangiography, ICG fluorescence and intraoperative ultrasound can help identify structures and prevent injury to the biliary tree. Bailout options such as subtotal cholecystectomy, cholecystostomy and placing drains and abandoning the procedure should be the last resort but have a role in preventing bile duct injury and referring to specialist centres. Emerging technology such as robotics has not been proven to be safe and effective in the difficult gallbladder and should be used with caution.

Key points for clinical practice

- Gallstones are a common cause of emergency general surgery workload, accounting for 30–40% of admissions in the UK
- Acute acalculous cholecystitis is a life-threatening inflammation of the gallbladder without stones, usually seen in severely ill patients, and caused by bile stasis and concentration leading to ischaemia, necrosis and perforation
- The diagnosis of acute cholecystitis requires the combination of symptoms, clinical signs and imaging investigations. The 2018 Tokyo guidelines provide an approach to diagnosing acute cholecystitis
- Management of acute cholecystitis depends on the severity – NICE guidelines advise that laparoscopic cholecystectomy is safe and effective in the management of acute cholecystitis within 7 days and should be offered in those that are fit for surgery

- Antibiotic therapy is an important aspect of treatment, with broad-spectrum antibiotics according to local hospital guidelines used, until the causative organism is identified
- Difficult cholecystectomy is described as an increased risk and incidence of complications compared to elective cholecystectomy, mainly due to repeated inflammatory attacks and distortion of the anatomy

REFERENCES

1. Royal College of Surgeons. (2013). Gallstones: Commissioning Guide. Available from https://www.rcseng.ac.uk/library-and-publications/rcs-publications/docs/gallstones-commissioning-guide/ [Last accessed 18 July 2025].
2. National Institute for Health and Care Excellence. Gallstone disease: diagnosis and management Clinical guideline Reference number: CG188; 2014. Available from https://www.nice.org.uk/guidance/cg188
3. Iqbal S, Khajinoori M, Mooney B. A case report of acalculous cholecystitis due to Salmonella paratyphi B. Radiol Case Rep. 2018; 13:1116–1118.
4. Yokoe M, Hata J, Takada T, et al. Tokyo Guidelines 2018: diagnostic criteria and severity grading of acute cholecystitis (with videos). J Hepatobiliary Pancreat Sci. 2018; 25:41–54.
5. Hwang H, Marsh I, Doyle J. Does ultrasonography accurately diagnose acute cholecystitis? Improving diagnostic accuracy based on a review at a regional hospital. Can J Surg 2014; 57:162.
6. Fuks D, Mouly C, Robert B, et al. Acute cholecystitis: preoperative CT can help the surgeon consider conversion from laparoscopic to open cholecystectomy. Radiology 2012; 263:128–138.
7. National Institute of Health and Care Excellence (NICE). (2014). Gallstone disease: Diagnosis and management. Available from www.nice.org.uk/guidance/cg188 [Last accessed 19 July 2025].
8. Yoshida M, Takada T, Kawarada Y, et al. Antimicrobial therapy for acute cholecystitis: Tokyo Guidelines. J Hepatobiliary Pancreat Surg 2007; 14:83.
9. Marne C, Pallarés R, Martín R, et al. Gangrenous cholecystitis and acute cholangitis associated with anaerobic bacteria in bile. Eur J Clin Microbiol 1986; 5:35–39.
10. El-Gendi A, El-Shafei M, Emara D. Emergency Versus Delayed Cholecystectomy After Percutaneous Transhepatic Gallbladder Drainage in Grade II Acute Cholecystitis Patients. J Gastrointest Surg 2017; 21:284–293.
11. Brodish RJ, Fink AS. ERCP, cholangiography, and laparoscopic cholecystectomy. The Society of American Gastrointestinal Endoscopic Surgeons (SAGES) opinion survey. Surg Endosc 1993; 7:3–8.
12. Skouras C, Jarral O, Deshpande R, et al. Is early laparoscopic cholecystectomy for acute cholecystitis preferable to delayed surgery?: Best evidence topic (BET). Int J Surg 2012; 10:250–258.
13. Ambe P, Weber SA, Christ H, et al. Cholecystectomy for acute cholecystitis. How time-critical are the so called "golden 72 hours"? Or better "golden 24 hours" and "silver 25-72 hour"? A case control study. World J Emerg Surg 2014; 9:60.
14. Bamber JR, Stephens TJ, Cromwell DA, et al. Effectiveness of a quality improvement collaborative in reducing time to surgery for patients requiring emergency cholecystectomy. BJS Open 2019; 3:802–811.
15. Wakabayashi G, Iwashita Y, Hibi T, et al. Tokyo Guidelines 2018: surgical management of acute cholecystitis: safe steps in laparoscopic cholecystectomy for acute cholecystitis (with videos). J Hepatobiliary Pancreat Sci 2018; 25:73–86.
16. Sugrue M, Sahebally SM, Ansaloni L, et al. Grading operative findings at laparoscopic cholecystectomy- a new scoring system. World J Emerg Surg 2015; 10:1–8.
17. Sgaramella LI, Gurrado A, Pasculli A, et al. The critical view of safety during laparoscopic cholecystectomy: Strasberg Yes or No? An Italian Multicentre study. Surg Endosc 2021; 35:3698.
18. Strasberg SM, Brunt LM. Rationale and use of the critical view of safety in laparoscopic cholecystectomy. J Am Coll Surg 2010; 211:132–138.
19. Törnqvist B, Strömberg C, Akre O, et al. Selective intraoperative cholangiography and risk of bile duct injury during cholecystectomy. Br J Surg 2015; 102:952–958.
20. Hope WW, Fanelli R, Walsh DS, et al. SAGES clinical spotlight review: intraoperative cholangiography. Surg Endosc 2017; 31:2007–2016.

21. Sheffield KM, Riall TS, Han Y, et al. Association between cholecystectomy with vs without intraoperative cholangiography and risk of common duct injury. JAMA 2013; 310:812–820.
22. Abelson JS, Afaneh C, Rich BS, et al. Advanced laparoscopic fellowship training decreases conversion rates during laparoscopic cholecystectomy for acute biliary diseases: a retrospective cohort study. Int J Surg 2015; 13:221–226.
23. Philips PA, Amaral JF. Abdominal access complications in laparoscopic surgery. J Am Coll Surg 2001; 192:525–536.
24. Hanney RM, Carmalt HL, Merrett N, et al. Use of the Hasson cannula producing major vascular injury at laparoscopy. Surg Endosc 1999; 13:1238–1240.
25. Tzovaras G, Dervenis C. Vascular injuries in laparoscopic cholecystectomy: an underestimated problem. Dig Surg 2006; 23:370–374.
26. Sartelli M, Catena F, Biancafarina A, et al. Use of floseal hemostatic matrix for control of hemostasis during laparoscopic cholecystectomy for acute cholecystitis: a multicenter historical control group comparison (the GLA study gelatin matrix for acute cholecystitis). J Laparoendosc Adv Surg Tech A 2014; 24:837–841.
27. Strasberg SM, Pucci MJ, Brunt LM, et al. Subtotal Cholecystectomy-"Fenestrating" vs "Reconstituting" Subtypes and the Prevention of Bile Duct Injury: Definition of the Optimal Procedure in Difficult Operative Conditions. J Am Coll Surg 2016; 222:89–96.
28. Ngoi SS, Goh P, Kok K, et al. Needlescopic or minisite cholecystectomy. Surg Endosc 1999; 13:303–305.
29. Ng WT, Kong CK, Wong YT. One-wound laparoscopic cholecystectomy. Br J Surg 1997; 84:1627.
30. Arezzo A, Scozzari G, Famiglietti F, et al. Is single-incision laparoscopic cholecystectomy safe? Results of a systematic review and meta-analysis. Surg Endosc 2013; 27:2293–2304.
31. Marescaux J, Dallemagne B, Perretta S, et al. Surgery without scars: report of transluminal cholecystectomy in a human being. Arch Surg 2007; 142:823–826.
32. Milone M, Vertaldi S, Bracale U, et al. Robotic cholecystectomy for acute cholecystitis: Three case reports. Medicine 2019; 98:e16010.
33. Strosberg DS, Nguyen MC, Muscarella P, et al. A retrospective comparison of robotic cholecystectomy versus laparoscopic cholecystectomy: operative outcomes and cost analysis. Surg Endosc 2017; 31:1436–1441.
34. Kane WJ, Charles EJ, Mehaffey JH, et al. Robotic compared with laparoscopic cholecystectomy: A propensity matched analysis. Surgery 2020; 167:432.

Section 5

Intestinal surgery

Chapter 10

Management of rectal injuries

Deborah Keller, Richard Cohen, James J Crosbie

ABSTRACT

Rectal injuries occur in both military and civilian practice. The mechanism and extent of injury vary considerably. However, a knowledge of the anatomy of the rectum is essential, particularly its relation to the peritoneal cavity. The majority of rectal injuries are extraperitoneal in the lower part of the rectum and can often be managed without the need for laparotomy or bowel resection. Intraperitoneal injuries of the upper rectum can cause peritonitis leading to sepsis and require early resuscitation and treatment. The traditional 4 Ds approach – *d*ebridement, *d*iversion, *d*rainage and *d*istal rectal washout – has been superseded by treatment tailored to the patient's specific rectal injury and any other concomitant injuries or comorbidities. A diverting stoma is not mandatory for all cases but may still be a useful option for those with significant contamination, sphincter disruption or serious comorbidities or haemodynamic instability. Options for repair will be discussed in this chapter.

INTRODUCTION

The management of rectal injuries was historically based on long-standing wartime practices. The immediate need for damage control procedures to improve mortality in military situations became the norm for rectal injuries in civilians as well, despite differences in the patients and injury mechanisms. Management continues to be refined with improved technology, experience and evidence-based research. Old dogmas, such as the 4 Ds of rectal injury, avoiding definitive repair or resection in the damage control setting and a mandatory colostomy, are no longer universal truths. A knowledge of the current

---

Deborah Keller MS MD, Professor, School of Biological and Health Systems Engineering, Arizona State University, Adjunct Professor, Department of Surgery, Mayo Clinic Arizona, Program Chair, Innovation in Medical and Patient Care Technologies (IMPACT) Program, Mayo Clinic and Arizona State Alliance for Healthcare, Phoenix, Arizona, USA
E-mail: debbykeller@gmail.com (for correspondence)

Richard Cohen MS FRCS, Professor of Surgery, Department of Targeted Intervention, University College London, Gower Street, London
E-mail: richardchohen@btinternet.com (for correspondence)

James J Crosbie MB BCh BAO MSc FRCSI (General Surgery), Consultant Colorectal Surgeon, University College London Hospital, London, UK
E-mail: j.crosbie@nhs.net (for correspondence)

guidelines and literature is needed to ensure the best management is utilised to optimise patient outcomes. In this chapter, the history and evolution of rectal injury management will be reviewed.

HISTORY OF RECTAL INJURY CARE

The management of injuries during wartime had a great influence on the treatment of all traumatic injuries. Understanding the history of rectal injury management is important, as these traditions continue to have great influence on current practice. In the 1860s, patients with colon and rectal injuries were managed expectantly and mortality was nearly universal. During World War I, surgical management became the norm for rectal injuries, with an ensuing reduction in mortality to between 60 and 75% [1]. During World War II, Sir William Ogilvie directed British surgeons to perform faecal diversion for all colorectal injuries, a command that was soon mimicked by the US Surgeon General, who similarly mandated colostomy or 'exteriorisation' for all combat colorectal injuries [2,3]. With universal diversion, immediate mortality rates further declined to between 53 and 59% [1,2]. Hence, diversion became the dogma for rectal injuries, even in postwar civilian surgery, despite the dramatic differences in patient and injury patterns. During the Vietnam War, Lavenson and Cohen introduced distal rectal washout, with the thinking that the washing out of faecal debris would prevent pelvic contamination. This further reduced the mortality rate and popularised the 'four Ds' as the standard treatment of rectal injuries [4]:
1. Debridement
2. Diversion
3. Drainage
4. Distal rectal washout

The experience gained from these military battles led to the practice that all rectal injuries required debridement, diversion, drainage and distal rectal washout. Modern combat changed over the years, with the most recent Iraq and Afghanistan conflicts reporting head and neck injuries were more common than thoracic, bowel and extremity, because of the increased use of body armour and personnel protective equipment [5]. A rise in explosive injury patterns was seen with the increasing use of improvised explosive device (IED), within operations in Iraq and Afghanistan [5,6]. With this change in weapons and tactics, rectal injury patterns also changed, with the highest percentage of injuries reported to arise from explosive devices – nearly two-thirds of patients – with firearms accounting for the remainder [7].

PARADIGM SHIFT AND CIVILIAN MANAGEMENT

Civilian experience paralleled the military rectal injury management algorithms, despite vast differences in the patients, injury mechanisms and treatment options available. To this end, the famous surgeon Dr Michael DeBakey stated, from lessons learned in World War II, *'All the circumstances of war surgery thus do violence to civilian concepts of traumatic surgery'* [8]. Many factors have led to changes in management for all rectal injury patients, including better transport time, resuscitation, transfusion, antibiotics and improved surgical techniques. Research and experience further refined current treatment algorithms.

Surgeons returning from World War II adopted mandatory colostomy for all rectal injuries, which became standard practice, even for civilians. However, this practice was questioned as early as the 1950s. Woodhall and Ochsner published a case series which showed success in highly selected cases of primary repair, with a mortality rate of only 9% [9]. In 1979, Stone and Fabian published the first randomised, controlled, unblinded study comparing primary repair versus mandatory colostomy, in 139 patients with penetrating colorectal injuries. The authors had substantial exclusion criteria, including faecal contamination, devastating injuries, shock, treatment delay or extensive blood loss. However, within the selected cohort, primary repair proved to be superior to colostomy, with significantly lower infection rates, morbidity, postoperative length of stay and costs [10]. This landmark study marked the evolution of management of colorectal injuries, distinguishing civilian treatment from combat scenarios. Multiple subsequent studies expanded on this seminal work and continued to advance the field.

ANATOMY OF THE RECTUM

Understanding the anatomy of the rectum is a key initial step to ensuring proper management. The management of rectal trauma has often been lumped in with colon trauma when, in fact, it is a distinct entity, with unique circumstances related to management and treatment, due to the anatomic nature of the rectum. In addition, rectal injuries are rarely seen in isolation, given the close proximity of other pelvic organs and vasculature, which can make management more difficult.

The rectum comprises the lower part of the gastrointestinal tract, up to approximately 15 cm from the anal verge (**Figure 10.1**). It is arbitrarily divided into three distinct parts – the upper, middle and lower rectum. From the anal verge, the lower rectum is 0–7 cm; middle rectum is 7–12 cm; and upper rectum is 12–15 cm. The upper rectum can be distinguished from the sigmoid colon as the three bands of taenia coalesce at the rectosigmoid junction, with an absence of taenia coli and epiploic appendages. The rectum is further divided into intra- and extraperitoneal sections by its relationship with the peritoneal reflection. The intraperitoneal portion includes the upper two-thirds anteriorly and the upper one-third

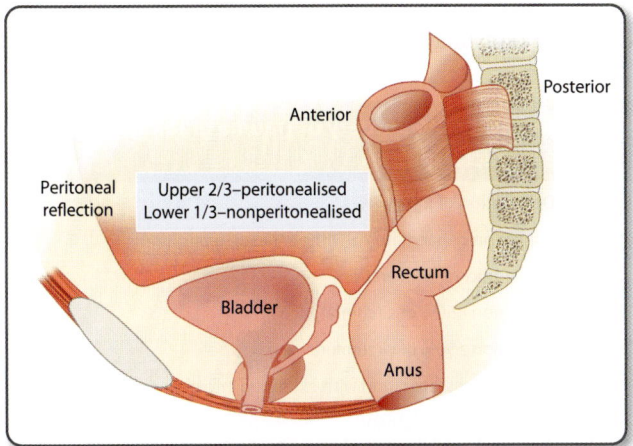

Figure 10.1 Anatomy of the rectum (male example).

laterally. The lower third of the rectum is extraperitoneal. The majority (93%) of penetrating rectal trauma occur in an extraperitoneal location, and 88% of these injuries occur in the lower one-third of the rectum [11].

AETIOLOGY

The aetiology of rectal injury differs across military and civilian scenarios. In all scenarios, however, the vast majority of rectal injuries are secondary to penetrating pelvic trauma, including iatrogenic, sexual-related and foreign body injuries. In military situations, the incidence of rectal injuries is reported around 5% [1]. These injuries involve much higher velocity weaponry, blast injuries, fragmentations and burns than their civilian counterparts. Nearly a quarter of war-related rectal injuries are due to explosive trauma. In civilian centres, the incidence of rectal trauma is reported between 1 and 3% [1]. The vast majority of injuries are caused by gunshot wounds (71–85%), then stab wounds (3–5%), with accidental or intentional impalement, iatrogenic injuries and rectal foreign bodies accounting for the rest. There has been a recent trend for gang-related assaults to deliberately produce rectal injuries rather than shooting to kill. These are so called 'bagging' assaults, such that the victim requires a stoma. This is intended to produce more 'shame' and less 'martyr' status for the victim, while avoiding the serious consequences of a murder charge, should the perpetrator be apprehended. Blunt trauma accounts for 5–10% of traumatic injuries. Of the blunt injury subset, many are secondary to open-book pelvic fractures, where the intrusion of sharp bony edges of anterior-posterior compression perforate the rectum [12,13]. The anus may be injured in a similar manner. The American Association for the Surgery of Trauma has published a grading scale for rectal injuries (**Table 10.1**) [14].

DIAGNOSIS

Recognition of rectal injuries requires a high level of suspicion in those evaluating any patient with a penetrating wound. This suspicion should increase with identification of penetrating wounds to the lower abdomen, pelvis, perineum, buttocks or thighs. Penetrating wounds should be counted and marked, such as with a paper clip taped adjacent to the penetration site, to help determine the missile trajectory. If the count is an odd number of penetrating wounds or there is no exit site for bullets, the physician should have heightened suspicion that a foreign body may remain internally. If any objects are

Grade	Type of injury	Description of injury
I	Haematoma	Contusion or haematoma without devascularisation
	Laceration	Partial-thickness laceration
II	Laceration	Laceration <50% of circumference
III	Laceration	Laceration ≥50% of circumference
IV	Laceration	Full-thickness laceration with extension into perineum
V	Vascular	Devascularised segment

Table 10.1 American Association for the Surgery of Trauma grading scale for rectal injuries

retained, these should not be removed until the patient is in a controlled environment, such as the operating room, no matter the location of the foreign body.

In patients who are hemodynamically stable, alert and oriented, obtaining a detailed history of the events surrounding their injury is essential. Questions pertinent to ask include the type of weapon, proximity of projectile when fired/stabbed and calibre of the weapon, if known. With all patients, it is crucial to attempt to obtain a brief history, including their past medical and surgical history, current medications and known drug allergies.

EVALUATION

With any traumatic injury, it is essential to identify immediate life-threatening injuries quickly. Therefore, a universal approach has been established by Advanced Trauma Life Support (ATLS) to follow in specific order: *A*irway maintenance, *B*reathing (ventilation), *C*irculation (including haemorrhage control), *D*isability (neurologic status) and *E*xposure. Airway assessment and management have the highest priority in any injured patient, irrespective of mechanism or injury location. It is essential to secure a patent airway first, before proceeding methodically, in appropriate order of A, B, C, D, E through the ATLS protocol. During the E portion of the primary survey, complete exposure of the patient is essential. The patient should be rolled to both sides (with appropriate cervical spine stabilisation), so as not to overlook penetrating injuries that may not be easily identifiable when lying in a supine position. The assessment should include an examination of the patient's back, axilla, flanks, perineum, buttocks and lower gluteal, anal and groin folds.

After the primary survey, focussed assessment with sonography for trauma (FAST), bedside ultrasonography examination, is considered the standard of care in the diagnostic assessment of a traumatic rectal injury patient. The suprapubic view, with visualisation of the pelvic cul-de-sac, is the most relevant for rectal trauma. The presence of fluid in this window may indicate intraperitoneal haemorrhage, hollow viscus injury, haemoperitoneum or ascites. The FAST scan is noted to have a sensitivity of 69.8% and a specificity of 92.1%; however, a threshold of at least 200 mL of fluid is reported necessary for the detection of intra-abdominal fluid [15]. Positive findings in a stable patient can be evaluated further with computed tomography (CT), while positive findings in an unstable patient necessitate emergent abdominal exploration. FAST has replaced diagnostic peritoneal lavage (DPL) in the contemporary evaluation of patients with suspected rectal injury, although DPL may be useful if CT is unavailable, or the patient is in the operating theatre for a prolonged period for other injuries. With DPL, the presence of gross blood or faecal matter on aspiration, or >500 white cells/>1,00,000 red cells on lavage analysis are highly suggestive of intra-abdominal injury and should prompt abdominal exploration.

During the secondary survey, physical examination findings of pelvic instability, blood at the urethral meatus, soft-tissue defect of the perineum or penetrating injury near the pelvis should raise suspicion for rectal trauma. A universal digital rectal examination (DRE) has been removed from the secondary trauma survey. DRE has low sensitivity to rule out injury and a high false-negative rate, estimated at approximately 51% and 63–67%, respectively [16,17]. The variability in detection rates is likely secondary to the evaluator's experience in detecting injury [18]. The nonselective use of a DRE alters management in only 1.2% of trauma evaluations; however, this number can increase up to 11% when the clinician's pretest suspicion is high. A nonselective DRE can be detrimental to patients, increasing the size of an existing soft tissue injury, converting a partial thickness to a full thickness injury or creating a defect or false tract in the friable tissue. It can also be a hazard for the practitioner, potentially exposes them to injury, transmission of infectious disease and even litigation for assault [16]. However, there are some situations where a DRE has utility. Careful DRE by an experienced practitioner is recommended in the setting of an open pelvic fracture and high-velocity trauma with sacral and pubic fractures, to assess for a gross defect in the rectal vault, in light of questionable physical examination findings, or as confirmation of diagnostic suspicion. Concerning findings for rectal injury on DRE include a palpable defect in the rectal wall, gross luminal blood, decreased anal sphincter tone, palpable bony fragments or a high-riding prostate [19]. These findings mandate further evaluation. Other clinical tests, such as intraoperative examination with sigmoidoscopy, either rigid or flexible, may diagnose rectal injury with improved yield and accuracy over DRE. If the location of the injury is not identifiable, blood seen on proctosigmoidoscopy has a sensitivity of 71% overall for the diagnosis of rectal injury and a sensitivity as high as 88% for extraperitoneal rectal injury [20]. Proctoscopy is an important step in the evaluation of rectal injuries. It can allow documentation of the size and extent of the patient's injury. It can also distinguish between an intra- and extraperitoneal rectal injury, which can avoid the morbidity of a negative laparotomy if extraperitoneal. Most commonly, proctoscopy does not detect a distinct injury, but demonstrates less conclusive findings, such as the presence or absence of intraluminal blood, prompting further evaluation. However, there is controversy on where to perform the proctoscopy. Some providers advocate for proctoscopy in the trauma bay, although lack of bowel preparation, an inexperienced examiner, an uncooperative patient and associated injuries may decrease the sensitivity of proctoscopy. It may also create a worse injury if performed in the face of injury with poor visualisation. We recommend that stable patients, with obvious abnormalities on physical examination, should be evaluated with proctoscopy in the operating room.

Patients with hemodynamic instability on initial trauma evaluation should proceed immediately to surgical exploration. Stable patients go to imaging for a better picture of the injury pattern. CT with IV contrast is the most useful adjunct for evaluation in the stable trauma patient, to help identify or rule out injuries. In patients with a normal physical examination, but heightened suspicion for rectal trauma (e.g. widened pubic symphysis, penetrating injury near the rectum and blood at the urethral meatus), a pelvic CT offers a non-invasive evaluation for rectal injury. This can also be done sequentially with CT cystography during Foley catheter insertion, when there is a concern for bladder injury or haematuria, to rule out associated bladder or genitourinary injury. These injuries accompany up to one-third of rectal injuries. CT scan with bladder and rectal contrast is indicated for preoperative planning in stable patients. The most sensitive finding on CT in rectal injury is a wound tract that extends adjacent to the bowel, while the most specific are extravasation of intraluminal contrast, a full-thickness wall defect, foci of asymmetric extraluminal free air and haemorrhage within the bowel wall [21]. Additional secondary findings, which suggest a rectal injury, include rectal wall thickening, perirectal fat stranding and unexplained intraperitoneal free fluid [19,21]. A retrospective review of 10 patients injured in combat demonstrated that CT was able to detect each rectal injury but had a 20% false-positive rate [19]. Pararectal air was the most common finding on CT. Triple-contrast CT (oral, rectal and intravenous) is reported to be equally efficacious for detecting rectal trauma as proctoscopy in paediatric patients, but there is inadequate evidence in adults to support or refute the routine use of intraluminal contrast [19,21]. The use of rectal contrast is institution dependent and may not adequately evaluate the distal rectum, due to occlusion by the device's balloon. However, we recommend triple-contrast CT in adults, when feasible, for the improved intraluminal visualisation of possible injuries.

Stable patients, with a normal physical examination and CT, can be observed clinically or discharged. A positive finding on CT warrants further evaluation with proctoscopy, unless the injury is clearly intraperitoneal, prompting surgical management. Certain injury patterns, such as transpelvic or buttock gunshot wounds, need thorough investigation, even in the absence of rectal blood. Most anal injuries are obvious on external inspection, although occult sphincter disruption may occasionally occur.

DIFFERENTIAL DIAGNOSIS

Suspicion for rectal injury should increase with any identification of a pelvic fracture from blunt injury or penetrating wound to the lower abdomen, pelvis, perineum, buttocks or thighs. With the identification of trauma to this region, the differential diagnosis must distinguish intra- versus extraperitoneal rectal injury and determine if there is concomitant vascular or bladder injury. Nearly any major vasculature or viscera may be injured and subsequently must be excluded, with the identification of a penetrating injury.

TREATMENT ALGORITHM

In a haemodynamically unstable patient, with massive blood loss, acidosis, hypothermia and coagulopathy, expedient operative exploration with a damage control laparotomy (DCL) should be performed. The DCL can allow stabilisation of an unstable, coagulopathic or hypothermic patient, who would not otherwise tolerate definitive repair at the initial operation. During the initial exploration for penetrating trauma, control of gross spillage with quick suturing or stapling should occur rapidly, as soon as exsanguinating haemorrhage is stopped. The colon can be left in discontinuity at the initial exploration and creation of a colostomy is not necessary. The abdomen can be temporarily closed using nonstick plastic drapes or a Bogota bag, and a suction method of collecting fluid can be fashioned. Once restoration of normothermia and correction of acidosis and coagulopathy are accomplished, the patient can return to the operating room for further treatment, based on their stability.

In a haemodynamically stable patient, the anatomy of the rectum actually dictates the management of rectal injuries.

Intraperitoneal

The management of intraperitoneal wounds is the same as colon injuries. In general, most patients with intraperitoneal injuries undergo direct repair or resection with or without proximal diversion. Technically, the colon needs to be fully mobilised above suspected injuries, with particular care paid to the flexures and rectosigmoid junction; extensive rectal mobilisation is not recommended. In penetrating trauma, paracolic haematomas must be fully explored; this is less important for blunt injuries unless there are other signs of perforation, such as soiling or retroperitoneal emphysema. Primary repair can be safely accomplished with little difference between single- and double-layered suture techniques or hand-sewn versus stapled anastomoses [22,23]. Perforations that are within a few centimetres of each other are best treated by removing the intervening bridge of tissue and performing a single repair. Adherence to the standard principles of no tension, good tissue approximation and adequate blood supply are critical. There is no need for colonic lavage, even when a left-sided anastomosis is constructed. In nearly all cases of penetrating intraperitoneal rectal injury, the skin is left open, with planned delayed primary closure or secondary closure with a vacuum-assisted closure device. The patient should also receive broad-spectrum antibiotics covering gram-negative and anaerobes for at least 24 hours.

If the injury is non-destructive (<50% of the circumference of the intraperitoneal rectum), it can undergo primary repair. Randomised trials and high-quality data have conclusively shown the safety and efficacy of primary repair in patients with grade II injuries (**Table 10.1**), even in the presence of risk factors such as hypotension, multiple transfusions and gross spillage [24–26]. In fact, the primary repair groups had significantly fewer complications than the colostomy group. Small perforations can also be safely closed without proximal diversion, either transanally, if low enough, or from an abdominal approach, if minimal rectal mobilisation is required. If perforations cannot be safely closed or the injury is inaccessible, proximal diversion is still required [13,27]. If the wound is destructive (>50% circumferential involvement), the rectum requires resection to viable, healthy tissue. Primary anastomosis is preferred in patients who are reasonably healthy and stable, as colostomy creation and closure are associated with significant cost, morbidity and compromised quality of life [28,29]. The concept of mandatory colostomy has been long discarded, diversion is not associated with improved outcomes [30]. Following the Stone and Fabian randomised prospective trial that revolutionised this concept in colorectal trauma, there have been multiple studies showing that faecal diversion is not necessary, except in the setting of various transfusion requirements or hypotension [23]. In 2001, the American Association for the Surgery of Trauma conducted a prospective multicentre study on penetrating bowel injuries, comparing diversion or primary repair. This study demonstrated lower mortality in the primary repair arm (0% vs. 1.3%) with no relationship between the repair technique and abdominal complications [31]. Severe faecal contamination, transfusion of four or more units of blood within the first 24 hours and single-agent antibiotic prophylaxis were independent risk factors for abdominal complications. When considering diversion, one must also take into account all of the complications of stomas, including readmission, parastomal hernias, stenosis, retraction and metabolic imbalance, which range from 17 to 55%, as well as the complications related to stoma reversal, which range from 5 to 25% [32–36]. Despite the evidence, diversion is still frequently performed in cases of rectal trauma. The American Association for the Surgery of Trauma performed a multi-institutional retrospective study of 785 patients who sustained a traumatic rectal injury from 2004 to 2015, finding rectal injuries were intraperitoneal in 32% [37]. Most patients with intraperitoneal injuries underwent direct repair or resection with proximal diversion, although patients managed with diversion developed significantly more complications.

Extraperitoneal

The standard of care for most extraperitoneal rectal injuries is selective faecal diversion. Each of the traditional 'three Ds' has been challenged in the modern civilian management of rectal extraperitoneal trauma. Over the past few decades, there have been numerous studies demonstrating no benefit in presacral drainage or distal rectal washout. The practice of distal rectal washout forces faecal material into the injured tissues, which leads to increased incidence of contamination [13,38,39]. Liquefaction of the stool column, with subsequent spread into the pelvic spaces, has been touted as a potential negative consequence of vigorous rectal irrigation in traumatic injuries [13]. Several studies on routine presacral drainage showed the extensive disruption of normal tissue planes required had no benefit [13,40].

In a multi-institutional retrospective study of Level 1 Trauma Centres in the US, Brown et al. (2018) found that extraperitoneal rectal injuries occurred in 58% of patients, while both intra- and extraperitoneal injuries occurred in 9% [37]. There were significantly more abdominal complications in patients who received a presacral drain ($p = 0.004$), or distal rectal washout ($p = 0.002$). After multivariate analysis, distal rectal washout [3.4 (1.4–8.5), $p = 0.008$] and presacral drain [2.6 (1.1–6.1), $p = 0.02$] were independent risk factors for abdominal complications. While these additional manoeuvres are independently associated with a three-fold increase in abdominal complications, 20% of patients still received a presacral drain and/or distal rectal washout [37]. However, closed suction drains placed in the pelvis after mobilisation and repair of mid-rectal injuries at laparotomy may still be useful, as clean tissue planes are not violated.

For penetrating non-destructive extraperitoneal rectal injuries, the Eastern Association of the Surgery of Trauma practice management guidelines conditionally recommend proximal diversion for management of these injuries, while conditionally recommending the avoidance of routine presacral drains and distal rectal washout [41]. If a patient is stable, without peritoneal signs, and suspected of having an isolated extraperitoneal rectal injury, laparoscopy can be used for evaluation. If there is no evidence of intraperitoneal injury, then a loop sigmoid colostomy may be easily constructed [42].

For penetrating, destructive, extraperitoneal rectal trauma (>50% circumferential involvement), associated pelvic fractures or concomitant vascular injuries that can compromise the blood supply to the rectum causing anastomotic failure, faecal diversion is recommended as the safest option [43]. Blunt trauma accounts for 1–2% of rectal trauma and is usually secondary to an anterior-posterior compression mechanism, causing an open book pelvic fracture [44]. These injuries require faecal diversion. For anal injuries that are not destructive, wounds can be repaired primarily; routine proximal faecal diversion is not required. For destructive perineal wounds, appropriate debridement and proximal diversion are paramount. A vacuum-assisted wound closure device can be used on the perineum if serial debridement is ongoing. Marking of the ends of the sphincters with nonabsorbable sutures can aid later reconstruction.

A proposed algorithm for management of rectal trauma is shown in **Figure 10.2**.

CONCLUSION

The aetiology of rectal injury differs across military and civilian scenarios with, in the past few decades, a paradigm shift in management for civilians. After a trauma evaluation, the patient can be classified as stable or unstable, with further investigation or damage control surgery as needed. In stable patients, the anatomy of the rectum – either intra- or extraperitoneal – will guide management. Intraperitoneal injuries can be considered for primary repair or resection with primary anastomosis, depending on the degree of tissue destruction. Proximal diversion is not necessary in all cases. Extraperitoneal injuries can usually be managed with proximal diversion and routine presacral drains. Distal rectal washout has no benefit. A knowledge of the current guidelines and emerging literature can help ensure the best management is utilised to optimise patient outcomes.

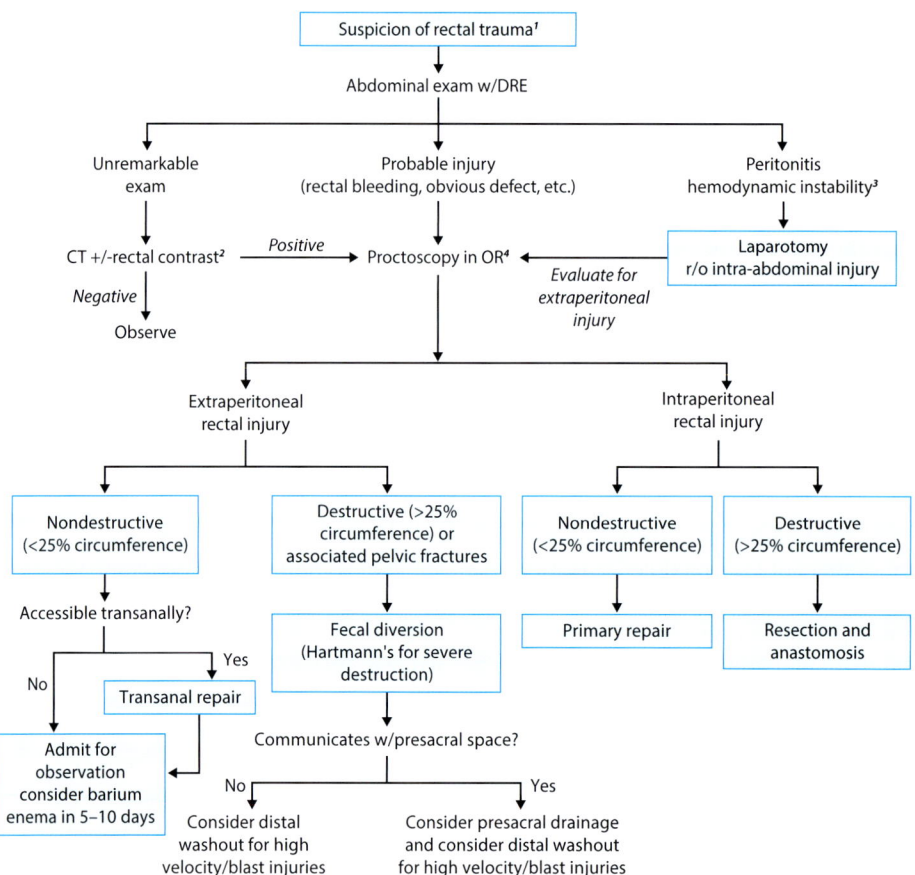

Figure 10.2 Algorithm of management of rectal trauma.

[1] Widened pubic symphysis, anteroposterior pelvic fracture, blood at the urethral meatus, transpelvic gunshot wound, impalement
[2] Wound tract extending to the rectal vault (most sensitive); contrast extravasation, transmural defect, extraluminal gas, bowel wall hemorrhage (more specific) also consider bowel wall thickening, fat stranding, infiltration, or unexplained intraperitoneal free fluid
[3] Consider diagnostic peritoneal lavage
[4] Consider custography. Gastrozafin enema, and plain film as indicated

Key points for clinical practice

- A colostomy is not always necessary, but diversion should be considered in patients undergoing DCL, or who have significant preinjury comorbidities or haemodynamic derangement
- Rectal injuries are not universally managed by the 4 Ds. Presacral drainage and distal washout are no longer recommended
- Diversion alone, without direct repair, is sufficient to treat isolated extraperitoneal rectal injuries
- Primary repair is appropriate for accessible rectal injuries and for all non-destructive colonic injuries near the rectum
- Resection and anastomosis are the treatment of choice for most destructive colonic injuries near the rectum
- Anal trauma lends itself to delayed reconstruction

REFERENCES

1. Steele SR, Maykel JA, Johnson EK. Traumatic injury of the colon and rectum: the evidence vs dogma. Dis Colon Rectum 2011; g54:1184–1201.
2. Ogilvie WH. Abdominal wounds in the Western Desert. Bull U S Army Med Dep 1946; 6:435–445.
3. Imed PR. War surgery of the abdomen. Surg Gynecol Obstet 1945; 81:608–616.
4. Lavenson GS, Cohen A. Management of rectal injuries. Am J Surg 1971; 122:226–230.
5. Owens BD, Kragh JF, Wenke JC, et al. Combat wounds in operation Iraqi Freedom and operation Enduring Freedom. J Trauma 2008; 64:295–299.
6. Ramasamy A, Hill AM, Clasper JC. Improvised explosive devices: pathophysiology, injury profiles and current medical management. J R Army Med Corps 2009; 155:265–272.
7. Al-Doghan IEM, Majeed YH, Jasim HA. War rectal injuries with its complications during civil violence in Iraq. Int J Surg Open 2019; 21:17–20.
8. DeBakey ME. Military surgery in World War II; a backward glance and a forward look. N Engl J Med 1947; 236:341–350.
9. Woodhall JP, Ochsner A. The management of perforating injuries of the colon and rectum in civilian practice. Surgery 1951; 29:305–320.
10. Stone HH, Fabian TC. Management of perforating colon trauma: randomization between primary closure and exteriorization. Ann Surg 1979; 190:430–436.
11. Weinberg JA, Fabian TC, Magnotti LJ, et al. Penetrating rectal trauma: management by anatomic distinction improves outcome. J Trauma 2006; 60:508–13; discussion 513.
12. Morken JJ, Kraatz JJ, Balcos EG, et al. Civilian rectal trauma: a changing perspective. Surgery 1999; 126:693–8; discussion 698.
13. Velmahos GC, Gomez H, Falabella A, et al. Operative management of civilian rectal gunshot wounds: simpler is better. World J Surg 2000; 24:114–118.
14. Moore EE, Cogbill TH, Malangoni MA, et al. Organ injury scaling, II: Pancreas, duodenum, small bowel, colon, and rectum. J Trauma 1990; 30:1427–1429.
15. Engles S, Saini NS, Rathore S. Emergency Focused Assessment with Sonography in Blunt Trauma Abdomen. Int J Appl Basic Med Res 2019; 9:193–196.
16. Esposito TJ, Ingraham A, Luchette FA, et al. Reasons to omit digital rectal exam in trauma patients: no fingers, no rectum, no useful additional information. J Trauma 2005; 59:1314–1319.
17. Porter JM, Ursic CM. Digital rectal examination for trauma: does every patient need one. Am Surg 2001; 67:438–441.
18. Smith DS, Catalona WJ. Interexaminer variability of digital rectal examination in detecting prostate cancer. Urology 1995; 45:70–74.
19. Johnson EK, Judge T, Lundy J, et al. Diagnostic pelvic computed tomography in the rectal-injured combat casualty. Mil Med 2008; 173:293–299.
20. Hargraves MB, Magnotti LJ, Fischer PE, et al. Injury location dictates utility of digital rectal examination and rigid sigmoidoscopy in the evaluation of penetrating rectal trauma. Am Surg 2009; 75:1069–1072.
21. Anderson SW, Soto JA. Anorectal trauma: the use of computed tomography scan in diagnosis. Semin Ultrasound CT MR 2008; 29:472–482.
22. Law WL, Bailey HR, Max E, et al. Single-layer continuous colon and rectal anastomosis using monofilament absorbable suture (Maxon): study of 500 cases. Dis Colon Rectum 1999; 42:736–740.
23. Demetriades D, Murray JA, Chan LS, et al. Handsewn versus stapled anastomosis in penetrating colon injuries requiring resection: a multicenter study. J Trauma 2002; 52:117–121.
24. Chappuis CW, Frey DJ, Dietzen CD, et al. Management of penetrating colon injuries. A prospective randomized trial. Ann Surg 1991; 213:492–7; discussion 497.
25. Sasaki LS, Allaben RD, Golwala R, et al. Primary repair of colon injuries: a prospective randomized study. J Trauma 1995; 39:895–901.
26. Gonzalez RP, Falimirski ME, Holevar MR. Further evaluation of colostomy in penetrating colon injury. Am Surg 2000; 66:342–6; discussion 346.
27. Levine JH, Longo WE, Pruitt C, et al. Management of selected rectal injuries by primary repair. Am J Surg 1996; 172:575–8; discussion 578.
28. Berne JD, Velmahos GC, Chan LS, et al. The high morbidity of colostomy closure after trauma: further support for the primary repair of colon injuries. Surgery 1998; 123:157–164.
29. Pachter HL, Hoballah JJ, Corcoran TA, et al. The morbidity and financial impact of colostomy closure in trauma patients. J Trauma 1990; 30:1510–1513.

30. Nance ML, Nance FC. A stake through the heart of colostomy. J Trauma 1995; 39:811–812.
31. Demetriades D, Murray JA, Chan L, et al. Penetrating colon injuries requiring resection: diversion or primary anastomosis? An AAST prospective multicenter study. J Trauma 2001; 50:765–775.
32. Hendren S, Hammond K, Glasgow SC, et al. Clinical practice guidelines for ostomy surgery. Dis Colon Rectum 2015; 58:375–387.
33. Robertson JP, Puckett J, Vather R, et al. Early closure of temporary loop ileostomies: a systematic review. Ostomy Wound Manage 2015; 61:50–57.
34. Chow A, Tilney HS, Paraskeva P, et al. The morbidity surrounding reversal of defunctioning ileostomies: a systematic review of 48 studies including 6,107 cases. Int J Colorectal Dis 2009; 24:711–723.
35. Krouse RS, Grant M, Wendel CS, et al. A mixed-methods evaluation of health-related quality of life for male veterans with and without intestinal stomas. Dis Colon Rectum 2007; 50:2054–2066.
36. Clemens MS, Heafner TA, Watson JD, et al. Quality of Life in United States Veterans With Combat-Related Ostomies From Iraq and Afghanistan. Mil Med 2016; 181:e1569–e1574.
37. Brown CVR, Teixeira PG, Furay E, et al. Contemporary management of rectal injuries at Level I trauma centers: The results of an American Association for the Surgery of Trauma multi-institutional study. J Trauma Acute Care Surg 2018; 84:225–233.
38. Tuggle D, Huber PJ. Management of rectal trauma. Am J Surg 1984; 148:806–808.
39. Burch JM, Feliciano DV, Mattox KL. Colostomy and drainage for civilian rectal injuries: is that all. Ann Surg 1989; 209:600–10; discussion 610.
40. Gonzalez RP, Falimirski ME, Holevar MR. The role of presacral drainage in the management of penetrating rectal injuries. J Trauma 1998; 45:656–661.
41. Bosarge PL, Como JJ, Fox N, et al. Management of penetrating extraperitoneal rectal injuries: An Eastern Association for the Surgery of Trauma practice management guideline. J Trauma Acute Care Surg 2016; 80:546–551.
42. Navsaria PH, Shaw JM, Zellweger R, et al. Diagnostic laparoscopy and diverting sigmoid loop colostomy in the management of civilian extraperitoneal rectal gunshot injuries. Br J Surg 2004; 91:460–464.
43. Cleary RK, Pomerantz RA, Lampman RM. Colon and rectal injuries. Dis Colon Rectum 2006; 49:1203–1222.
44. Giannoudis PV, Grotz MR, Tzioupis C, et al. Prevalence of pelvic fractures, associated injuries, and mortality: the United Kingdom perspective. J Trauma 2007; 63:875–883.

Chapter 11

Recent advances in intestinal transplantation

Jang I Moon, Kishore Iyer

ABSTRACT

Intestinal transplantation is a viable treatment option for patients with irreversible intestinal failure, experiencing complications of parenteral nutrition. Small bowel may be transplanted alone or in combination with liver and/or other parts of the gastrointestinal tract. Multidisciplinary care, with attention to both medical and surgical management, is essential. Improvements in surgical procedures, perioperative care and postintestinal transplantation management have made intestinal transplantation safer and more effective. The identification of donor-specific antibodies through new techniques has also improved clinical outcomes. The relatively small number of intestinal transplant procedures is an obstacle to substantive research and establishment of more effective immunosuppressive therapy. Severe acute rejection remains a major cause of postoperative mortality and morbidity including graft loss. Improvement in long-term survival is essential to expand the indications for this surgical option to be offered to a wider range of intestinal failure patients.

INTRODUCTION

Successful intestinal transplantation (ITx) was first reported by David Grant and colleagues in 1990, as a life-saving procedure for patients suffering from intestinal failure and life-threatening complications of parenteral nutrition (PN) [1]. The number of ITx procedures slowly increased, reaching a peak of 198 transplantations in 2007. Since then, the annual number of ITx procedures has steadily decreased, with only 82 procedures performed in the US in 2022 [2]. ITx remains the least common solid organ transplantation procedure. According to the annual report of the Scientific Registry of Transplant Recipient (SRTR), advances in PN and improved intestinal rehabilitation are the leading reasons for the decrease in the number of ITx procedures [3]. However, ITx still remains a viable treatment

---

Jang I Moon MD, Associate Professor of Surgery and Attending Transplant Surgeon, Recanati Miller Transplant Institute, Mount Sinai Hospital, New York, US
E-mail: jang.moon@mountsinai.org (for correspondence)

Kishore Iyer MBBS MSc FRCS(England) FACS, Professor of Surgery, Pediatrics and Global Health, Director, Intestinal rehab and Transplant Program, Recanati Miller Transplant Institute, Mount Sinai Hospital, New York, US
E-mail: kishore.iyer@mountsinai.org (for correspondence)

option for patients with intestinal failure, experiencing life-threatening complications of PN. In fact, recent improvements in clinical outcomes have made ITx more attractive as a potential treatment option for patients with intestinal failure, even in the absence of PN-related complications. There have been significant improvements in the last 5 years, due to a better understanding of this uncommon transplant procedure. This chapter describes general aspects of ITx, with an emphasis on recent improvements in both the operative surgery and postoperative care of small bowel transplant patients.

DEFINITION OF INTESTINAL TRANSPLANT

Intestinal transplantation refers to any transplantation procedure, which uses a visceral allograft that includes the small intestine.

The most common forms of ITx include isolated small bowel ITx, liver-intestine combinations and multivisceral transplantation (MVT). However, theoretically, ITx can be performed with many different combinations of visceral allografts (**Figure 11.1**). Organ retrieval is based on the vascular territory of the necessary organ. The major difference among the various forms of ITx relates to the inclusion or exclusion of the liver. The presence or absence of a liver allograft affects the surgical procedure, immunological reaction, development of acute rejection and clinical outcomes – essentially every aspect of transplantation. In this chapter, ITx without liver allograft will be described as the basic model of ITx.

Intestinal transplantation is defined as a transplantation using visceral composite allograft, which includes small intestine. Theoretically, ITx can be performed in different allograft combinations.

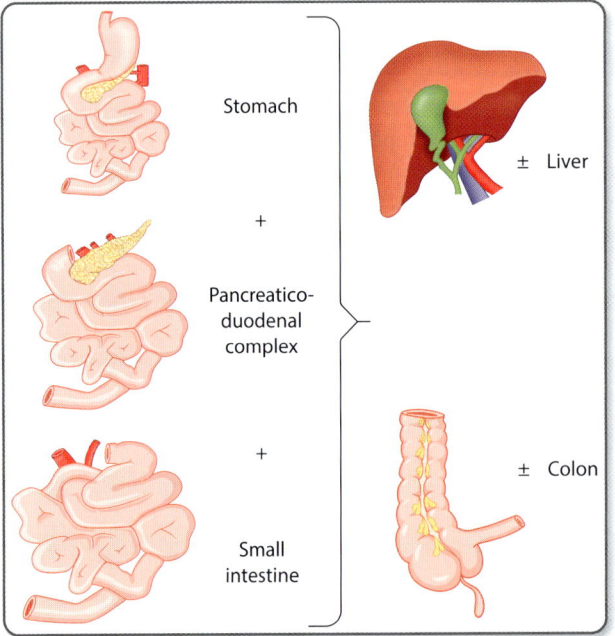

Figure 11.1 Definition of intestinal transplantation (ITx).

INDICATIONS FOR INTESTINAL TRANSPLANT

It is important to emphasise that the traditional indications for ITx are not related to a specific underlying disease but rather to intestinal failure broadly, accompanied by failure or significant complications while on PN. When the Centres for Medicare and Medicaid Services (CMS) first approved ITx in the US in 2000, they required fulfilment of two conditions before consideration of ITx:
1. Presence of irreversible intestinal failure, which, for practical purposes, is refractory PN-dependency
2. Presence of life-threatening complications of PN, i.e. PN-failure

The majority of patients presenting for ITx have intestinal failure secondary to short bowel syndrome, which may be due to a variety of causes including mesenteric ischaemia, inflammatory bowel disease (predominantly, but not exclusively Crohn's disease), trauma and surgical resection often in the setting of extensive abdominal adhesions, or very complex enteroatmospheric fistulae. Patients with non-reconstructible gastrointestinal tracts, often in the aftermath of surgical misadventure, constitute an important and possibly growing indication for ITx. About 25–30% of patients being considered for ITx have intestinal failure related to functional causes such as idiopathic pseudo-obstruction, other dysmotility syndromes, total intestinal aganglionosis, etc. In children, the major underlying causes of short bowel are necrotising enterocolitis and congenital anomalies, including gastroschisis and midgut volvulus. It should be noted that the precise aetiology leading to intestinal failure has only limited significance in the consideration of ITx, even if it might impact some technical considerations in operative planning. As ITx outcomes have steadily improved, especially over the last decade, the indications for ITx have expanded with ITx now being considered for quality of life reasons.

PRETRANSPLANT EVALUATION, PATIENT SELECTION AND INDICATIONS FOR INTESTINAL TRANSPLANT

First and foremost, pretransplant evaluation should include a process to confirm the necessity of permanent PN, i.e. to confirm irreversible intestinal failure. Maximum effort should be made to restore continuity of the gastrointestinal (GI) tract, recruit unused remnant bowel, attempt bowel lengthening procedures, if possible, and consider pharmacological treatment [4]. Once the patient is confirmed to have irreversible or refractory intestinal failure, the second critical step is to determine if ITx is justified, due to presence of PN-related complications or unacceptable quality of life on PN (**Figure 11.2**).

Historically, intestinal failure patients, who were stable on PN, were not considered ITx candidates unless there were life-threatening complications. ITx was justified only for intestinal failure patients suffering from PN-related life-threatening complications, such as repeated catheter-related sepsis, liver failure or loss of vascular access for central venous catheter placement. Recent improvements in patient survival after ITx provide an opportunity to revisit these classical indications. The Scientific Registry of Transplant Recipients (SRTR) annual report clearly demonstrates survival improvement for ITx in the US [2]. In the early 2000s, 1-year patient survival was 80%, but recent reports indicate almost 90% patient survival in isolated ITx. Some centres of excellence are consistently reporting over 90% survival in isolated ITx cases [4,5]. As the SRTR annual report illustrates, combined ITx, including a liver allograft, results in poorer patient survival than

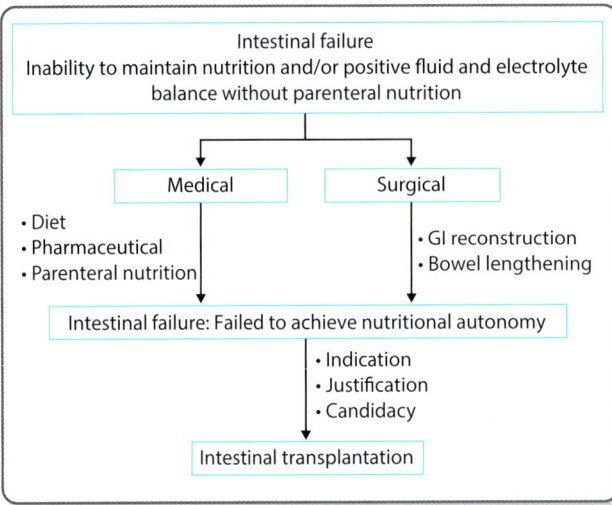

Figure 11.2 Intestinal rehabilitation and transplantation. Algorithm to treat intestinal failure patients and select intestinal transplantation candidates. GI, gastrointestinal.

isolated ITx. Therefore, early ITx before liver failure supervenes seems to be justifiable. Patients with ultra-short gut syndrome (SGS), who appear to have poor outcomes on PN and marked impairment of quality of life, are now often considered early for ITx before the onset of PN-related complications. The patient with a stapled-off duodenum or duodenostomy status after an abdominal catastrophe is extremely difficult to maintain on PN. This patient group is entirely different from most SGS patients, who are often stable and can enjoy a good quality of life on PN. Before further deterioration, such as renal failure supervenes, ITx can be performed in these ultra-SGS patients with the expectation of good clinical outcomes.

An important indication for ITx is non-resectable soft tissue tumours, such as desmoid tumours and mesenteric lymphangiomas at the root of the mesentery. Non-resectability of mesenteric root tumours is often determined by the relation of the tumour to the origin of the superior mesenteric artery, although in the case of very large desmoid tumours, it may also be related to diffuse encroachment of the tumour to the mesenteric border of the bowel, along its entire length. It is important to emphasise that early referral of such patients to ITx centres may allow more aggressive attempts at tumour resection, while preserving adequate bowel length, using techniques such as *ex-vivo* resection and autotransplantation, which is very much part of the transplant armamentarium. In such cases, having rapid access to allotransplantation is a critical prerequisite for success to achieve long-term survival with acceptable tumour recurrence rates. Tumour recurrences are predictably not in the allograft intestine and can be managed in most cases with suppressive medical treatment or limited surgical intervention.

There are also expanded indications for ITx unrelated to the presence of intestinal failure. MVT in liver cirrhosis, with complete portomesenteric thrombosis, was first reported in 2009 with good survival [5]. Since then, MVT has become standard practice to rescue liver cirrhosis patients who do not have a patent portomesenteric vein for liver transplantation. Including an intestinal allograft in this type of transplantation is not due to intestinal failure but for technical reasons, related to confluent portomesenteric venous thrombosis and lack of suitable portal venous inflow for successful isolated liver replacement. Even though the indication for transplantation in this subset of patients is end-stage liver failure, rather than intestinal failure, it is still classified as ITx conforming with the definition of ITx above.

DONOR SELECTION AND ORGAN RECOVERY

There has been limited progress in donor selection criteria or surgical techniques for organ recovery in the past 5 years, with a few exceptional advances. Since there is no biochemical marker to assess intestinal function, function of other organs such as the liver or kidney, donor hemodynamic status and acid-base balance are used as indirect proxies for preservation of intestine function and to identify suitable intestinal donors. A recent development in this area is the size match between the donor and recipient. A small graft is preferred for uncomplicated abdominal wall closure. More than a decade ago, abdominal wall transplantation was proposed to address the difficult issue of abdominal wall closure in some recipients, although this novel technique has not gained wide acceptance for several reasons [6]. There is no small-for-size syndrome in ITx, demonstrating that the donor-recipient weight ratio can go as low as 30% without affecting clinical outcomes, including achievement of nutritional autonomy [7]. Using an allograft from a smaller donor can facilitate abdominal wall closure and reduce the need for abdominal wall transplantation.

Organ recovery is always conceptualised as the successful procurement of an en-bloc composite graft. As described above, ITx can be performed with various types of allograft, depending on specific recipient pathology and circumstances. No matter which organs are included in the ITx graft, all organs are recovered as a single unit, with a technique that does not impact other solid organ recovery (**Figure 11.3**).

All types of intestinal allografts are recovered as an en-bloc organ based on vasculature.

A challenging situation occurs when intestine and pancreas have been allocated to separate recipients. The shared vascular anatomy in this scenario results in the intestinal

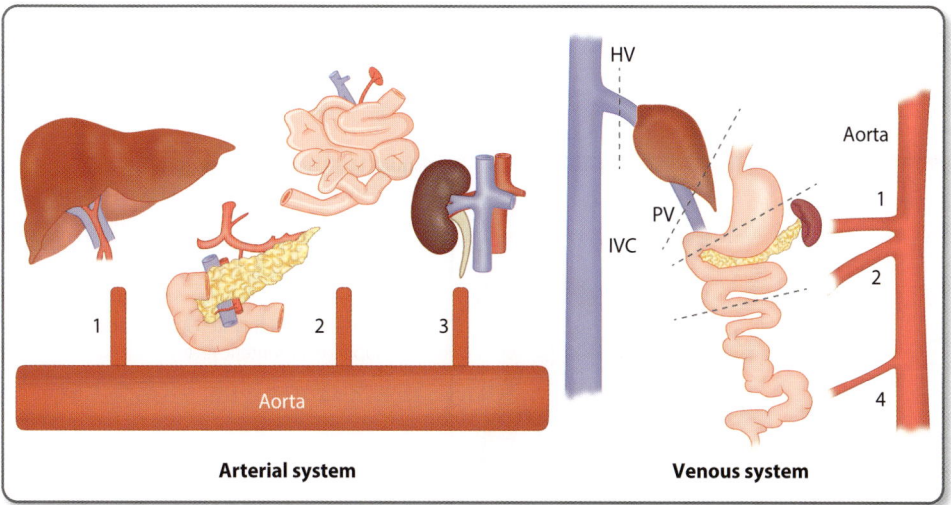

Figure 11.3 Concept of abdominal organ cluster. 1 – coeliac trunk; 2 – superior mesenteric artery; 3 – renal artery; 4 – inferior mesenteric artery. HV, hepatic veins; IVC, inferior vena cava; PV, portal vein.

graft having a shorter vascular stump, which necessitates extension vascular grafts on the superior mesenteric artery and vein, for safe vascular anastomoses. Recovery of vessels from the same donor at the time of intestinal procurement is critically important for possible vascular reconstruction. Donor iliac vessels and neck arteries provide excellent vascular grafts for arterial reconstruction (**Figure 11.4**).

The use of virtual crossmatch has become mandatory for the past 5 years, to avoid early onset of acute rejection related to the presence of preformed antibodies to donor antigens [8,9]. It has been reported that such donor-specific antibodies (DSAs) are strongly correlated with the development of acute rejection and poor graft survival [10]. Recent advances in immunologic tests, such as the single antigen bead assay, have given an opportunity to perform virtual crossmatch with relative ease. This test requires donor human leukocyte antigen (HLA) typing and recipient single antigen bead assay profiles. The virtual crossmatch can supplant the need for physical crossmatch, at the time of organ offer, since the latter can be challenging in ITx due to time constraints. A significant proportion of ITx candidates are highly sensitised to HLA antigens because of their past medical and surgical history, such as repeated transfusions or bloodstream infections. It has become standard practice to list unacceptable HLA antigens based on recipient single antigen bead assay profiles and to avoid a donor against whom the recipient demonstrates preformed anti-HLA antibodies, at the time of the virtual crossmatch. In addition to virtual crossmatch, there may be a role for desensitisation and attenuation of preformed antibodies in highly sensitised recipients [11]. However, more data is needed to confirm the effectiveness of desensitisation. These relatively new approaches suggest that avoiding and adopting approaches to manage DSA is a critically important strategy to improve clinical outcomes after ITx.

Until recently, HLA mismatch between the donor and recipient has not been considered a significant factor in donor selection, with no clear evidence that it impacts clinical outcome. However, there is an emerging view that HLA mismatch could be a risk factor for the clinical outcome of ITx. Recent improvements in survival after ITx, by avoiding other overwhelming risk factors, have provided an opportunity to re-examine the impact of HLA mismatch. It is hoped that further studies will reveal the correlation between clinical outcome and HLA mismatch and allow further improvements in immunological outcomes after ITx.

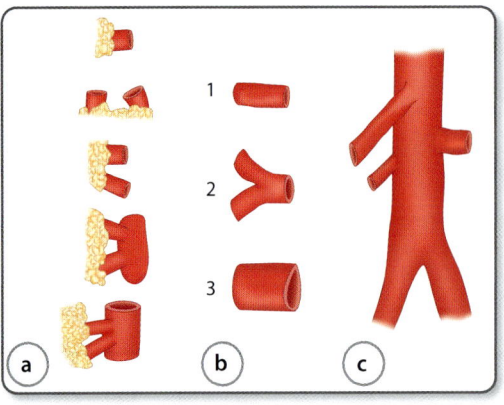

Figure 11.4 Various options for allograft arterial stump and arterial conduits. (a) Possible permutations of arterial pedicle stump on allograft. (b) Donor arterial conduits: 1 – donor iliac; 2 – donor brachiocephalic trunk; 3 – segment of donor aorta. (c) Recipient aorta with SMA and renal arteries. The allograft is usually implanted into infrarenal aorta. SMA, superior mesenteric artery.

SURGICAL PROCEDURE AND ANAESTHESIA

The basic surgical procedure for ITx has remained the same since its inception. The procedure can be divided into the following stages:
- Completion enterectomy (if necessary)
- Vascular anastomoses
- Gastrointestinal tract reconstruction
- Supplementary procedures – including stoma creation and abdominal wall closure.

The extent of completion enterectomy is determined by the recipient's GI anatomy. The purpose of completion enterectomy is to obtain adequate space for the intestinal allograft and to secure healthy and functional GI tract stumps for GI reconstruction. In cases of global GI dysmotility syndromes, it is ideal to remove as much of the native GI tract as possible, which usually includes partial gastrectomy, while retaining a short pancreaticobiliary pedicle and a short sigmoid colon. To preserve the native colon, attention needs to be given to preserving arterial inflow and venous outflow. However, it is not always possible to leave a long segment of the native colon when there is a failure to preserve these vascular structures.

Orthotopic transplantation is not always feasible, or safe, due to difficulties in identifying and preserving reasonable length and/or quality superior mesenteric artery and vein. As a result, many centres use the infrarenal aorta for arterial inflow. The mesenteric vein of the graft is typically drained into the recipient's inferior vena cava instead of the portal vein, which is not physiologic but is generally a safe procedure (**Figure 11.5**).

Systemic venous drainage can sometimes cause elevated serum ammonia and encephalopathy (akin to the situation with meso-caval shunts performed for portal hypertension). However, these issues can be easily controlled with conservative care, without further consequences that can impact clinical outcome [12]. The use of extension vascular conduits is common in facilitating vascular anastomoses without complications. Therefore, it is crucial to recover vascular grafts (artery and vein) during organ retrieval surgery, to enable safe and easy vascular anastomoses.

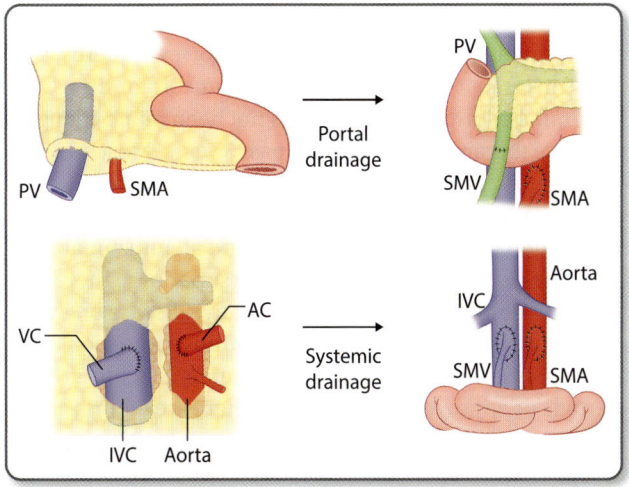

Figure 11.5 Portal and systemic drainage of intestinal allograft. Aorta, infrarenal aorta; IVC, inferior vena cava; PV, portal vein; SMA, superior mesenteric artery; SMV, superior mesenteric vein; VC, venous conduit from donor; AC, arterial conduit from donor.

The GI anastomosis in ITx follows general surgical principles. Compared to older techniques, the current trend is to simplify the procedure. Creating a stoma for frequent allograft surveillance used to be viewed as the gold standard but this concept has recently been challenged. There is evidence that ITx can be performed without stoma creation, which will be discussed further in the section below on graft surveillance [13,14].

Anaesthetic management during ITx has improved with increased understanding of the physiologic changes during the various ITx procedures. Significant haemodynamic derangement is rare, with postreperfusion syndrome occurring in <10% of cases. With accumulated experience in isolated ITx (i.e. liver-excluding), anaesthetic management is now standardised, without requiring the intensive resources required for liver transplantation [15].

APPLICATION OF INTESTINAL TRANSPLANTATION SURGICAL TECHNIQUE

The surgical techniques developed and refined for ITx have provided important options for treating pathologic lesions of the root of the mesentery. This surgical approach was first reported two decades ago and select centres have adopted it to treat these difficult problems [16]. After evisceration of the abdominal organs, including the pathologic lesion, the mesenteric root becomes approachable, and the lesion can then be safely removed *ex vivo* in a bloodless field. The ITx surgical technique then provides an opportunity for autotransplantation of the eviscerated abdominal organ, with the patient serving as his or her own intestinal donor.

IMMUNOSUPPRESSION

Unlike other solid organ transplantations, a standardised immunosuppressive protocol has not yet been established in the field of ITx. The relatively small number of ITx procedures is one of the major obstacles to studying and developing such a strategy. Immunosuppressive therapy after ITx is highly variable among individual centres and continues to diverge, as confirmed by recent reports [17]. There are sporadic reports of using new immunosuppressive agents in different clinical scenarios. However, there are not enough cases to achieve consensus in immunosuppressive protocols for the highly immunogenic intestinal allograft. Unfortunately, there has not been much change or improvement in immunosuppressive therapy after ITx in the past 5 years. Most ITx centres use induction immunosuppression with wide variation. Corticosteroids, antithymocyte globulin or interleukin-2 receptor blockers are the most common induction immunosuppressive therapies, in addition to rituximab, infliximab and alemtuzumab. However, it is not clear whether any one of the induction regimens is superior to the others in preventing acute rejection, post-transplant lymphoproliferative disease or graft versus host disease. Tacrolimus is the mainstay of maintenance immunosuppression, used mainly in combination with corticosteroids or mycophenolate mofetil. Acute rejection is treated with corticosteroids or antithymocyte globulin. There are reports of clinical experience using various combinations or new agents to treat refractory acute rejection [17–21]. However, fragmented experience of small numbers of cases prevents development of consensus opinions, or even standard best practices, in immunosuppressive management of ITx.

GRAFT SURVEILLANCE AND ACUTE REJECTION

Intestinal allografts are known to be highly immunogenic compared to other solid organ allografts. The incidence of acute rejection within the first year after ITx is reported to be around 35%; this has not changed for the past decade, despite advances in immunosuppression. Acute rejection is not only closely related to graft loss but also to mortality. If it is not diagnosed and treated in a timely manner, acute rejection remains one of the most important risk factors for adverse clinical outcomes after ITx. Since there is no reliable biochemical marker to assess intestinal function, frequent surveillance endoscopy and biopsy has traditionally been considered the only meaningful method for graft surveillance [22]. Each ITx centre has its own surveillance endoscopy protocol and, due to the frequency of endoscopy, the creation of a stoma for ease of access has been standard practice for ITx. More recent thinking suggests that such frequent routine surveillance endoscopy and biopsy may not confer a survival benefit and that endoscopy and biopsy for diagnosis only when symptoms, clinical signs or biochemical findings prompt investigation, may be sufficient to maintain graft survival [13]. This approach has resulted in a significant decrease in the number of endoscopies and biopsies performed after ITx, which calls into question the necessity of routine stoma creation during ITx [14].

Donor-specific antibodies have been shown to be a risk factor for the development of acute rejection [23,24]. As described above, virtual crossmatch has become a standard practice to select donors and avoid DSA-related acute rejection. An interesting feature that requires further study is the precise relationship between DSA and acute rejection. There are diagnostic criteria for antibody-mediated acute rejection but, most episodes of acute rejection in the setting of positive DSA do not fulfil these criteria and instead manifest as acute cellular rejection. The immunologic mechanisms which trigger acute cellular rejection, in the presence of positive DSA, merit further study [24,25]. Most cases of mild and moderate acute rejection can be treated with steroid boluses or antithymocyte globulin, regardless of the presence or absence of DSA. However, when acute rejection is severe, the risk of graft loss is high and, there is currently no uniformly effective treatment for severe acute rejection [26]. If there were innovations in the treatment of severe acute rejection, clinical outcomes would improve and ITx could become standard practice for treating patients with intestinal failure, even in the absence of PN-related complications.

POST-INTESTINAL TRANSPLANTATION MANAGEMENT AND CLINICAL OUTCOMES

Post-ITx management should focus on achieving nutritional autonomy with freedom from PN and improving the patient's quality of life, in addition to ensuring patient survival. To achieve these goals, physicians must understand the clinical behaviour of ITx patients and develop a monitoring strategy for recipients. It is convenient to divide post-transplant management into short- and long-term care, based on frequent clinical events at each stage. Unfortunately, ITx remains a rare form of solid organ transplantation and the post-transplant management experience is fragmented among centres.

The short-term period after ITx can be arbitrarily defined as the 1st year after the surgery, including the immediate post-transplant period. During this period, caregivers must pay attention to transplant surgery-related complications, organ-specific management, the development of acute rejection, immunosuppression and the pre-existing comorbidities of the recipients. ITx is essentially major abdominal surgery and it shares common postsurgical complications with other major laparotomy operations. In addition to these common surgical complications, ITx carries a few specific complications. Of these, vascular complications, which can have catastrophic consequences, are fortunately uncommon. Allograft arterial thrombosis is a typical example. When it occurs, graft loss is almost inevitable. However, early diagnosis and timely treatment can avoid mortality and provide an opportunity for a second transplant.

Another specific complication is abdominal cavity infection. Small bowel transplantation is a clean-contaminated operation, which raises the risk of abdominal infection after transplantation, particularly against a background of heavy immunosuppression. Moreover, transplant candidates usually have a history of multiple abdominal surgeries, resulting in ultimate intestinal failure. Many of these patients harbour occult abdominal sepsis secondary to the original pathology and repeated abdominal surgery. The best treatment is prevention. When a transplant candidate presents with significant abdominal infection, achieving source control of sepsis before considering transplantation is critical. This 'tidy-up-treatment' usually requires major abdominal surgery, which may also provide an opportunity to restore the continuity of the GI tract or to allow access to ITx in a well-optimised candidate. Inevitably, it has the unfortunate but still beneficial role of disqualifying some patients for ITx as described above.

Organ-specific management is mainly focussed on nutritional therapy. All recipients are on PN before transplant surgery, and the purpose of ITx is to switch from parenteral to enteral nutrition. However, it is not always an easy task due to cold ischaemia, reperfusion injury and surgical injury to the nervous and lymphatic system of the intestinal allograft. Transplanted small bowel often exhibits impaired peristalsis and poor absorption of long-chain fatty acids. Enteral feeding can be started with a low osmolality, low fat and low lactose diet. Tube feeding formula with medium-chain fatty acids is often recommended, where supplemental tube feeding is employed. High stoma output or frequent bowel movements with loose stool are common. Antidiarrhoeal agents, such as loperamide and diphenoxylate with atropine, are useful to avoid excessive volume and electrolyte loss. The development of chylous ascites is a short-term surgical complication, related to the disruption without reconstitution of the lymphatic system of the intestinal allograft. As enteral feeding advances, chylous ascites develops in 10–20% of recipients. Treatment involves stopping enteral feeding and resuming PN, which usually allows complete resolution in 2–4 weeks.

Patients usually have a complex medical and surgical history. Nearly all candidates suffer from malnutrition with macro- and micronutrient deficiencies. Careful assessment and customised management cannot be emphasised enough for a successful outcome after ITx. Optimal management of pre-existing comorbidities is an important factor for a successful ITx [27]. Long-term management after ITx typically involves medical care and requires extensive experience and a multidisciplinary approach. While most recipients achieve nutritional autonomy with freedom from PN and return to normal life after a year, maintaining a positive fluid and electrolyte balance can be challenging. If the recipient has a stoma, reversal should be considered to prevent unnecessary fluid loss, further exacerbating the risk of long-term chronic kidney injury. Chronic rejection can also cause fluid-electrolyte imbalances but its diagnosis requires a full-thickness biopsy, which involves challenging open abdominal surgery and transplant bowel resection. In cases of chronic rejection, a second ITx is currently the only solution. In addition, post-transplant lymphoproliferative disorder (PTLD), often related to infection with Epstein–Barr virus (EBV), is a concerning complication in long-term care, especially in children. Outcomes for PTLD post-ITx have improved considerably, related in part to improved ability to monitor for EBV-viraemia and improved modalities for customised treatment, based on the status of EBV, CD20 receptor and cell type, all while maintaining some immunosuppression to preserve the allograft.

Patient and graft survival after ITx have significantly improved over the decades. However, there has been no noticeable change in the past 5 years. Graft survival for younger recipients (under 18 years old) is slightly better than for adult recipients (18 years old or older). 1-year patient survival is superior in isolated ITx compared to liver-included ITx, at 86.4% and 75.2%, respectively, the gap narrowing to 61.2% and 58.1%, respectively, after 5 years [3]. Short-term survival has markedly improved. Further study and effort to improve long-term survival are needed. With >32 years of history, ITx has progressed beyond being standard of care for patients with intestinal failure who also have PN-failure. ITx has become a valuable life-saving therapy for patients who have suffered an abdominal catastrophe even in the absence of classically defined intestinal failure.

CONCLUSION

Intestinal transplantation has emerged as the standard of care for patients with intestinal failure who also suffer from life-threatening parenteral nutrition-related complications. The procedure may also be performed, albeit much less frequently for quality of life reasons. Intestinal transplant should be viewed as any transplant that includes the small intestine as part of a composite graft. It can hence be performed in different combinations of organs depending on the pathology and the residual anatomy. The technical procedures involved are now well characterised and can be performed in consistent fashion. Immune surveillance remains a challenge for a graft with a heavy immunologic burden at high risk of rejection. While short-term and medium-term outcomes are excellent, long term outcomes continue to lag behind those of other organ transplants.

Key points for clinical practice

- Intestinal transplantation refers to any transplantation procedure, which uses a visceral allograft that includes the small intestine
- Pretransplant evaluation should include a process to confirm irreversible intestinal failure.
- Intestinal transplantation may be justified due to presence of PN-related complications or unacceptable quality of life on PN
- The use of virtual crossmatch has become mandatory for the past 5 years to avoid early onset of acute rejection related to the presence of preformed antibodies to donor antigens.
- Intestinal allografts are known to be highly immunogenic compared to other solid organ allografts
- Acute rejection must be diagnosed and treated in a timely manner in order to prevent graft loss and/or mortality

REFERENCES

1. Grant D, Wall W, Mimeault R, et al. Successful small-bowel/liver transplantation. Lancet 1990; 335:181–184.
2. Organ Procurement and Transplantation Network. National data. Available from https://optn.transplant.hrsa.gov/data/view-data-reports/national-data/ [Last accessed 24 July 2025].
3. OPTN/SRTR. (2021). Annual Data Report: Intestine. Available from https://srtr.transplant.hrsa.gov/annual_reports/2021/Intestine.aspx. [Last accessed 24 July 2025]
4. Iyer K, Moon J. Adult intestinal transplantation in the United States. Curr Opin Organ Transplant 2020; 25:196–200.
5. Vianna R, Kubal C, Mangus R, et al. Intestinal and multivisceral transplantation at Indiana University: 6 years' experience with 100 cases. Clin Transpl 2009; 219–228.
6. Levi DM, Tzakis AG, Kato T, et al. Transplantation of the abdominal wall. Lancet 2003; 361:2173–2176.
7. Moon J, Schiano T, Burnham A, et al. Small-for-size syndrome does not occur in intestinal transplantation without liver containing grafts. Transplantation 2018; 102:1300–1306.
8. Cheng EY, DuBray BJ, Farmer DG. The impact of antibodies and virtual crossmatching on intestinal transplant outcomes. Curr Opin Organ Transplant 2017; 22:149–154.
9. Moon JI, Ko HM, Iyer KR. Enhanced virtual crossmatch in intestinal transplantation: association with outcomes and application in practice. Korean J Transplant 2021; 35:230–237.
10. Cheng EY, Everly MJ, Kaneku H, et al. Prevalence and clinical impact of donor-specific alloantibody among intestinal transplant recipients. Transplantation 2017; 101:873–882.
11. Santeusanio AD, Moon J, Nair V, et al. Is there a role for desensitization in intestinal transplantation? Prog Transplant 2019; 29:275–278.
12. Berney T, Kato T, Nishida S, et al. Portal versus systemic drainage of small bowel allografts: comparative assessment of survival, function, rejection, and bacterial translocation. J Am Coll Surg 2022; 195:804–813.
13. Moon J, Schiano TD, Iyer KR. Routine surveillance endoscopy and biopsy after isolated intestinal transplantation-Revisiting gold standard. Clin Transplant 2019; 33:e13684.
14. Moon J, Zhang H, Waldron L, et al. "Stoma or no stoma": first report of intestinal transplantation without stoma. Am J Transplant 2020; 20:3550–3557.
15. Zerillo J, Kim S, Hill B, et al. Anesthetic management for intestinal transplantation: a decade of experience. Clin Transplant 2017; 31:e13085.
16. Tzakis AG, Tryphonopoulos P, DeFaria W, et al. Partial abdominal evisceration, ex vivo resection, and intestinal autotransplantation for the treatment of pathologic lesions of the root of the mesentery. J Am Coll Surg 2033; 197:770–776.
17. Weiner J, Llore N, Ormsby D, et al The First Collective Examination of Immunosuppressive Practices Among American Intestinal Transplant Centers. Transplant Direct. 2023; 9:e1512.
18. Rao B, Jafri SM, Kazimi M, et al. A case report of acute cellular rejection following intestinal transplantation managed with Adalimumab. Transplant Proc 2016; 48:536–538.
19. Narang A, Xi D, Mitsinikos T, et al. Severe late-onset acute cellular rejection in a pediatric patient with isolated small intestinal transplant rescued with aggressive immunosuppressive approach: A case report. Transplant Proc 2019; 51:3181–3185.
20. Fujiwara S, Wada M, Kudo H, et al. Effectiveness of Bortezomib in a patient with acute rejection associated with an elevation of donor-specific HLA antibodies after small-bowel transplantation: Case report. Transplant Proc 2016; 48:525–527.
21. De Greef E, Avitzur Y, Grant D, et al. Infliximab as salvage therapy in paediatric intestinal transplant with steroid- and thymoglobulin-resistant late acute rejection. J Pediatr Gastroenterol Nutr 2012; 54:565–567.
22. Crismale JF, Mahmoud D, Moon J, et al. The role of endoscopy in the small intestinal transplant recipient: A review. Am J Transplant 2021; 21:1705–1712.
23. Cheng EY, Kaneku H, Farmer DG. The role of donor-specific antibodies in intestinal transplantation: Experience at the University of California Los Angeles and literature review. Clin Transpl 2014; 153–159.
24. Wozniak LJ, Venick RS. Donor-specific antibodies following liver and intestinal transplantation: Clinical significance, pathogenesis and recommendations. Int Rev Immunol 2019; 38:106–117.
25. Rumbo M, Oltean M. Intestinal transplant immunology and intestinal graft rejection: From basic mechanisms to potential biomarkers. Int J Mol Sci 2023; 24:4541–4558.
26. Huard G, Schiano T, Moon J, et al. Severe Acute Cellular Rejection after Intestinal Transplantation is Associated with Poor Patient and Graft Survival. Clin Transplant 2017; 31:e12956.
27. Sivaprakasam R, Hidenori T, Pither C, et al. Preoperative comorbidity correlates inversely with survival after intestinal and multivisceral transplantation in adults. J Transplant 2013; 202410.

Section 6

Vascular surgery

Chapter 12

Modern management of aortic dissection

Sven Tan, Richard White, W Rhodri Thomas, Mohamad Bashir, Ian Williams

ABSTRACT

Advances in surgical technology and perioperative care have revolutionised the management of aortic dissection in the modern era. Various classification systems for aortic dissection have been described, but the most commonly used is that of Stanford, where the site of the primary entry tear (proximal or distal to the origin of the left subclavian artery) defines type A or B, respectively. The gold-standard treatment for Stanford type A aortic dissection remains open surgical repair, despite the development of endovascular devices for use in the proximal aorta. Type B aortic dissection is now increasingly recognised as a dynamic and progressive disease process, with the use of pre-emptive endovascular repair in patients with uncomplicated disease increasing. Surgical repair of type B dissection is recommended primarily for younger patients and those with chronic disease or a connective tissue disorder.

INTRODUCTION

Aortic dissection (AD) represents a dynamic clinical entity that is associated with high mortality rates and is challenging to identify and treat. AD is characterised by the development of a tear in the aortic tunica intima, allowing pressurised blood to enter between intimal and medial layers. This creates a false lumen (FL) which runs adjacent to

---

Sven Tan MSc Student, Critical Care, William Harvey Research Institute, Queen Mary University of London, UK
E-mail: s.z.c.tan@smd19.qmul.ac.uk (for correspondence)

Richard White BSc (Medical Sciences) MBChB FRCR, Interventional Radiologist, University Hospital of Wales, Heath Park, Cardiff, UK
E-mail: Richard.White3@wales.nhs.uk (for correspondence)

W Rhodri Thomas FRCR, Interventional Radiologist, University Hospital of Wales, Heath Park, Cardiff, UK
E-mail: Wiliam.R.Thomas@wales.nhs.uk (for correspondence)

Mohamad Bashir MD PhD, Clinical Professor of Cardiovascular Surgery, Neurovascular Research Laboratory, Faculty of Life Sciences and Education, University of South Wales, UK
E-mail: Mohamad.bashir@southwales.ac.uk (for correspondence)

Ian Williams MD FRCS, Vascular Surgeon, University Hospital of Wales, Heath Park, Cardiff, UK
E-mail: i.williams250@btinternet.com (for correspondence)

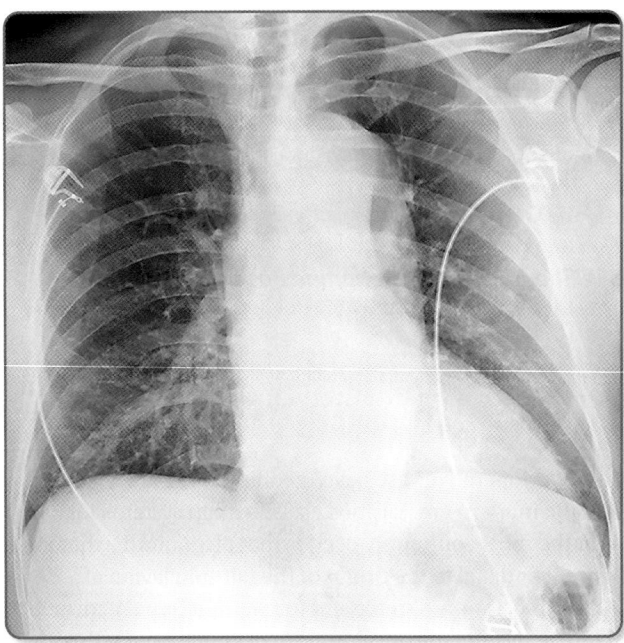

Figure 12.1 Chest X-ray showing widened mediastinum.

the true lumen (TL), separated by the dissection membrane. AD is, therefore, differentiated from other forms of acute aortic syndrome, such as penetrating atherosclerotic ulcer (PAU) or intramural haematoma (IMH), by the presence of a pressurised FL [1]. Continued perfusion of the FL results in its anterograde or retrograde propagation away from the primary tear site; this increases the risk of rupture, complications and mortality [1]. Unsurprisingly, patients with acute AD that suffer aortic rupture exsanguinate quickly and die before reaching hospital. The presentation is invariably with sudden onset severe chest pain, which is described as a tearing sensation. This can spread to the abdomen and lower back, depending on the propagation of the dissection flap. Other less common presentations include syncope, weakness in the legs or even stroke-like symptoms. Routine investigations may show a widened mediastinum (**Figure 12.1**) but for a definitive diagnosis, computed tomography is required.

CLASSIFICATION OF AORTIC DISSECTION

The location of the primary entry tear in AD determines the subsequent clinical evolution of the disease entity. Notably, the most proximal entry tear may not necessarily be the primary entry tear (e.g. in the case of retrograde dissection with distal re-entry tears) [1]. Various classifications for AD are used in literature and clinical practice; classically, the Stanford classification of AD is determined by the location of the primary entry tear and the regions of the aorta affected. The Stanford classification defines cases according to the location of the most proximal involvement. Stanford Type A dissections are those involving any part of the aorta proximal to the origin of the left subclavian artery (LSCA) and Type B dissections are those arising distal to the LSCA origin.

Another commonly used classification system is that of DeBakey, which separates the Stanford Type A into those affecting the ascending aorta only from those that cross the arch [2].

Other classification systems have divided the thoracic and abdominal aorta into 11 zones, 6 of which are within the thoracic cavity [3,4]. These are zones 0 to 5 and are invaluable in describing the area of the thoracic aorta, where a stent may be placed, and which vital branches might require coverage, to ensure a durable seal. This was published by the Society for Vascular Surgery (SVS) Ad Hoc Committee on thoracic endovascular aortic repair (TEVAR) reporting guidelines in 2010. AD acuity is described as acute (<2 weeks), subacute (2 weeks to 3 months) or chronic (>3 months) [1].

WHY IS AORTIC DISSECTION ASSOCIATED WITH HIGH MORTALITY RATES?

The incidence of acute AD varies considerably and is estimated to be between 3 and 16 cases per 1,00,000 individuals each year [1]. The Rochester Epidemiology Project suggested an overall age- and sex-adjusted incidence of acute aortic syndrome of 7.7 cases per 1,00,000 person-years; acute AD is the most common form of acute aortic syndrome [5]. The true incidence of AD is underestimated: an unknown number of patients die out-of-hospital from AD. Up to 7% of out-of-hospital cardiac arrests (OHCAs) are attributed to AD, and the mortality rate associated with OHCA due to AD is 100% [6].

Aortic rupture is a predominant complication of AD. Intimal-medial separation and formation of the perfused FL weaken the aortic wall considerably and predispose to unfavourable morphological changes (e.g. aneurysmal dilatation). Refractory systolic hypertension is a common finding in patients with acute AD: the increased hemodynamic shear force exerted on the weakened aortic wall predisposes to rupture [7].

Acute aortic valve regurgitation is the most common complication of AD involving the ascending aorta [1]. It is caused by detachment of the valve commissures from the aortic wall (due to retrograde separation of the intimal and medial layers), incomplete valve closure due to root dilatation or prolapse of the dissection membrane through the valve [1]. Even in the absence of aortic rupture, acute aortic regurgitation and pump failure increase the risk of mortality considerably.

Malperfusion syndrome is thought to occur in 40–50% of patients with AD and potentiates coronary, cerebral, spinal, visceral and lower body ischaemia [7]. Variable protrusion of the dissection membrane into the ostium of an aortic branch vessel, dependent on changes in FL pressurisation with the cardiac cycle, causes dynamic malperfusion of the downstream organ bed and, therefore, variable symptoms [8]. In contrast, static protrusion of the dissection membrane into the branch ostium causes thrombosis of the vessel, resulting in ischaemia of the branch's organ bed [8]. Visceral malperfusion syndromes are more commonly seen in AD affecting the descending thoracic aorta (DTA), while coronary malperfusion may be seen in ascending AD.

Type A

Stanford type A AD (TAAD) is analogous to DeBakey types I and II AD, referring to dissection of the ascending aorta with the primary entry tear located along the ascending aorta or aortic root (**Figure 12.2**) [9]. Acute TAAD is thought to carry the worst prognosis (approximately 1% mortality rate per hour) and typically warrants urgent open surgical repair (OSR). It should be noted that ascending AD, originating from an entry tear in the aortic arch or DTA, is referred to as retrograde type A thoracic

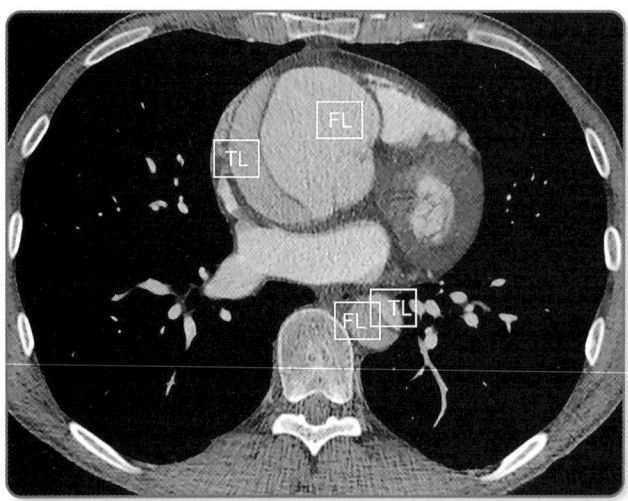

Figure 12.2 77-cm aortic root dilatation with type A aortic dissection which has propagated distally into the descending thoracic aorta. TL, true lumen; FL, false lumen.

AD (rather than TAAD) and carries a 2% attrition rate per hour, due to the likelihood of cardiac tamponade secondary to rupture or transudation, aortic regurgitation and malperfusion syndromes [1].

Type B

Stanford type B AD (TBAD) refers to dissection of the descending aorta with or without involvement of the abdominal aorta, in the absence of aortic arch or ascending aortic disease [1]. Acute TBAD is traditionally further subdivided into complicated (co-TBAD) and uncomplicated (un-TBAD) forms, depending on the presence or absence of refractory pain, refractory hypertension, early aortic expansion, malperfusion syndrome and signs of aortic rupture [10]. These criteria are, however, based on broad consensus rather than clinical evidence, and indeed factors such as refractory pain or hypertension both leave room for subjective interpretation. Un-TBAD can often be managed with conservative medical therapy, while co-TBAD typically requires endovascular or surgical repair [10].

Non-A non-B

Non-A non-B AD refers to aortic arch dissection without ascending aortic involvement and is further subdivided into descending-entry type if the entry tear is distal to the LSCA or arch-entry type if the entry tear is between the LSCA and innominate artery (IA) [11]. This subgroup of AD is uncommon and associated with a high risk of rupture, evolution to retrograde type A thoracic AD, and end-organ malperfusion.

Stanford type A aortic dissection

Up to 66% of AD cases are Stanford type A. Acute TAAD represents a challenging surgical emergency [12]. The risk of mortality associated with acute TAAD increases by 1–2% each hour. Nonoperative management of acute TAAD is associated with a 60% mortality rate [9]. Key complications of acute TAAD include aortic rupture, cardiac tamponade, aortic regurgitation and malperfusion. Notably, the definitive operative management of acute TAAD (the current gold-standard) is itself also associated with high mortality and morbidity rates; complications such as stroke, spinal cord injury (SCI), recurrent laryngeal nerve (RLN) palsy and renal dysfunction are common [13].

Surgical management

Open surgical repair of acute TAAD is life-saving and remains the gold-standard treatment [9]. The rationale behind OSR is to exclude the primary entry tear, prevent continued FL pressurisation, induce FL thrombosis, ensure visceral perfusion and promote positive TL remodelling. OSR is maximally invasive and is associated with a rising turn-down rate, as patients are declared unfit for OSR given the need for cardiopulmonary bypass (CPB) and hypothermic circulatory arrest (HCA) [14]. Notably, some patients with retrograde type A thoracic AD may be treated definitively with TEVAR of the DTA [1]. Similarly, patients who have suffered iatrogenic catheter induced TAAD limited to the aortic, root may be treated with nonoperative management [1].

There exists a spectrum of approaches to the surgical repair of the ascending aorta, such as ascending-only 'limited' replacement, hemiarch reconstruction (HAR) and total arch reconstruction (TAR). However, there have hitherto been no randomised controlled trials (RCTs) evaluating the efficacies of each technique; the decision to undertake limited or extensive aortic arch reconstruction is chiefly informed by patient characteristics and disease extent [9].

Perioperative care

The use of CPB and HCA in proximal aortic surgery afford the surgeon a bloodless operative field, while simultaneously protecting the brain and viscera against hypoxic damage [15]. Cannulation strategies for instituting CPB vary considerably between patient, surgeon and centre; femoral, axillary or innominate cannulations are the most common [9]. Following the initiation of CPB, the circuit is cooled to the desired temperature [≤24°C for deep HCA (DHCA), or ≥24°C for moderate HCA], in addition to topical cooling of the head with packed ice. Core temperature is monitored via a probe in the urinary bladder. Adjunctive cerebral perfusion techniques, such as antegrade cerebral perfusion (ACP), retrograde cerebral perfusion (RCP) or integrated cerebral perfusion, are employed to protect the brain during intervals of circulatory arrest [15]. These involve cannulation of the arterial supply (in ACP) or venous outflow (in RCP) of the brain. The brain can then be perfused with oxygenated blood in isolation, once HCA is established.

There is currently no consensus on the optimal approach to neuroprotection in aortic arch surgery. A 2023 review found that DHCA alone, though associated with favourable short-term outcomes in cases where the duration of HCA did not exceed 30 minutes, was associated with an increased risk of perioperative stroke and mortality, when HCA duration exceeded 30 minutes [16]. DHCA without ACP or RCP has been identified as a risk factor for perioperative stroke and is associated with poorer long-term survival rates compared to DHCA plus ACP or RCP and is no longer recommended for the operative treatment of TAAD [17,18]. There exists limited evidence to suggest the superiority of RCP or ACP over the other [16]. Prospective investigations remain scarce and limited by their small cohort size. Both techniques are, therefore, endorsed by the American Association for Thoracic Surgery [16]. ACP has established itself among European centres, as it can be used in conjunction with moderate HCA (leading to shorter rewarming and overall CPB durations), the brain is perfused in the physiological anterograde manner and RCP has been associated with limited benefits for longer (> 60 minutes) cases [9].

Limited aortic arch repair

In cases where the primary entry tear is isolated to the ascending aorta, replacement thereof with a vascular graft proximally anastomosed to the sinotubular junction is performed [1]. Depending on whether the entry tear extends to the aortic arch, the surgeon may opt to extend the distal anastomosis by performing a bevelled anastomosis, or hemiarch replacement [9]. The distal anastomosis may be strengthened with a multilayer reconstruction using felt or by buttressing with folded redundant adventitia. A high-quality suture line is crucial for preventing new intimal tears, postoperative bleeding and to ensure durability [9]. Open distal anastomosis, under CPB and HCA, has been associated with improved survival outcomes and aortic remodelling than clamped distal anastomosis [19,20]. However, clamped distal anastomosis without HCA may be preferred at lower-volume centres [9].

Isolated replacement of the ascending aorta may be sufficient in patients with functional aortic valves and normal aortic root diameters. Patients with aortic root dilatation, coronary artery ostial involvement or aortic valve dysfunction usually require a concomitant Bentall procedure [1]. However, valve-sparing root replacement should be considered in patients <50 years old with root dilatation [21].

Patients undergoing limited aortic arch repair for TAAD may require complex reoperation in the future. Hemiarch repair has been associated with significantly better freedom from reintervention rates at 10 years than ascending-only repair [22]. The question of balancing the risks and benefits associated with limited versus extended repair, therefore, remains a topic of debate.

Extended aortic arch repair

Extended aortic arch repair may be indicated in patients with TAAD, wherein the primary tear extends beyond that which would be replaced by HAR, when such intervention would not fully restore physiological TL flow, or in the case of non-A non-B AD. Extended repair should also be considered in patients with malperfusion syndromes, or in younger patients with connective tissue disorders (e.g. Marfan syndrome) [23]. Extended repair in acute TAAD typically refers to total arch replacement (TAR), which involves complete resection of the ascending aorta and arch, with either complete or partial arch vessel debranching and reimplantation.

The frozen elephant trunk (FET) technique is the preeminent form of TAR and involves the use of a specialised two-part endoprosthesis comprised of a proximal portion, designed for replacement of the ascending aorta and arch and a distal stented portion, intended for insertion into the remaining native DTA, past the distal anastomosis. The distal 'frozen' stent-graft promotes favourable downstream aortic remodelling and facilitates hybrid TEVAR for complete stabilisation of the DTA [13]. Additionally, occlusion or dissection of the arch vessels may not be relieved by limited aortic arch repair, whereas TAR provides a useful platform for arch branch reconstruction and secondary TEVAR [24,25]. Thrombosis of the FL occurs in up to 85% of patients post-FET [26]. Furthermore, the use of a continuous arch graft and distal stent-graft eliminates the risk of endoprosthesis migration and type I endoleak.

The surgical technique of the FET procedure is discussed at length in the literature [24,27,28]. Once anaesthetic preparations are complete, access is gained via median sternotomy and the desired vessels are cannulated. A femoral guidewire may be positioned in the DTA to aid identification of the TL [28]. CPB, cardioplegia, hypothermia and the chosen cerebral perfusion method are instituted, and the patient is heparinised. The diseased portion of the aorta is then resected and the aortic root and DTA are inspected. Concomitant repair to the aortic root or valve may be performed [27,29]. The stent-graft of the FET endoprosthesis is then advanced, anterograde, down the remaining distal aorta, with care taken to ensure TL patency and dissection membrane integrity. The distal anastomosis site may vary between patient, centre and surgeon; it can be performed distal to the LSCA, along the aortic arch, or at the level of the IA take-off [24]. Most commercially available FET endoprostheses feature a dedicated cuff positioned between the proximal graft and stent-graft, to facilitate distal anastomosis [13]. Following distal anastomosis, the arch vessels are reimplanted via the island technique or to the endoprosthesis' branches (devices with adjustable branch arm length simplify challenging LSCA anastomosis) [13]. Some FET devices feature a dedicated fourth branch to allow reperfusion of the lower body, after distal anastomosis [13]. Proximal anastomosis can then be completed. It is crucial to meticulously de-air the endoprosthesis following each anastomosis. Following implantation of the FET device, the patient may be rewarmed, circulation restarted and protamine administered.

The FET procedure is known to be associated with longer CPB durations than most cardiac surgical procedures. Tan et al. (2022) reported average CPB and DHCA durations of 202 ± 72 and 69 ± 50 minutes respectively in their series of 931 patients treated with the Thoraflex Hybrid endoprosthesis (Terumo Aortic, Scotland, UK) [13]. Over 30,000 hybrid TAR procedures involving FET devices have been carried out [30]. Early mortality ranges from 1.5 to 17.2% across various devices and centres [30]. Long-term outcomes following the FET procedure are also favourable: Tan et al. (2022) reported a 94% event-free survival rate at 84 months postoperative [11]. Multicentre studies have shown that extensive FL thrombosis can be achieved in up to 85% of patients following FET, and that neurological complication rates can be as low as 1.9% [13,26].

However, the risks associated with prolonged CPB and HCA durations should be considered carefully before proceeding with TAR. Additionally, stenting of the DTA is associated with a risk of SCI, with more extensive stenting increasing the risk thereof significantly.

Endovascular management of type A aortic dissection

Given the invasiveness and physiologically demanding nature of open TAR, the turn-down rate associated therewith is as high as 40% and continues to increase [14]. TEVAR of the ascending aorta and aortic arch represents a promising alternative treatment for patients deemed unsuitable for open TAR. Aortic arch TEVAR would, in comparison, be minimally invasive (requiring only femoral access) and conducted under general anaesthesia, without the need for CPB or HCA. Endografts purpose-built for on-label use in the aortic arch are now available [31,32]. Fenestrations, branches or chimneys are used to ensure patency of the arch vessels, and many such endografts, such as the RELAY Branched series (Terumo Aortic, Scotland, UK), are custom-made to maximise the likelihood of technical success [31].

Aortic arch TEVAR should be avoided in patients with unfavourable anatomy. Such contraindications include primary entry tears within 20 mm of the sinotubular junction, lack of suitable access vessels, proximal landing zone diameter <38 mm, aortic valve involvement and the presence of coronary artery bypass grafts anastomosed to the ascending aorta [14,33].

The mediolateral and anteroposterior curvatures of the aortic arch and DTA may inhibit torque control over guidewires; buddy wires or through-and-through catheterisation may, therefore, be required [34]. The risk of endograft misalignment or malorientation is also greater than in traditional TEVAR, as the windsock effect is most pronounced under the maximal hemodynamic pressures of the ascending aorta [35]. Intraluminal instrumentation, or the manipulation of diseased proximal aorta, also presents a risk of particulate embolisation or arch vessel coverage – this risk is greater in patients with more proximal landing zones [31]. Care must be taken not to cause extension of the dissection into the arch vessels, as this may cause static or dynamic cerebral malperfusion.

Early data on the use of aortic arch TEVAR is promising, with multicentre analyses from Europe reporting 2.7% mortality, 4.1% disabling stroke, 5.4% non-disabling stroke and 19.6% reintervention rates [31]. Additionally, technical success rates of 99.3% have been reported, with 80.2% of patients exhibiting target vessel patency 24 months postoperative [32].

Medical management of type A aortic dissection

Optimal medical therapy (OMT) is not a substitute for curative surgery in TAAD. Rather, its role is to optimise patients with TAAD for theatre by decreasing as much as possible the hemodynamic shear force exerted on the dissection membrane [9]. This serves to reduce FL pressurisation and the risk of rupture. Initial medical therapy should be informed by each patient's clinical presentation, and complications (e.g. aortic regurgitation or malperfusion syndrome) should be alleviated where possible.

Anti-impulse therapy involves optimising heart rate, blood pressure and maximal changes in left ventricular (LV) pressure (also termed dP/dt_{max}) during systole [36]. α- and β-blockers are commonly used to achieve hemodynamic optimisation (blood pressure ≤120/80 mmHg, heart rate <70 beats/min), with angiotensin-converting enzyme inhibitors, angiotensin receptor antagonists and dihydropyridine calcium channel blockers available as alternatives [10]. Notably, a similar approach is taken to the medical management of un-TBAD (Section 3).

Stanford type B aortic dissection

Type B AD refers to dissection of the distal thoracic aorta (DTA) with or without involvement of the abdominal aorta. Importantly, the aortic arch and ascending aorta are unaffected (**Figure 12.3**). TBAD is less common than TAAD and may sometimes follow a comparatively benign clinical course, requiring only medical therapy [1]. The management of TBAD depends largely on whether the dissection is considered complicated or uncomplicated – misdiagnosing co-TBAD as un-TBAD may have disastrous consequences.

Classification of acute type B aortic dissection

The classification of acute TBAD into co- and un-TBAD represents an area of ongoing debate. Current SVS and Society of Thoracic Surgeons (STS) guidelines (from 2020 and 2021 respectively) define TBAD as complicated when occurring in the presence of clinically or radiologically apparent aortic rupture or malperfusion syndrome [37]. This distinction provides a binary view of what is a dynamic and progressive disease entity. Current guidelines recommend that patients with co-TBAD undergo TEVAR, while patients with un-TBAD be managed conservatively, with anti-impulse therapy [5]. This begs the question how best are patients, not definitely complicated or uncomplicated, treated?

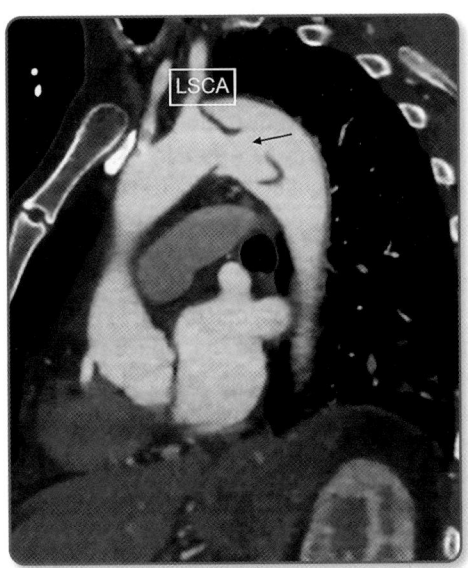

Figure 12.3 Computerised tomogram of a 54-year-old man presenting with acute chest pain. This shows a type B aortic dissection with the entry tear just distal to the origin of the left subclavian artery. LSCA, left subclavian artery; arrow, entry tear.

Additionally, the SVS and STS guidelines point to a third group of 'high-risk' un-TBAD patients, who exhibit clinical features suggestive of imminent deterioration, development of malperfusion syndrome and aortic rupture (i.e. progression to co-TBAD) [7]. Bashir et al. (2023) have defined these as – maximal aortic diameter >40 mm, FL diameter >22 mm, single entry tears >10 mm, primary entry tears proximal to the LSCA and a free-floating TL [38]. Whether patients with 'high-risk' un-TBAD (without malperfusion syndrome or aortic rupture) would benefit from early TEVAR is a question widely investigated and discussed in the literature. The landmark ADSORB trial found that early TEVAR (in addition to anti-impulse therapy) led to improved aortic remodelling (decreased maximal FL diameters and higher FL thrombosis rates), compared to OMT alone [39]. Similarly, the INSTEAD trial argued that early TEVAR in un-TBAD led to a reduction in aortic event-related mortality, disease progression and improved FL thrombosis rates compared to anti-impulse therapy alone, despite there being no significant difference in all-cause mortality [40]. Research into the use of biomarkers, such as monocyte to high-density lipoprotein cholesterol ratio, to identify patients with un-TBAD that would benefit from pre-emptive TEVAR, is ongoing [38].

Optimal medical therapy for type B aortic dissection

Anti-impulse therapy is the initial treatment plan for un-TBAD not at risk of deterioration to co-TBAD and is described above. A stepwise approach to the management of un-TBAD, which ensures identification of the primary entry tear, status of the LSCA, aortic dimensions and excluding organ malperfusion or imminent rupture, is crucial [7]. Once hemodynamic optimisation is achieved and the patient is successfully stabilised, follow-up imaging and assessment postdischarge is essential [7].

Endovascular repair for type B aortic dissection

Thoracic endovascular aortic repair is the mainstay treatment for TBAD in patients with favourable anatomy, for whom medical management alone would be insufficient

(**Figure 12.4**). TEVAR is efficacious in achieving rupture control, entry tear exclusion, restoration of TL flow, FL obliteration and in reducing visceral ischaemic time (in addition to being far less invasive and associated with fewer short-term mortalities and complications than OSR) [7]. In 2013, the US Food and Drug Administration expanded the indications for TEVAR to include traumatic aortic transection and TBAD [41].

Preoperative planning involves thorough imaging assessment of the landing zone, thoracic aortic tortuosity, coverage length, LSCA involvement and access sites, to ensure anatomical compatibility with TEVAR. For example, 20 mm of healthy aortic wall either side of the endograft and a TL diameter between 16 and 42 mm are usually required [41]. Patients with challenging anatomy may be treated with scalloped, fenestrated or branched endografts (or considered for OSR), and brachiofemoral through-and-through guidewire access may also be used. The use of physician-modified grafts is increasing, as these are especially useful in cases where the landing zone is suboptimal [41]. Patients with atherosclerotic or tortuous iliofemoral arteries may require preoperative balloon angioplasty to treat any stenosis prior to stent deployment [41].

The predominant complications of TEVAR are SCI, stroke, endoleak and access site injury. Both TEVAR and OSR are associated with a similar incidence of SCI of around 2–10%, which is primarily the result of inadequate collateral perfusion of the spinal cord, secondary to intercostal artery coverage or atheroembolism of aortic plaques to the segmental arteries [39,41]. More extensive DTA coverage by the endograft is also associated with a greater risk of SCI [42]. Prevention methods include mean arterial pressure optimisation, lumbar cerebrospinal fluid drainage and intrathecal papaverine [43].

The incidence of postoperative stroke ranges from 1.2 to 8.2% and may occur due to manipulation of the aortic arch, causing particulate embolism or a reduction in global cerebral perfusion due to aortic coverage (e.g. coverage of the LSCA without preoperative

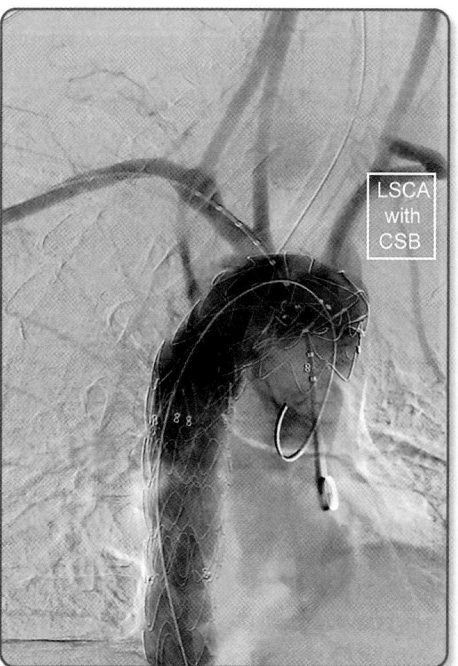

Figure 12.4 Thoracic stent graft placed in zone 2 occluding the origin of the LSCA. A left CSB has been performed. A plug was subsequently inserted into the LSCA proximal to the origin of the VA. LSCA, left subclavian artery; CSB, carotid subclavian bypass; VA, vertebral artery.

extra-anatomical bypass), perioperative hypotension or prolonged operative duration [31,44]. Screening patients for a dominant left vertebral artery, routine preoperative LSCA revascularisation and the use of fenestrated, scalloped or branched endografts serve to reduce the risk of TEVAR-induced stroke [45].

Endoleak refers to continued pressurisation of the diseased aortic segment, despite placement of an endograft. Reintervention is invariably the treatment for an endoleak, while percutaneous methods are typically effective, open surgical reoperation may be required. Type II endoleak – where the diseased segment is perfused by retrograde flow from a branch vessel – is the most common form of endoleak associated with TEVAR [46]. Type I endoleak results from inadequate proximal (Ia) or distal (Ib) sealing. Type III and IV endoleaks result from graft defects and graft porosity respectively – these have now become rare complications due to advances in endograft material [41].

Vascular access remains a limiting factor for patient eligibility, even though this can be modified by preoperative balloon angioplasty, predominantly of the iliac arteries. Preoperative assessment of iliofemoral artery morphology and ankle-brachial pressure index are essential [41]. Early complications such as arterial dissection, rupture, perforation or distal embolisation may warrant rapid conversion to OSR.

Open surgical repair for type B aortic dissection

The popularity of OSR for TBAD has declined in favour of percutaneous, minimally invasive and endovascular alternatives. However, OSR remains a viable option for patients with co-TBAD that are anatomically unsuitable for TEVAR, patients with un-TBAD and predictors of poor outcomes, younger patients (OSR is associated with less late aneurysmal changes) and patients with chronic dissection with late malperfusion syndromes [47,48]. Most frequently, OSR is indicated in chronic TBAD: TEVAR for chronic TBAD is associated with more variable aortic remodelling rates than acute TBAD, notably TEVAR has been demonstrated to not reduce aortic rupture risk or increase life expectancy in chronic TBAD [48]. In contrast, OSR totally ameliorates the risk of aneurysm-related death in chronic TBAD, by entirely replacing the diseased segment of aorta [48].

The surgical technique for OSR in TBAD varies considerably depending on the extent and nature of disease, patient-specific characteristics, local practice and surgeon preference. For example, Trimarchi et al. (2006) evaluated the clinical outcomes of 82 patients undergoing TBAD OSR in 2006 and reported that 69.3% of patients underwent descending aortic replacement, 20.6% underwent partial arch replacement, 9% received concomitant visceral or iliac artery stenting and 48% of patients required HCA [49].

Modern surgical techniques and improvements in perioperative care have led to better postoperative mortality and morbidity rates in OSR for TBAD. A 2014 systematic review of contemporary and historical series reported a pooled 11.1% 30-day mortality rate [48]. The incidences of postoperative stroke, SCI, renal dysfunction and reintervention were 5.6%, 4.9%, 11.9% and 9.9%, respectively. Contemporary series also demonstrated significantly improved reintervention rates and medium-term outcomes [48].

Although TEVAR is associated with better short-term procedural outcomes in TBAD than OSR, it should be noted that successful OSR eliminates the risk of unfavourable late aortic remodelling in the repaired segment and may, therefore, represent a more suitable option for younger patients, or those with connective tissue disorders. Furthermore, in the endovascular era, patients who ultimately undergo OSR for TBAD are very likely to have more extensive disease – 48.5% of patients in the aforementioned systematic review required thoracoabdominal (rather than simply thoracic) repair [48].

CONCLUSION

The advances in imaging techniques and endovascular intervention has meant the treatment of AD has changed over the last 30 years. For TBAD (after initial blood pressure and pain control) close attention to the imaging performed and subtle changes can change the treatment options. This has meant there are three categories for TBAD: complicated, uncomplicated and high risk. The place of TEVAR for the latter two categories remains uncertain as does the timing and optimum length of coverage of the aorta.

For TAAD open surgery remains the gold standard though there have been stent grafts used with strict adherence to morphological criteria. The treatment of ascending aortic and non-A non-B AD has seen the development of branched thoracic grafts enabling the arch vessels to be perfused avoiding extra-anatomical bypass. Future aortic dilatation is common and the use of FET have enabled landing zones to be used in the future thus avoiding redo surgery and left thoracotomy. All patients with AD need careful radiological assessment mindful of the fact changes to the aorta can occur rapidly. Many patients with AD will have connective tissue disorders such as Marfans and Ehlers Danlos syndrome where open surgery may be appropriate for optimum long term results.

Key points for clinical practice

- The classification of AD is yet to be standardised – while the Stanford classification is widely used, other systems have been recently employed
- Aortic dissection a deadly disease due to malperfusion syndrome, valvular dysfunction and aortic rupture
- Type A dissection most often requires surgical intervention, while type B dissection can be managed medically or via endovascular repair
- The medical management of type A dissection essentially serves as a 'bridge' to definitive, life-saving surgical repair
- Patients presenting with uncomplicated type B dissection may be at a high risk of deterioration and, therefore, could benefit from being managed as 'complicated TBAD' patients
- Open surgical repair of TBAD is effective for chronic TBAD, younger patients and patients with connective tissue disorders, as it ameliorates the risk of late aortic changes
- Anti-impulse therapy, stabilisation and close follow-up with serial imaging are sufficient for patients with uncomplicated type B AD without any high-risk features

REFERENCES

1. Carrel T, Sundt TM, von Kodolitsch Y, et al. Acute aortic dissection. Lancet 2023; 401:773–788.
2. DeBakey ME, Henly WS, Cooley DA, et al. Surgical management of dissecting aneurysms of the aorta. J Thorac Cardiovasc Surg 1965; 49:130–149.
3. Fillinger MD, Greenberg RK, McKinsey JF, et al. Society for Vascular Surgery Ad Hoc Committee on TEVAR Reporting Guidelines. Reporting standards for thoracic endovascular aortic repair (TEVAR). J Vasc Surg 2010; 52:1022–1033.
4. Upchurch GR, Escobar GA, Azizzadeh A, et al. Society for Vascular Surgery clinical practice guidelines of thoracic endovascular aortic repair for descending thoracic aortic aneurysms. J Vasc Surg 2021; 73:55S–83S.

5. DeMartino RR, Sen I, Huang Y, et al. Population-based assessment of the incidence of aortic dissection, intramural hematoma, and penetrating ulcer, and its associated mortality from 1995 to 2015. Circulation 2018; 11:e004689.
6. e Melo RG, Machado C, Caldeira D, et al. Incidence of acute aortic dissections in patients with out of hospital cardiac arrest: A systematic review and meta-analysis of observational studies. IJC Heart Vasc 2022; 38:100934.
7. MacGillivray TE, Gleason TG, Patel HJ, et al. The Society of Thoracic Surgeons/American Association for Thoracic Surgery clinical practice guidelines on the management of type B aortic dissection. J Thorac Cardiovasc Surg 2022; 163:1231–1249.
8. Crawford TC, Beaulieu RJ, Ehlert BA, et al. Malperfusion syndromes in aortic dissections. Vasc Med 2016; 21:264–273.
9. Malaisrie SC, Szeto WY, Halas M, et al. 2021 The American Association for Thoracic Surgery expert consensus document: surgical treatment of acute type A aortic dissection. J Thorac Cardiovasc Surg 2021; 162:735–758.
10. Tadros RO, Tang GH, Barnes HJ, et al. Optimal treatment of uncomplicated type B aortic dissection: JACC review topic of the week. J Am Coll Cardiol 2019; 74:1494–1504.
11. Rylski B, Pérez M, Beyersdorf F, et al. Acute non-A non-B aortic dissection: incidence, treatment and outcome. Eur J Cardiothorac Surg 2017; 52:1111–1117.
12. Evangelista A, Isselbacher EM, Bossone E, et al. Insights from the international registry of acute aortic dissection: a 20-year experience of collaborative clinical research. Circulation 2018; 137:1846–1860.
13. Tan SZ, Jubouri M, Mohammed I, et al. What is the long-term clinical efficacy of the Thoraflex™ hybrid prosthesis for aortic arch repair? Front Cardiovasc Med 2022; 9:12.
14. Nordon IM, Hinchliffe RJ, Morgan R, et al. Progress in endovascular management of type A dissection. Eur J Vasc Endovasc Surg 2012; 44:406–410.
15. Tan SZ, Singh S, Austin NJ, et al. Duration of Deep Hypothermic Circulatory Arrest (DHCA) for aortic arch surgery: is it a myth, fiction, or scientific leap? J Cardiovasc Surg 2022; 63:243–253.
16. Pitts L, Kofler M, Montagner M, et al. Cerebral Protection Strategies and Stroke in Surgery for Acute Type A Aortic Dissection. J Clin Med 2023; 12:2271.
17. Czerny M, Fleck T, Zimpfer D, et al. Risk factors of mortality and permanent neurologic injury in patients undergoing ascending aortic and arch repair. J Thorac Cardiovasc Surg 2003; 126:1296–1301.
18. Wiedemann D, Kocher A, Dorfmeister M, et al. Effect of cerebral protection strategy on outcome of patients with Stanford type A aortic dissection. J Thorac Cardiovasc Surg 2013; 146:647–655.e1.
19. Lawton JS, Liu J, Kulshrestha K, et al. The impact of surgical strategy on survival after repair of type A aortic dissection. J Thorac Cardiovasc Surg 2015; 150:294–301.
20. Malvindi PG, Modi A, Miskolczi S, et al. Open and closed distal anastomosis for acute type A aortic dissection repair. Interact Cardiovasc Thorac Surg 2016; 22:776–783.
21. Rosenblum JM, Leshnower BG, Moon RC, et al. Durability and safety of David V valve-sparing root replacement in acute type A aortic dissection. J Thorac Cardiovasc Surg 2019; 157:14–23.
22. Moon MR, Sundt III TM, Pasque MK, et al. Does the extent of proximal or distal resection influence outcome for type A dissections? Ann Thorac Surg 2001; 71:1244–1249.
23. Larsen M, Trimarchi S, Patel HJ, et al. Extended versus limited arch replacement in acute Type A aortic dissection. Eur J Cardiothorac Surg 2017; 52:1104–1110.
24. Tan SZ, Lopuszko A, Munir W, et al. Aortic proximalization—Zone 0 versus Zone 2: A concept or true challenge?. J Cardiac Surg 2021; 36:3319–3325.
25. Hostalrich A, Porterie J, Boisroux T, et al. Outcomes of Secondary Endovascular Aortic Repair After Frozen Elephant Trunk. J Endovasc Ther 2025; 32:148–158.
26. Shrestha M, Bachet J, Bavaria J, et al. Current status and recommendations for use of the frozen elephant trunk technique: a position paper by the Vascular Domain of EACTS. Eur J Cardiothorac Surg 2015; 47:759–769.
27. Yamamoto H, Kadohama T, Yamaura G, et al. Total arch repair with frozen elephant trunk using the "zone 0 arch repair" strategy for type A acute aortic dissection. J Thorac Cardiovasc Surg 2020; 159:36–45.
28. Leone A, Di Marco L, Coppola G, et al. Open distal anastomosis in the frozen elephant trunk technique: initial experiences and preliminary results of arch zone 2 versus arch zone 3. Eur J Cardiothorac Surg 2019; 56:564–571.
29. Jakob H, Shehada SE, Dohle D, et al. New 3-zone hybrid graft: first-in-man experience in acute type I dissection. J Thorac Cardiovasc Surg 2022; 163:568–574.
30. Leone A, Murana G, Coppola G, et al. Frozen elephant trunk—the Bologna experience. Ann Cardiothorac Surg 2020; 9:220.

31. Tan SZ, Surkhi AO, Singh S, et al. Favorable neurological outcomes in thoracic endovascular aortic repair with RELAY™ branched—An international perspective. J Cardiac Surg 2022; 37:3556–3563.
32. Singh S, Surkhi AO, Tan SZ, et al. RELAYTM branched–international results of vessel patency and reintervention. Front Cardiovasc Med 2022; 9:962884.
33. Malkawi AH, Hinchliffe RJ, Yates M, et al. Morphology of aortic arch pathology: implications for endovascular repair. J Endovasc Ther 2010; 17:474–479.
34. Kölbel T, Rostock T, Larena-Avellaneda A, et al. An externalized transseptal guidewire technique to facilitate guidewire stabilization and stent-graft passage in the aortic arch. J Endovasc Ther 2010; 17:744–749.
35. Nienaber CA, Kische S, Rehders TC, et al. Rapid pacing for better placing: comparison of techniques for precise deployment of endografts in the thoracic aorta. J Endovasc Ther 2007; 14:506–512.
36. Nienaber CA, Clough RE. Management of acute aortic dissection. Lancet 2015; 385:800–811.
37. Lombardi JV, Hughes GC, Appoo JJ, et al. Society for Vascular Surgery (SVS) and Society of Thoracic Surgeons (STS) reporting standards for type B aortic dissections. Ann Thorac Surg 2020; 109:959–981.
38. Bashir M, Tan SZ, Jubouri M, et al. Uncomplicated Type B Aortic Dissection: Challenges in Diagnosis and Categorisation. Ann Vasc Surg 2023; 94:92–101.
39. Brunkwall J, Kasprzak P, Verhoeven E, et al. Endovascular repair of acute uncomplicated aortic type B dissection promotes aortic remodelling: 1 year results of the ADSORB trial. Eur J Vasc Endovasc Surg 2014; 48:285–291.
40. Nienaber CA, Rousseau H, Eggebrecht H, et al. Randomized comparison of strategies for type B aortic dissection: the INvestigation of STEnt Grafts in Aortic Dissection (INSTEAD) trial. Circulation 2009; 120:2519–2528.
41. Chen SW, Lee KB, Napolitano MA, et al. Complications and management of the thoracic endovascular aortic repair. Aorta 2020; 8:49–58.
42. Jiang SM, Ali Hassan SM, Nguyen G, et al. Zone 0 frozen elephant trunk for type A retrograde acute aortic dissection following endovascular stenting of the arch. J Cardiac Surg 2021; 36:2124–2126.
43. Lima B, Nowicki ER, Blackstone EH. Spinal cord protective strategies during descending and thoracoabdominal aortic aneurysm repair in the modern era: the role of intrathecal papaverine. J Thorac Cardiovasc Surg 2012; 143:945–952.e1.
44. Grabenwöger M, Alfonso F, Bachet J. Thoracic endovascular aortic repair (TEVAR) for the treatment of aortic diseases: a position statement from the European Association for Cardio-Thoracic Surgery (EACTS) and the European Society of Cardiology (ESC), in collaboration with the European Association of Percutaneous Cardiovascular Interventions (EAPCI). Eur Heart J 2012; 33:1558–1563.
45. Sattah AP, Secrist MH, Sarin S. Complications and perioperative management of patients undergoing thoracic endovascular aortic repair. J Intensive Care Med 2018; 33:394–406.
46. Terzi F, Rocchi G, Fattori R. Current challenges in endovascular therapy for thoracic aneurysms. Expert Rev Cardiovasc Ther 2016; 14:599–607.
47. Mitchell RS. Operative Repair of Type B Aortic Dissection. Oper Tech Thorac Cardiovasc Surg 2009; 14:136–149.
48. Tian DH, De Silva RP, Wang T, et al. Open surgical repair for chronic type B aortic dissection: a systematic review. Ann Cardiothorac Surg 2014; 3:340.
49. Trimarchi S, Nienaber CA, Rampoldi V, et al. Role and results of surgery in acute type B aortic dissection: insights from the International Registry of Acute Aortic Dissection (IRAD). Circulation 2006; 114:I357–I364.

Chapter 13

The role of tranexamic acid in reducing surgical bleeding

John Houghton, Ian Roberts, Robert Sayers

ABSTRACT

Results from randomised trials show that perioperative use of tranexamic acid (TxA) significantly reduces surgical bleeding, without increasing the risk of vascular occlusive events. The POISE-3 (Perioperative Ischaemia Evaluation 3) trial confirmed prior evidence that TxA given at the start of noncardiac surgical procedures reduces the risk of major bleeding events by about 25%. Also consistent with previous research, the POISE-3 trial found a very low probability of any increase in thromboembolic events. Since TxA prevents bleeding, it should be given prior to skin incision for maximal effect. Wider use of TxA will improve surgical safety by reducing the risk of major blood loss and reducing unnecessary blood transfusion.

INTRODUCTION

Tranexamic acid (TxA) is an antifibrinolytic that acts on the plasmin fibrinolysis pathway. It inhibits fibrin clot degradation and, therefore, can reduce bleeding. Major perioperative bleeding occurs in 10–15% of patients undergoing noncardiac surgery [1,2]. It is strongly associated with 30-day mortality, and is the largest single contributor to postoperative death following noncardiac surgery (17% of deaths) [1]. Recent evidence shows that TxA use in surgery can reduce major bleeding and the use of blood products, and reduce perioperative deaths.

HISTORY

The research leading to the discovery of TxA in the 1950s and 1960s was undertaken by Japanese husband and wife medical researchers, Drs Utako and Shosuke Okamoto.

John Houghton MBChB MD MRCS, Clinical Lecturer, University of Leicester, Leicester, UK
E-mail: john.houghton@nhs.net (for correspondence)

Ian Roberts MB BCh PhD, Professor of Clinical Epidemiology and Public Health, London School of Hygiene and Tropical Medicine, London, UK
E-mail: Ian.Roberts@lshtm.ac.uk (for correspondence)

Robert Sayers MD FRCS, Professor of Vascular Surgery, University of Leicester, Leicester, UK
E-mail: rs152@leicester.ac.uk (for correspondence)

The motivation for their research was to find a drug that could reduce maternal deaths from postpartum haemorrhage. During the 1950s, they discovered that the amino acid lysine inhibits the activation and conversion of plasminogen to plasmin. Recognising that inhibition of plasmin formation, and subsequent reduction of fibrinolysis and clot stabilisation, might be a potential therapeutic target to reduce bleeding, they discovered that a synthetic lysine derivative, Epsilon aminocaproic acid (EACA), has a strong antifibrinolytic effect [3]. Following this success, they discovered a more potent inhibitor of plasmin activation, 4-amino-methyl-cyclohexane-carboxylic acid (AMCHA) [4]. Further research demonstrated that only the trans isomer of AMCHA had an antifibrinolytic effect: trans-AMCHA – or TxA [5]. These findings were independently corroborated by a Swedish team in 1965 [6].

Despite the success of their laboratory-based research, the Okamotos were unable to persuade their obstetric colleagues to undertake a clinical trial to determine the clinical effectiveness of TxA in the treatment of postpartum haemorrhage [7]. While Utako lived to see the start of the World Maternal Antifibrinolytic (WOMAN) trial, she died in 2016 shortly before the results of the trial were reported, that did indeed demonstrate TxA reduces maternal mortality from postpartum haemorrhage [8].

MECHANISM OF ACTION OF TRANEXAMIC ACID

Blood vessel injury during tissue damage (e.g. surgery or trauma) triggers a cascade of physiological responses – vasoconstriction, platelet plugging and coagulation, resulting in the formation of a fibrin clot formation. However, blood vessel rupture also triggers fibrinolysis. Plasminogen binds to specific lysine molecules in the fibrin molecule, via lysine binding sites, where it is activated into plasmin which causes fibrin degradation [3]. Endothelial damage causes the release of tissue-type plasminogen activator (tPA), which also binds to fibrin via lysine-binding sites, inducing localised fibrinolysis at the site of injury. Natural plasmin inhibitors exist, such as plasminogen activator inhibitors 1 and 2, and α2-antiplasmin [9,10]. These enzymes work in normal homeostatic balance to stabilise clot formation to prevent both bleeding and excessive clot formation.

Tranexamic acid is a competitive inhibitor of plasminogen, binding to the lysine-binding sites on the plasminogen protein and preventing its activation to plasmin, thereby reducing fibrinolysis [3]. As a potent antifibrinolytic, TxA can reduce fibrinolysis by blocking conversion of plasminogen to plasmin and, therefore, reduce bleeding.

Tranexamic acid can be given orally or intravenously; however in the context of surgery, it is important that the loading dose is given prior to the first incision and release of tPA, to inhibit excessive plasmin activation, as TxA acts upon its precursor plasminogen. In POISE-3 trial, a 1g intravenous loading dose was given at anaesthetic induction (i.e. prior to the first incision) followed by a further 1g intravenous bolus at the end of the procedure [2].

While oral, intravenous and even topical TxAs have an excellent safety profile, it should be noted that inadvertent intrathecal administration of TxA (e.g. during epidural anaesthesia for caesarean section) carries a significant mortality and morbidity risk. TxA is highly neurotoxic and intrathecal injection induces rapid onset of seizures with a 50% mortality rate [11].

THE PERIOPERATIVE ISCHAEMIA EVALUATION 3 TRIAL AND OTHER EVIDENCE

There is considerable evidence that favours both the efficacy and safety of TxA – the most important safety concern is that of thrombosis. The most recent evidence comes from the POISE-3 trial. POISE-3 was a multicentred trial (114 hospital in 22 countries) that randomised 9,535 adults aged ≥45 years, undergoing noncardiac surgery and deemed at risk for bleeding and cardiovascular complications [2]. Patients were eligible if they were anticipated to be admitted for at least one night postoperatively and met the criteria to identify those at risk of bleeding and cardiovascular complications [12]. Importantly, patients were excluded if use of TxA perioperatively was already planned.

Participants were randomised to receive 1 g of TxA or placebo immediately prior to the first skin incision (within 20 minutes before) and at the end of the procedure (at wound closure). TxA (1 g) or a matched volume of 0.9% saline (placebo) was given as a bolus via injection or infusion over 10 minutes. Patients undergoing cardiac surgery or intracranial neurosurgery were excluded. 37% of patients underwent a general surgery procedure, 23% orthopaedic and 15% vascular [2].

There were two major endpoints – a primary composite efficacy outcome of life-threatening bleeding, major bleeding or bleeding into a critical organ within 30 days (composite bleeding outcome) and a primary composite safety outcome of myocardial injury, non-haemorrhagic stroke, peripheral arterial thrombosis or symptomatic proximal venous thromboembolism within 30 days (composite cardiovascular outcome). The results are summarised in **Table 13.1**. The safety outcome was assessed using the non-inferiority principle – this tests whether the new treatment (TxA) is not worse than the current treatment (placebo). In order to establish non-inferiority, an arbitrary value for the upper boundary of the 97.5% confidence interval (CI) was set at <1.125 and the p value was set at < 0.025.

The results demonstrated a significant benefit of TxA in preventing major bleeding events, within 30 days of surgery. There were fewer bleeding events (composite bleeding

Table 13.1 Summary of results from POISE-3 trial (Devereaux et al. 2022)

	Placebo	TxA	HR (CI) or p value
Patients	4,778	4,757	
*Bleeding events at 30 days (composite bleeding outcome)	561 (11.7%)	433 (9.1%)	0.76 (0.67–0.87)
*Thrombotic events at 30 days (composite cardiovascular outcome)	639 (13.9%)	649 (14.2%)	1.02 (0.92–1.14)
Bleeding associated with death	541 (11.3%)	416 (8.7%)	0.76 (0.67–0.87)
Major bleeds	496 (10.4%)	363 (7.6%)	0.72 (0.63–0.83)
Major bleed according to ISTH criteria	415 (8.7%)	315 (6.6%)	0.75 (0.65–0.87)
Transfusion ≥1 unit packed red cells	574 (12.0%)	449 (9.4%)	0.77 (0.68–0.88)
SAE	242 (5.1%)	263 (5.5%)	$p = 0.16$

*Primary outcomes
(CI, confidence interval; HR, hazard ratio; ISTH, International Society on Thrombosis and Haemostasis; SAE, serious adverse events)

outcome) in the TxA group (433 patients; 9.1%) than the placebo group (561 patients; 11.7%). This translates to a 24% reduction in bleeding risk with TxA [hazard ratio (HR) 0.76; 95% CI 0.67, 0.87]. This was largely due to a significant reduction in major bleeds (resulting in a postoperative haemoglobin ≤70 g/L; a transfusion of ≥1 unit of red blood cells; or led to an intervention) from 10.4% in the placebo group to 7.6% in the TxA group (HR 0.72; 95% CI 0.63, 0.83).

The composite cardiovascular outcome (primary safety endpoint) was similar in the two groups. A total of 649 (14.2%) of the TxA group and 639 (13.9%) of the placebo group had one or more of the thrombotic events that made up the composite cardiovascular outcome, within 30 days of surgery (HR 1.02; 95% CI 0.92, 1.14). The incidence of the individual perioperative thrombotic events that made up the composite cardiovascular outcome (myocardial infarction, non-haemorrhagic stroke, peripheral arterial thrombus or symptomatic proximal venous thromboembolism), were similar across both the TxA and placebo groups. However, although the thrombosis rate was similar in the two groups, inferiority was not established.

Another area of potential concern for surgeons, when assessing the relevance of POISE-3 to clinical practice, is the results from the subgroup analysis [2]. Significant benefits of TxA administration were recorded for urology, spinal, orthopaedic and general surgical procedures. Although there was no statistically significant reduction in major bleeding in the vascular surgery subgroup, the results were consistent with the overall effect.

The POISE-3 supports many other studies that show benefits of TxA in preventing major surgical bleeding [13–15]. However, the question of thrombosis risk is likely to be a concern for surgeons and requires further consideration.

Another recent trial that addressed this issue was the ATACAS (Aspirin and Tranexamic Acid for Coronary Artery Surgery) trial, which is important because it investigated TxA in patients undergoing coronary artery surgery [13]. Cardiac surgery was one of the two surgical specialties not covered by POISE-3, the other being intracranial neurosurgery [2]. In ATACAS, 4,631 patients undergoing coronary surgery were randomised to TxA ($n = 2,311$) or placebo ($n = 2,320$) [13]. The primary outcome was a composite of death and thrombosis (non-fatal myocardial infarction, stroke, pulmonary embolus, renal failure or bowel infarction), within 30 days of operation. The primary outcome occurred in 386 patients in the TxA group (16.7%) and 420 patients in the placebo group (18.1%) [relative risk (RR) 0.92; 95% CI 0.81–1.05; $p = 0.22$]. Transfused blood products were lower in the TxA group (4,331 vs. 7,994, $p < 0.001$). Major bleeding or cardiac tamponade requiring reoperation was also significantly lower in the TxA group (1.4% vs. 2.8%, $p = 0.001$) but seizures were more common in the TxA group (0.7% vs. 0.1%, $p = 0.002$). The results of ATACAS (summarised in **Table 13.2**) show a reduced risk of bleeding, but no increased risk of death or thrombotic complications after surgery.

In addition, two recent meta-analyses have investigated the safety of TxA and found that TxA did not appear to increase the risk of thrombotic events. Murao et al. (2021) investigated 234 studies in 1,02,681 patients with traumatic, surgical, obstetric, intracranial or gastrointestinal (GI) bleeding [16]. There was no evidence that TxA increased the risk of thrombotic events (RR 1.00; 95% CI 0.93, 1.08), venous thromboembolism (RR 1.04; 95% CI 0.92, 1.17), acute coronary syndrome (RR 0.88; 95% CI 0.78, 1.00) or stroke (RR 1.12; 95% CI 0.98, 1.27).

A similar meta-analysis was performed by Taeuber et al. (2021) that investigated the association of TxA with thromboembolic events and mortality in 216 studies of 1,25,550

Table 13.2 Summary of results from ATACAS trial (Myles et al. 2017)

	Placebo	TxA	RR (CI) or p value
Patients	2,320	2,311	
*Death and thrombosis (composite primary outcome)	420 (18.1%)	386 (16.7%)	0.92 (0.81–1.05)
Transfused blood products	7,994	4,331	$p < 0.001$
Major bleeds/cardiac tamponade requiring reoperation	65 (2.8%)	32 (1.4%)	$p = 0.001$
Myocardial infarction	300 (12.9%)	269 (11.6%)	0.84 (0.70–1.00)
Seizures	2 (0.1%)	15 (0.7%)	$p = 0.002$

*Primary outcome
(CI, confidence interval; RR, relative risk)

patients undergoing surgical procedures [17]. There were 1,020 thromboembolic events in the TxA group (2.1%) and 900 in the control group (2.0%). There was no association between TxA and risk of thromboembolic events such as venous thromboembolism, pulmonary embolism, venous thrombosis, myocardial infarction or ischaemia and cerebral infarction or ischaemia (risk difference 0.001; 95% CI –0.001, 0.002; $p = 0.49$). In addition, use of TxA reduced overall mortality significantly and reduced mortality associated with bleeding significantly.

ECONOMIC AND RESOURCE UTILISATION IMPACTS OF PERIOPERATIVE TRANEXAMIC ACID

The National Institute of Health and Care Excellence (NICE) published guidance on Blood Transfusion in November 2015 (updated in March 2022) [18]. The section regarding alternatives to blood transfusion for patients having surgery (Section 1.1) states – patients undergoing surgery that are expected to have at least moderate blood loss (>500 mL) should be offered perioperative TxA. The guidance also advises that cell salvage should not be routinely used without TxA.

These recommendations are based on an extensive meta-analysis and network meta-analysis, in addition to a cost-effectiveness analysis, performed by the multidisciplinary Guideline Development Group [18]. Pairwise, meta-analyses demonstrated that TxA was related to lower risk of needing blood transfusion (RR 0.71; 95% CI 0.63, 0.81), lower mean number of units of red blood cells transfused (0.83 lower; 95% CI 1.17 lower, 0.5 lower) and lower risk of postoperative mortality (RR 0.52; 95% CI 0.31, 0.87), when compared to standard treatment in patients undergoing high risk surgery (anticipated blood loss >1,000 mL). Results were similar for patients undergoing moderate risk surgery (anticipated blood loss >500 mL), with lower risk of needing blood transfusion (RR 0.45; 95% CI 0.38, 0.52) and lower mean number of units of red blood cells transfused (0.88 lower; 95% CI 1.22 lower, 0.54 lower). Results were replicated in the network meta-analyses and TxA use, either with or without cell salvage, was consistently ranked higher than standard treatment in the rank-o-grams in patients undergoing surgery, with both moderate- and high-risk for blood loss. Use of TxA was ranked the most cost-effective option to reduce blood transfusion among individuals undergoing surgery with both moderate (£169 savings per patient) and high risk (£212 savings per patient) based on 2015 costings [18].

Alongside this guidance, NICE published their Blood Transfusion Quality Standard (QS138) in December 2016 [19]. Quality standard 2 in QS138 states – 'Adults who are having surgery and are expected to have moderate blood loss are offered TxA' and suggests that the measure of quality for this standard is the proportion of all patients undergoing surgery with moderate risk of blood loss (anticipated >500 mL blood loss). The 2021 National Comparative Audit of NICE QS138 published by NHS Blood and Transplant audited records of 4,679 patients from 153 NHS hospital sites [20]. A total of 1,079/1,599 (67.5%) of patients with expected moderate blood loss (>500 mL) received perioperative TxA. Published estimates suggest that compliance with NICE guidelines and QS138 would save over 15,000 major perioperative bleeds and save 33,000 units of blood, at significant cost savings to the NHS [21].

These potential savings of blood products are of even greater significance in low- and middle-income countries, where resources of blood products are far scarcer. Published modelling of the impact of TxA on reducing bleeding events in sub-Saharan Africa estimates that the use of TxA is an extremely cost-effective method of reducing perioperative mortality [22].

TRANEXAMIC ACID USE IN TRAUMA PATIENTS

The use of TxA in the context of trauma is well established and recommended in UK and international guidelines [23,24]. The recommendations are largely based on the results of the CRASH-2 (Clinical Randomisation of an Antifibrinolytic in Significant Haemorrhage 2) trial [25].

The CRASH-2 trial recruited 20,211 adult patients (274 participating hospitals from 40 different countries) with significant haemorrhage (defined as systolic blood pressure <90 mmHg and/or heart rate >100 beats/min), or at high risk or significant haemorrhage, and were within 8 hours of injury [25]. Included patients were randomised to receive either 1 g loading dose of intravenous TxA (infused over 10 minutes) followed by a further 1 g of TxA infused over 8 hours or matching placebo infusions (0.9% saline). The primary outcome measure was in-hospital death within 28 days of injury. All-cause mortality (primary outcome) was 14.5% in the TxA group versus 16.0% for placebo [absolute risk reduction 1.5%; risk ratio (RR) 0.91 (95% CI 0.85, 0.97); $p = 0.0035$]. Deaths due to bleeding were also lower among those receiving TxA [4.9% vs. 5.7%; RR 0.85 (95% CI 0.76, 0.96); $p = 0.0077$]. No difference in vascular occlusive events was observed between the TxA and placebo groups and incidence of myocardial infarction was lower among those receiving TxA [0.3% vs. 0.5%; RR 0.64 (0.42, 0.97); $p = 0.035$].

The results from CRASH-2 (summarised in **Table 13.3**) also demonstrate the importance of early administration of TxA in trauma. A retrospective, exploratory analysis of CRASH-2 data by the study authors sought also to investigate the effect of timing of TxA treatment on deaths from bleeding [26]. Treatment within 1 hour of injury showed a significant reduction in deaths from bleeding among the TxA group [5.3% vs. 7.7%; RR 0.68 (95% CI 0.57, 0.82); $p < 0.0001$] with a similar benefit of TxA with those treated between 1 and 3 hours of injury [4.8% vs. 6.1%; RR 0.79 (95% CI 0.64, 0.97); $p = 0.03$]. However, in patients treated >3 hours after injury, TxA significantly increased the risk of death due to bleeding compared to placebo [4.4% vs. 3.1%; RR 1.44 (95% CI 1.12, 1.84); $p = 0.004$]. The precise mechanism for

Table 13.3 Summary of results from CRASH-2 trial (Shakur et al. 2010)

	Placebo	TxA	RR (CI) or p value
Patients	10,115	10,096	
*All-cause mortality	1,613 (16.0%)	1,463 (14.5%)	0.91 (0.85–0.97) p = 0.0035
Deaths due to bleeding	574 (5.7%)	489 (4.9%)	0.85 (0.76–0.96) p = 0.0077
Any vascular occlusive event	201 (2.0%)	168 (1.7%)	0.84 (0.68–1.02) p = 0.084 ns
Deep vein thrombosis	41 (0.4%)	40 (0.4%)	0.98 (0.63–1.51) p = 0.21 ns
Myocardial infarction	300 (12.9%)	269 (11.6%)	0.64 (0.42–0.97) ns
Overall mortality in those treated >3 hours after injury			1.00 (0.86–1.17) ns

*Primary outcome
(CI, confidence interval; ns, non-significant; RR, relative risk)

this observation is unclear. Trauma patients with hyperfibrinolysis have the highest early mortality; however, fibrinolytic shutdown is a more common presentation and develops within the first 3 hours of injury, which may explain the lack of overall mortality benefit in TxA given >3 hours postinjury [27]. The development of thrombotic disseminated coagulopathy, which can occur in the late phase of trauma, or a higher prevalence of hypoxia and acidosis in those >3 hours postinjury leading to coagulopathy which may be exacerbated by TxA, are also possible explanations [26,28]. It is important to note, however, that there was no difference in overall mortality between TxA and placebo among those treated >3 hours after injury [RR 1.00 (95% CI 0.86, 1.17)] [25]. Because of these findings, UK NICE guidelines do not recommend the use of TxA in trauma >3 hours postinjury unless there is evidence of hyperfibrinolysis [23].

TRANEXAMIC ACID USE IN OBSTETRICS

The use of TxA has been trialled in a number of other contexts. The drug was initially developed to reduce maternal death from postpartum haemorrhage [29]. The WOMAN trial randomised 20,060 women (193 participating hospitals; 21 countries) aged ≥16 years with a clinical diagnosis of postpartum haemorrhage to receive either 1 g intravenous TxA (infused over 10 minutes) or a matched placebo infusion, followed by a further intravenous infusion of either 1 g TxA or placebo if bleeding continued after 30 minutes, or restarted within 24 hours of the first dose. TxA reduced the risk of death from bleeding within 6 weeks of delivery by 0.4% compared to placebo [1.5% vs. 1.9%; RR 0.81 (95% CI 0.65, 1.00); $p = 0.045$] but the observed reduction in all-cause mortality at 6 weeks of 0.3% was not statistically significant [2.3% vs. 2.6%; RR 0.88 (95% CI 0.74, 1.05); $p = 0.16$]. However, similarly to the results from CRASH-2, there was a significant reduction in all-cause mortality at 6 weeks with TxA versus placebo among women treated within 3 hours of delivery of 0.5% [1.2% vs. 1.7%; RR 0.69 (95% CI 0.52, 0.91); $p = 0.008$]. Subsequently, the World Health Organisation recommends the use of TxA as early as possible within 3 hours of onset of postpartum haemorrhage [30].

The TRAAP2 (Tranexamic Acid for Preventing Postpartum Haemorrhage Following a Caesarean Delivery) trial also demonstrated benefit in women undergoing caesarean section [31]. A total of 4,551 women were randomised to receive either a 1 g intravenous bolus of TxA or placebo (normal saline) over 30–60 seconds during the 3 minutes immediately after birth (after oxytocin or carbetocin administration and umbilical cord clamping). The primary outcome of postpartum haemorrhage (>1,000 mL estimated blood loss or red cell transfusion within 2 days postpartum) was experienced by 26.7% of women in the TxA group (2,222 included in the modified intention to treat analysis) versus 31.6% of women who received placebo (2,209 included) (adjusted risk ratio 0.84; 95% CI 0.75, 0.94; $p = 0.003$).

DOES TRANEXAMIC ACID STOP BLEEDING?: THE HALT-IT TRIAL

Tranexamic acid has not been shown to be effective for all causes of major haemorrhage. This may be due to its mechanism of action in preventing conversion of plasminogen to plasmin and, therefore, is time dependent and is most effective prior to blood vessel damage and tPA release [3]. As such, in settings where major haemorrhage is already established, long courses of TxA may not be beneficial in treating bleeding.

An example of this is GI bleeding. The HALT-IT (Haemorrhage Alleviation with Tranexamic Acid -Intestinal system) trial randomised 12,009 patients with significant upper or lower GI bleeding to receive a 1 g loading dose of TxA (in 100 mL 0.9% saline) by intravenous injection over 10 minutes followed by 3 g infusion (in 1,000 mL 0.9% saline) over 24 hours or placebo (0.9% saline 100 mL injection plus 1,000 mL infusion only) [32]. Significant bleeding was determined clinically as patients with a risk of death due to bleeding and included those with hypotension, tachycardia, signs of shock and those likely to need transfusion or urgent endoscopy or surgery. The primary outcome was death due to bleeding within 5 days of randomisation.

A total of 448 participants (3.8%) died due to bleeding within 5 days of randomisation (primary outcome measure) [32]. There was no difference in the primary outcome between the TxA and placebo groups (RR 0.99; 95% CI 0.82, 1.18). There was also no difference in all-cause mortality at 28 days in the two groups (RR 1.03; 95% CI 0.92, 1.16). Incidence of rebleeding at 24 hours (RR 1.00; 95% CI 0.65, 1.55), 5 days (RR 0.91; 95% CI 0.78, 1.07) and 28 days (RR 0.92; 95% CI 0.81, 1.05) were also similar in both groups. The use of TxA made no difference in the need for endoscopic, radiological or surgical intervention for GI bleeding, nor did use of transfused blood products differ between those receiving TxA and placebo.

There was a small but statistically significant increase in the combined venous thromboembolic events (deep venous thrombosis or pulmonary embolism), with an incidence of 0.8% observed in the TxA group compared to 0.4% in the placebo group (RR 1.85; 95% CI 1.15, 2.98) [32]. TxA was also associated with a small increase in seizures (0.6% vs. 0.4%; RR 1.73; 95% CI 1.03, 2.93).

In light of these results, the authors do not recommend that TxA is given to patients with GI bleeding, outside the context of a randomised control trial.

CONCLUSION

Tranexamic acid is an inexpensive, widely available and easy to administer drug with an excellent evidence base to support its use to prevent major haemorrhage, in multiple clinical settings. As such, TxA is listed in the WHO model list of essential medicines. In patients undergoing non-cardiac surgery where at least moderate blood loss (>500 mL) is anticipated, TxA reduces risk of serious bleeding by approximately 25%. TxA should be given immediately prior to surgery to prevent blood loss. Based on results from POISE-3, 1 g TxA given intravenously at induction of anaesthesia, followed by a second bolus during or after surgery, is recommended. Good evidence exists of cost-effectiveness of TxA in non-cardiac surgery. Widespread adoption of perioperative TxA in surgery anticipated blood loss >500 mL in the UK, in line with NICE guidance, would prevent thousands of perioperative bleeds and unnecessary blood transfusions annually.

Key points for clinical practice

- Tranexamic acid reduces the risk of serious bleeding by 25%
- The use of TxA is supported by the recent POISE-3 trial and NICE guidelines
- TxA has the potential to prevent 15,000 serious bleeds per year across the NHS
- TxA could save up to 33,000 units of blood being transfused per year in UK
- NICE recommends the use of TxA in adult patients with a predicted blood loss >500 mL

REFERENCES

1. Spence J, LeManach Y, Chan MTV, et al. Association between complications and death within 30 days after noncardiac surgery. CMAJ 2019; 191:E830–E837.
2. Devereaux PJ, Marcucci M, Painter TW, et al. Tranexamic Acid in Patients Undergoing Noncardiac Surgery. N Engl J Med 2022; 386:1986–1997.
3. Tengborn L, Blombäck M, Berntorp E. Tranexamic acid--an old drug still going strong and making a revival. Thromb Res 2015; 135:231–242.
4. Okamoto S, Okamoto U. Amino-Methyl-Cyclohexane-Carboxylic Acid: AMCHA. Keio J Med 1962; 11:105–115.
5. Okamoto S, Sato S, Takada Y, et al. An active stereo-isomer (trans-form) of AMCHA and its antifibrinolytic (antiplasminic) action in vitro and in vivo. Keio J Med 1964; 13:177–185.
6. Melander B, Gliniecki G, Granstrand B, et al. Biochemistry and toxicology of amikapron; the antifibrinolytically active isomer of AMCHA. (A comparative study with epsilon-aminocaproic acid). Acta Pharmacol Toxicol (Copenh) 1965; 22:340–352.
7. Watts G. Utako Okamoto. Lancet 2016; 387:2286.
8. WOMAN Trial Collaborators. Effect of early tranexamic acid administration on mortality, hysterectomy, and other morbidities in women with post-partum haemorrhage (WOMAN): an international, randomised, double-blind, placebo-controlled trial. Lancet 2017; 389:2105–2116.
9. Binder BR, Christ G, Gruber F, et al. Plasminogen activator inhibitor 1: physiological and pathophysiological roles. News Physiol Sci 2002; 17:56–61.
10. Sakata Y, Aoki N. Cross-linking of alpha 2-plasmin inhibitor to fibrin by fibrin-stabilizing factor. J Clin Invest 1980; 65:290–297.
11. Moran NF, Bishop DG, Fawcus S, et al. Tranexamic acid at cesarean delivery: drug-error deaths. Eur J Obstet Gynecol Reprod Biol 2022; 279:195-198.
12. Marcucci M, Painter TW, Conen D, et al. Rationale and design of the PeriOperative ISchemic Evaluation-3 (POISE-3): a randomized controlled trial evaluating tranexamic acid and a strategy to minimize hypotension in noncardiac surgery. Trials 2022; 23:101.

13. Myles PS, Smith JA, Forbes A, et al. Tranexamic Acid in Patients Undergoing Coronary-Artery Surgery. N Engl J Med 2017; 376:136-148.
14. Ker K, Edwards P, Perel P, et al. Effect of tranexamic acid on surgical bleeding: systematic review and cumulative meta-analysis. BMJ 2012; 344:e3054.
15. Kagoma YK, Crowther MA, Douketis J, et al. Use of antifibrinolytic therapy to reduce transfusion in patients undergoing orthopedic surgery: a systematic review of randomized trials. Thromb Res 2009; 123:687–696.
16. Murao S, Nakata H, Roberts I, et al. Effect of tranexamic acid on thrombotic events and seizures in bleeding patients: a systematic review and meta-analysis. Crit Care 2021; 25:380.
17. Taeuber I, Weibel S, Herrmann E, et al. Association of Intravenous Tranexamic Acid With Thromboembolic Events and Mortality: A Systematic Review, Meta-analysis, and Meta-regression. JAMA Surg 2021; 156:e210884.
18. National Institute of Health and Care Excellence. (2015). Blood transfusion: NICE guideline [NG24]. Available from https://www.nice.org.uk/guidance/ng24 [Last accessed 19 July 2025].
19. National Institute of Health and Care Excellence. (2016). Blood transfusion: Quality standard [QS138]. Available from https://www.nice.org.uk/guidance/qs138 [Last accessed 19 July 2025]
20. NHS Blood and Transplant. (2022). 2021 National Comparative Audit of NICE Quality Standard QS138. Available from https://nhsbtdbe.blob.core.windows.net/umbraco-assets-corp/25926/2021-nice-qs138-audit-report-generic.pdf [Last accessed 19 July 2025].
21. Grocott MPW, Murphy M, Roberts I, et al. Tranexamic acid for safer surgery: the time is now. Br J Surg 2022; 109:1182-3.
22. Guerriero C, Cairns J, Jayaraman S, et al. Giving tranexamic acid to reduce surgical bleeding in sub-Saharan Africa: an economic evaluation. Cost Eff Resour Alloc 2010; 8:1.
23. National Institute of Health and Care Excellence. (2016). Major trauma: assessment and initial management [NG39]. Available from https://www.nice.org.uk/guidance/ng39 [Last accessed 19 July 2025].
24. Spahn DR, Bouillon B, Cerny V, et al. The European guideline on management of major bleeding and coagulopathy following trauma: 5th edition. Crit Care 2019; 23:98.
25. Shakur H, Roberts I, Bautista R, et al. Effects of tranexamic acid on death, vascular occlusive events, and blood transfusion in trauma patients with significant haemorrhage (CRASH-2): a randomised, placebo-controlled trial. Lancet 2010; 376:23–32.
26. Roberts I, Shakur H, Afolabi A, et al. The importance of early treatment with tranexamic acid in bleeding trauma patients: an exploratory analysis of the CRASH-2 randomised controlled trial. Lancet 2011; 377:1096–101, 101.e1–2.
27. Hanley C, Callum J, Jerath A. Tranexamic acid and trauma coagulopathy: where are we now? Br J Anaesth 2021; 126:12–17.
28. Sawamura A, Hayakawa M, Gando S, et al. Disseminated intravascular coagulation with a fibrinolytic phenotype at an early phase of trauma predicts mortality. Thromb Res 2009; 124:608–613.
29. Brenner A, Ker K, Shakur-Still H, et al. Tranexamic acid for post-partum haemorrhage: What, who and when. Best Pract Res Clin Obstet Gynaecol 2019; 61:66–74.
30. World Health Organization (WHO). Updated WHO Recommendation on Tranexamic Acid for the Treatment of Postpartum Haemorrhage. Geneva, Switzerland: WHO; 2017. Licence: CC BY-NC-SA 3.0 IGO. WHO/RHR/17.21.
31. Sentilhes L, Sénat MV, Le Lous M, et al. Tranexamic Acid for the Prevention of Blood Loss after Cesarean Delivery. N Engl J Med 2021; 384:1623–1634.
32. HALT-IT Trial Collaborators. Effects of a high-dose 24-h infusion of tranexamic acid on death and thromboembolic events in patients with acute gastrointestinal bleeding (HALT-IT): an international randomised, double-blind, placebo-controlled trial. Lancet 2020; 395:1927–1936.

Index

Note: Page numbers in **bold** or *italic* refer to tables or figures respectively.

A

Abandoning procedure 133
Abdomen 57, 60, 63, 145
Abdominal cavity 60
    infection 160
Abdominal closure 61, *66*
Abdominal compartment syndrome 58, 67
Abdominal complications 146, 147
Abdominal incision 60
    closure of 62
    major 60
Abdominal operation 57, 67
Abdominal organ cluster, concept of *155*
Abdominal peritonitis, persistent 65
Abdominal retraction anchor 65
Abdominal wall 60, 64, 65, *66*, 131
    closure 62-64
    defects 64
    hernia, large complex 64
    movement 62
    surgical treatment 65
    transplantation 155
Abemaciclib 82
Ablative therapies 110
Abscess 54
    formation 128
Acalculous cholecystitis 124
Acid-base balance 155
Acidosis 145
    correction of 145
Acute acalculous cholecystitis 124, 134
Acute aortic dissection 168
    classification of 172, 176
    open surgical repair of 169
Acute aortic regurgitation 167
Acute aortic syndrome 166
Acute cellular rejection 159
Acute cholecystectomy 126
    diagnosis of 124
Acute cholecystitis 117, 123-128
    diagnosis of 124, 134

    grades of 125
    imaging findings characteristic of 124
    management of 123, 126, 134
    mild 127
    moderate 127
    recent advances in management of 123
    severe 127
    traditional calculus 124
    treatment of 126, 134
Acute surgery units 53
Adhesions around gallbladder 129
Adipose tissue 75
Adjuvant endocrine treatment 77
Adriamycin 83
Advanced trauma life support 143
Aerobic exercise 23
Airway
    assessment 143
    maintenance 143
    management 143
Albeit anastrozole 79
Alcohol
    harm 27
    reduction 27
    use disorders identification test 27
Alemtuzumab 158
Allergy 54
Allograft arterial
    stump *156*
    thrombosis 160
Alpelisib 82
American Association for Surgery of Trauma 142, 146
    Grading Scale for Rectal Injuries **142**
American Association for Thoracic Surgery 169
American Hernia Societies 60
American Society of Anaesthesiologists 128
Amino acid lysine inhibits 180
Aminoglycosides 126
Amino-methyl-cyclohexane-carboxylic acid 180

Index

Ampicillin 126
Anaemia 25, 58, 60
   medical optimisation of **25**
Anaesthesia 8, 157
   epidural 180
   induction of 187
Anaesthetic gasses, inhaled 4
Anal
   injuries 147
   trauma 148
Analgesia 52, 55, 123
   intraoperative 54
   methods, novel 54
   postoperative 54
Anaphylactic reactions 75
Anastrozole 76, 78-83, 87
Androgens 75
Aneurysmal dilatation 167
Ankle-brachial pressure 175
Antegrade cerebral perfusion 169
Anterograde propagation 166
Antibiotic 54
   intravenous 123
   prophylaxis 146
   therapy 126, 127, 135
Anticancer
   activity 74
   effects, wide spectrum of 74
   treatments 78
Antidiarrhoeal agents 160
Anti-impulse therapy 172, 173
Anti-oestrogenic properties 74
Anti-oestrogens 74
Antithrombotic medication, reversal of 52
Antithymocyte globulin 158
Aorta 131, *157*
   abdominal 167, 168
   ascending 167, 169, 170
   infrarenal *157*
Aortic arch 168, 170, 171
   anteroposterior curvatures of 172
   dissection 168
   mediolateral curvatures of 172
   repair 170
      extended 170
   surgery 169
Aortic disease, ascending 168

Aortic dissection 165, 167, 168, *168*, 172, 176
   classification of 166
   endovascular management of 171
   endovascular repair for 173
   management of 165
   medical management of 172
   modern management of 165
   open surgical repair of 175
   type
      A 165, 168, 171, 172
      B 165, 172-174
Aortic expansion, early 168
Aortic plaques, atheroembolism of 174
Aortic regurgitation 168, 172
Aortic root 171
   dilatation *168*, 170
Aortic rupture 167, 176
   signs of 168
Aortic tunica intima 165
Aortic valve 171
   dysfunction 170
Aravind eye care systems 10
Aromatase
   expression 75
   inhibitors 74-76
Aromatisation 75
   peripheral 76
Arsenic 118
Arterial blood 126
Arterial conduit *157*
Arterial dissection 175
Arterial pedicle stump *156*
Artery
   hepatic 129
   innominate 168
Ascending aorta 167, 169, 170
   isolated replacement of 170
Ascites 143
Ascorbic acid 58
Aspirin 182
Aspirin and Tranexamic Acid for Coronary Artery Surgery trial **183**
Atherosclerotic ulcer, penetrating 166
Attack, acute 127
Atypical intraductal epithelial proliferation 109
Axilla 73
Axillary lymph node dissection 89

Axillary management 89
Axillary surgery considerations 89

B

Bacteria 123
Bariatric surgery candidates 120
Behaviour change, theories of 28
Bentall procedure 170
Beta-lactamase inhibitor 127
Bile
    concentration 124
    duct 129
        injury 121, 127, 129, 130
    stasis 124
Biliary colic 117, 128
Biliary disease 123, 134
Biliary drainage 127, 133
Biliary system 127
    anatomy of 130
Biologic mesh, prophylactic implantation of 64
Bisphosphates 104
Bisphosphonates 110
Bladder injury 145
Blast injuries 142
Bleeding 121, 131, 132, 186
    gangrenous 182
    severe 132
    vaginal 75
Blood
    loss, massive 145
    pressure 172, 176
        systolic 184
    products 179
    transfusion 179
        postoperative 58
    vessel injury 180
Blunt injury 145
Blunt trauma 58, 142, 147
Body mass index 24, 118, 128, 129
    high 128
Bogota bag 66, 145
Bone fractures 75
Bowel resection 139
Breast 73, 75
    cancer 73, 74, 77, 78, 103, 104, 106-109
        advanced 77
        cell proliferation 74
        diagnosis 74
        early 73, 77, 104
        growth 76
        local control of 105
        low-risk early-stage 107
        non-surgical systemic treatments for 104
        percutaneous treatment for 103
        size 105
        treatment 74, 76, 103, 104, 106
        triple-negative 73
    conservation surgery 73, 82, 83
        rates 88
    infection 107
    inflammation 107
    radiotherapy 106
    surgery 71
Breathing 62, 143
Bridging therapy 74
Broad-spectrum penicillin 127
Broken fascial sutures *59*
Buparlisib 82
Burst abdomen 57, *59*, 60, 61, *63*, 67
    complication of 60
    management of 57, 60
    presentation of 57
    prevention of 57, 60, 62
    risk factors for **58**
Buttock gunshot wounds 145

C

Caesarean section, epidural anaesthesia for 180
Caffeine 40
Calot's triangle 132
Cancers 73
    endometrial 74, 75
    gallbladder 118, 119
    prevention 117
Carbapenems 127
Carbetocin 186
Carbohydrate loading 52
Carbon
    dioxide production 20
    footprint 4
    ion 104
        therapy 105
    monoxide monitors 27

Carcinoma
    gallbladder 117, 118
    hepatocellular 107
    invasive
        ductal 106
        lobular 106
Cardiac surgery 182
Cardiac transplant 120
Cardiopulmonary bypass 169
Cardiopulmonary exercise testing
    variables 20, 22
    overview of **21**
Cardiopulmonary system, noninvasive assessment of 20
Cardiovascular complications 181
Cardiovascular disease 75
Cardiovascular observations 24
Cataract 75
Catastrophe, abdominal 161
Cavity
    abdominal 60
    peritoneal 130
Celecoxib 81
Cephalosporins
    fourth-generation 127
    oral 127
    second-generation 127
Cerebral infarction 183
Chemo-endocrine score 86
Chemotherapy 73, 110
    adjuvant 78
    neoadjuvant 73
Chest
    complications 58
    X-ray *166*
Cholangiography 130
    intraoperative 130, 134
    use of 130
Cholangitis 128
Cholecystectomy 120, 123, 124, 126, 128-130, 132, 134
    acute laparoscopic 129
    difficult 128-130, 135, 143
    elective prophylactic 119
    emergency 123
    intraoperative difficulty scoring for 129
    laparoscopic 54, 120, 123, 126, 127, 134
    post-transplant 120
    routine prophylactic 119
    selective prophylactic 119
    subtotal 133
Cholecystitis 54, 118
    acute calculous 123
    emphysematous 125
    gangrenous 125
Cholecystostomy 124, 127, 133, 134
Cholelithiasis 117
Chole-QuIC project 127
Cholesterol-predominant stones 118
Chronic kidney injury 160
Circulation 143
Cirrhosis 58
Climate change 4
Clinical Randomisation of Antifibrinolytic in Significant Haemorrhage-2 trial **185**
Clot stabilisation 180
Coagulation 108
Coagulative necrosis 108
Coagulopathy 145
Coeliac trunk *155*
Cold ischaemia 160
Collagen, synthesis of 58
Colon
    injuries 140, 145
    trauma 141
Colorectal injuries 140
Colostomy 139, 140, 145, 148
Complete oestrogen receptor antagonists 77
Complete portomesenteric thrombosis 154
Comprehensive geriatric assessment 24, 30
Computed tomography 105, 166
    scan 53, 125
Congenital pancreaticobiliary maljunction 118
Conjunction 55
Connective tissue disorders 170
Consciousness, impaired level of 125
Continuous small-bites suturing technique 62, 67
Contusion 142
Coronary artery
    ostial involvement 170
    surgery 182
Coronary malperfusion 167
Corticosteroids 158
Coughing 62

COVID-19 pandemic 6, 7, 41, 74, 123, 128
C-reactive protein 124
    elevated 124
Crohn's disease 153
Cryoablation 103, 104, 106, 107
    devices 106
    probe 106
Cyclin-dependent kinase 4 and 6 inhibitors 77
Cyclophosphamide 80, 81, 83
Cystic duct 129

D

Damage control laparotomy 145
Day case surgery 18
Debridement 140
Deep vein thrombosis 75, 186
    prophylaxis 54
Defecation 62
Degarelix 83
Delayed dynamic abdominal closure device 65
Descending thoracic aorta 167, *168*
Desmoid tumours 154
Destructive perineal wounds 147
Devascularisation 142
Diabetes mellitus 25, 58, 60
    medical optimisation of **25**
Diagnostic peritoneal lavage 143
Diathermy, high-intensity 132
Disability 143
Dissection membrane 166
Distal
    embolisation 175
    rectal washout 140
    re-entry tears 166
    thoracic aorta 172
Disulfiram 28
Diverticulitis 54
Docetaxel 80, 81, 83
Donor
    aorta, segment of *156*
    arterial conduits *156*
    brachiocephalic trunk *156*
    iliac vessels 156, *156*
    specific antibodies 156, 159
Dopamine 28
Double diabolo 63
Double-blind 62
Doxorubicin 80

Drainage 140
Ductal carcinoma in situ 106
Duke University Preoperative Nutrition Score 26
Dunning-Kruger effect 45
Dynamic closure
    devices 65
    techniques 65
Dynamic vertical traction force
    application of 65
    principles of 65
Dysmotility syndromes 153

E

Early breast cancer 73, 77, 104
    management of 106, 110
Elective hernia surgery 65
Electrolyte management, preoperative 52
Electrosurgery 60
Emergency abdominal surgery, outcomes of 51
Emotion, effect of 40
Endocrine prognostic index 79
Endocrine therapy 73, 77, 78, 90, 104, 110
    types of 74
Endocrine treatment agents, adverse events of **75**
Endocrine-resistant disease 76, 82
Endoprosthesis 170
Endoscopic retrograde cholangiopancreatography 53
Endothelial damage 180
Energy
    conservation 8
    devices, minimising use of 131
Enhanced recovery after surgery guidelines 52
Enteral feeding 160
Enterectomy, completion 157
Enteroatmospheric fistulas 67
Epigastric vessels 132
Epirubicin 80, 81, 83
Epithelial atypia 109
Epithelial necrosis 108
Epsilon aminocaproic acid 180
Epstein–Barr virus 161
Erythema 108
Escherichia coli 127
Everolimus 82
Evisceration 57

Exemestane 79-81, 83
Extensive rectal mobilisation 145
Extraperitoneal rectal injury 144-147
    penetrating non-destructive 147
Extraperitoneal rectal trauma 147

F

Fascia 65
Fascial closure 61, 62
    primary *63*
Fascial dehiscence 57
Fascial healing 58, 61
Fat necrosis 107, 108
Fatigue 38, 75
Fatty acids
    long-chain 160
    medium-chain 160
Fever 121, 123, 124
Fibrin
    clot formation 180
    degradation 180
Fibrinolysis, subsequent reduction of 180
Flat epithelial atypia 109
Flexible sigmoidoscopy 53
Fluid
    electrolyte imbalances 160
    pericholecystic 125
Fluoroquinolones 127
    oral 127
Food and Drug Administration 77, 107
Fracture, pelvic 147
Frailty 25
    medical optimisation of **25**
Frozen elephant trunk 170
Fulvestrant 79, 81, 83
Functional aortic valves 170

G

Gallbladder 117, 123-125, 129, 130, *133*
    acute inflammation of 124
    appearance 129
    cancer 117-119
    carcinoma 117, 118
        development, high-risk factors for 118
    contracted 128
    distended 129
    fossa 132
    inflammation, painful 123
    retraction of 132
    symptomatic 54
    thick-walled 128
    wall thickness 128
Gallstone 117, 118, 123, 125, 134
    asymptomatic 117, 118
    disease 117
        long-standing 118
        symptomatic 123
    incidental 120
    pancreatitis 117
Gastrointestinal anastomosis 158
Gastrointestinal malignancy 58
Gastrointestinal tract 141, 153
    reconstruction 157
Gastroschisis 153
Gefitinib 80
Gene expression profiles 73
General surgery, principles of 1
Genitourinary injury 144
Gigli saw effect 62
Global anti-oestrogenic behaviour 77
Glucose management, preoperative 52
Gonadotropin-releasing hormone agonists 76
Goserelin 83
Graft surveillance 159
Graft versus host disease 158
Greenhouse gasses 4
Greenhouse warming potential 8

H

Haematological impairment 126
Haematoma 108, 131, 142
    injection site 75
    intramural 166
    paracolic 145
Haemodynamic instability 65
Haemoglobin 24
    glycosylated 24
Haemoperitoneum 143
Haemorrhage 132, 145, 184
    alleviation 186
    control 143
    intraperitoneal 143
    major 186, 187
    postpartum 180, 185, 186

Haemostats, absorbable 132
Halstead's radical mastectomy 104
Hazard ratio 181
Head and neck injuries 140
Headache 40, 75
Hemiarch reconstruction 169
Hemolytic disorders, chronic 120
Hepatic enzyme elevations 75
Hepatic impairment 126
Hepatobiliary surgery 115
Hernia
    incisional 58, 60, 61
    parastomal 146
    repair 65, 128
High American Society of Anaesthesiologists score 128
High-intensity focused ultrasound 106, 108
Hollow viscus injury 143
Hormone therapy 74
    primary 74
Hot gallbladder 134
Human leukocyte antigen 156
Hydration, importance of 39
Hypercholesterolaemia 75
Hyperplasia, endometrial 74, 75
Hypersensitivity 75
Hypertension 60
    intra-abdominal 67
    refractory 168
        systolic 167
Hypofractionated ablative external beam photon radiotherapy 105
Hypoperfusion 58
Hypotension 125, 146, 186
    postoperative 58
Hypothalamic-pituitary
    adrenal axis 21
    gonadal axis 76
Hypothermia 145
Hypothermic circulatory arrest 169

I

Iatrogenic injury 129, 142
Idiopathic pseudo-obstruction 153
Ileus, postoperative 58
Image-guided vacuum needle excision 104
Immune system 110
Immunosuppressive
    agents 158
    protocols 158
    therapy 158
Incisional hernia 58, 60, 61
    repair 64
    prevention of 62, 64
Indocyanine green 130
Induction therapy 73
Inefficient oestrogen synthesis inhibition 76
Infection 107, 121
Inferior mesenteric artery *155*
Inferior vena cava *155, 157*
Inflammation 107
    severe 129, 131
Inflammatory bowel disease 153
Inflammatory cell
    migration of 61
    recruitment 61
Inflammatory mass 125
Infliximab 158
Infusion, intravenous 185
Injury
    description of 142
    intra-abdominal 143
    intraperitoneal 139, 145, 147
    management of 140
    penetrating 144, 145
    surgical 160
    types of 142
Inspiratory muscle training 23
Integrated cerebral perfusion 169
Intensive care 52
Intercostal artery coverage 174
Interleukin-2 receptor blockers 158
International Society on Thrombosis and Haemostasis 181
Intestinal allograft 159
    portal drainage of *157*
    systemic drainage of *157*
Intestinal failure 151-154, *154*, 161
Intestinal system 186
Intestinal transplantation 151, 152, *152*, 153, *154*, 161
    recent advances in 151
    surgical technique, application of 158

Intestine function, preservation of 155
Intra-abdominal fluid 143
Intractable biliary colic 54
Intramuscular administration 77
Intraoperative care and pain relief protocols 51
Intraoperative communication tools 54
Intraoperative supportive care 54
Intraperitoneal adhesions 129
Intraperitoneal free fluid 144
Intraperitoneal rectal injury, penetrating 146
Intraperitoneal space 64
Intraperitoneal wounds, management of 145
Ionising radiation 104
Irreversible intestinal failure 151, 153
Ischaemia 183
    lower body 167
    mesenteric 153
Isolated tumour cells 89

J

James Reason's Swiss cheese theory 37
Jaundice 58, 121
    gallstone-related 54
Joint pain 75

K

Knotting 58

L

Labour standards assurance systems 11
Laceration 142
    partial-thickness 142
Laparoscopic cholecystectomy 54, 120, 123, 126, 127, 134
    recent advances in 134
Laparotomy 60-64, 139, 147
    decompressive 65
    emergency 57, 58, 62, 64
    exploratory *59*
    midline 62
    postoperative complication of 57
Lapatinib 81
Large bite technique 62
Laryngeal nerve palsy, recurrent 169
Laser 104
    ablation 106-108

Lean service delivery 6
Left subclavian artery 166, *174*
Lethargy 40
Letrozole 76, 78-85
    neoadjuvant 79
Linea alba 58
Liver
    cirrhosis 154
    injury 132
    sinusoids 132
    transplantation 158
    venous sinusoids 132
Lobular neoplasia 109
Local inflammation, signs of 124
Locoregional recurrence 82
Lumen
    false 165, *168*
    true 166, *168*
Lump formation 108
Lymph nodes 89
Lymphangiomas, mesenteric 154

M

Macmillan programme 18
Macronutrient deficiencies 160
Magnetic resonance
    cholangiopancreatography 125
    imaging scans 86, 105, 125
Malignancies 74
    secondary 74
Malnourishment 58
Malnutrition 60
    preoperative 24
Malperfusion syndrome 167, 168, 172, 176
Mammary tissue 74
Mammogram 108
Mammography 86
Marfan syndrome 170
Mechanical needle excision 109
Menopausal symptoms 75, 76
Mental fatigue 38
Mesh augmentation, role of 63
Metabolic imbalance 146
Micronutrient deficiencies 160
Microwave ablation 106, 108
Micturition 62
Midgut volvulus 153
Minimally invasive percutaneous methods 104

Minute ventilation 20
Mobilisation, delayed 55
Monofilament suture, absorbable 61
Multicentre insect 62
Multidisciplinary teams 53, 88
Multiple transfusions 146
Multivisceral transplantation 152
Murphy's sign 124
Muscles, internal oblique 65
Musculoaponeurosis 60
Musculoskeletal aches 76
Musculoskeletal syndrome 76
Mycophenolate mofetil 158
Myocardial infarction 182, 183
Myocardial injury 181

N

Nasogastric intubation 52
National Cancer Database 88
National Confidential Enquiry on Perioperative Deaths 52
National Health Service 4
National Institute for Health and Care Excellence 8, 183
    guidelines 126
Natural orifice cholecystectomy 134
Nausea 75
Neck arteries 156
Necrotic tumour cell death 106
Necrotising enterocolitis 153
Negative pressure wound therapy 65
Neoadjuvant endocrine therapy 73, 74, 82
    randomised trials of **80, 83**
Neoadjuvant therapy 73, 87, 88
Neoadjuvant treatment 73, 87
Noncardiac surgery 179
Non-steroidal inhibitors, third-generation 76
Nutrition 24
Nutritional status 39

O

Obesity 26, 58, 119, 130
Oblique muscle, external 65
Obstruction, intestinal 58
Oedema 65, 131
    peripheral 75

Oesophagogastroduodenoscopy 53
Oestradiol 75
Oestrogen 75
    deprivation 76
    hormone receptor 73
    production 76
    receptor 74
        expression 85
    suppressor 76
Oestrogenic properties 74
Oliguria 125
Omental adhesions 132
Onlay mesh 64
Oophorectomy 76
Open Hasson technique 131
Optimal emergency care 53
Optimal medical therapy 172, 173
Optimisation, rationale for 25
Organ
    failure 125
    recovery 155
    specific management 160
    support 126
    transplants 161
Orthotopic transplantation 157
Osteopenia 76
Osteoporosis 75, 76
Out-of-hospital cardiac arrests 167
Ovarian function 76
    suppression 76
Ovarian stimulation 76
Over time surgical techniques 104
Oxygen
    consumption 20
    partial pressure of 126
Oxytocin 186

P

Paclitaxel 80
Pain 108, 124
    biliary 118, 121
    control 176
    joint 75
    management 18, 124
    musculoskeletal 75
    refractory 168
    relief, preoperative 53

Palbociclib 81, 83
Pancreatitis 54, 118, 119, 128
Parenteral nutrition 151
    long-term 120
Pelvic cul-de-sac 143
Pelvic
    organs 141
    trauma, penetrating 142
Pelvis 145
Penicillin 127
Percutaneous ablative 110
    approaches 109
    techniques 111
Percutaneous vacuum needle excision 110
Perineum 145
Perioperative ischaemia evaluation 3 trial 179, 181, **181**
Perioperative thrombotic events 182
Peripheral arterial thrombosis 181
Peritoneal incisions 60
Peritoneal reflection 141
Peritonitis 58, 64, 139
Personal protective equipment 40
Pesticides 118
Pfannenstiel incision *59*
Photons 104
Physiotherapy 52, 55
Piperacillin 126
Placebo 80-83
Plasmin 186
    fibrinolysis pathway 179
    formation 180
    inhibitors, natural 180
Plasminogen 186
    activator inhibitors 180
    protein 180
Platelet count 126
Pneumonitis, interstitial 75
Pneumoperitoneum 131
Point-of-care testing 51
    machines 53
Point-of-care ultrasound 53
Polypropylene mesh 64
Polyps 74
    endometrial 75
Portal vein *155*, 157, *157*
Portomesenteric venous thrombosis 154

Positron emission tomography 108
    scans 86
Post-cholecystectomy syndromes 119, 121
Post-intestinal transplantation management 159
Postpartum haemorrhage 180, 185, 186
    following caesarean delivery trial 186
Post-transplant lymphoproliferative
    disease 158
    disorder 161
Preanaesthetic medication 52
Preoperative nutrition therapy *26*
Presacral drainage 148
Proctoscopy 144, 145
Proctosigmoidoscopy 144
Progesterone 79
Prophybiom 64
Prophylactic
    biological mesh reinforcement versus standard closure of stoma site trial 64
    cholecystectomy 117, 119
Prosthesis 37
Protein denaturation 108
Proteolysis-targeting chimeras 77
Prothrombin time 126
Protons
    beam therapy 105
    ions 104
Pubic symphysis 144
Pulmonary embolism 75, 183, 186

Q

Quality of life 22

R

Radial scar 109
Radiofrequency ablation 106, 107
Radiotherapy 58, 104, 105
    ablative 104-106
    advanced 105
Raised blood inflammatory markers 123
Raloxifene 74, 75
Randomised controlled trials 61, 169
Rectal bleeding 54
Rectal extraperitoneal trauma 146

Rectal foreign bodies 142
Rectal injury 139-145, 148
    aetiology of 142, 147
    care, history of 140
    diagnosis of 144
    intraperitoneal 145
    majority of 139
    management of 139, 140
    recognition of 142
Rectal trauma 145
    management of 141, 147, *148*
    penetrating 142
Rectal wall thickening 144
Rectosigmoid junction 145
Rectum 139
    anatomy of 139, 141, *141*
    intraperitoneal 146
Red blood cells 182, 183
Refractory intestinal failure 153
Rehabilitation, intestinal *154*
Renal artery *155*
Renal dysfunction 169
Renal impairment 125
Reperfusion injury 160
Residual cancer burden 84
Respiratory impairment 126
Retrograde cerebral perfusion 169
Retromuscular mesh placement 64
Retromuscular plane 64
Retroperitoneal emphysema 145
Right hypochondrial mass 124
Rituximab 158
Robotic cholecystectomy 134
Robotic procedures 7

S

Salmonella typhi carriage, chronic 118
Sarcomas 74
Sarcopenia 26, 58
Scalpel 60
Scarpa's fascia 65
Sciatica, injection site-related 75
Selective oestrogen receptor
    covalent antagonists 77
    degraders 74-76
    downgraders 74, 76
    modulators 74, 75
        antagonistic effect of 74

Sentinel lymph node biopsy 89
Sepsis 52, 129, 139
    intraperitoneal 58
    monitor for 52
    screen for 52
    severe 127
Seroma formation 104
Serosanguinous fluid, drainage of 58
Sexual dysfunction 76
Shared decision making 18, 29, 30
    concept of 53
Shock, signs of 186
Sickle cell disease 120
Sigmoid colostomy 147
Sigmoidoscopy 144
Single-incision laparoscopic surgery
    cholecystectomy 134
Sinotubular junction 170
Six-minute walk test 20, 22
Skin retraction 107
Small bite technique 62
Sneezing 62
Society for Vascular Surgery 167
Society of Thoracic Surgeons 172
Solid organ transplant recipients 120
Spinal cord injury 169
Stanford classification 176
Static abdominal wall closure 65
Stenosis 146
Steroidal inactivator exemestane 76
Steroids 58
Stoma closure 64
Stone
    characteristics 118
    diameter 119
    volume, high 118
Stress, effect of 40
Stroke 75, 169
    non-haemorrhagic 181, 182
    perioperative 169
Subcutaneous tissue 60, *66*
Subtotal cholecystectomy 133
    types of 133, *133*
Superior mesenteric
    artery *155*, *157*
    vein *157*
Surgery 51, 180
    abdominal 120

de-escalation 88
emergency 49, 51, 53, 54, 58
intestinal 137
risk assessment for 52
Surgical disease prevention 6
Surgical outcomes risk tool 19
Surgical site infection 59
Surgical team performance 35
Surgical wound 65
spontaneous opening of 57
Sustainable surgery, principles of 5
Sutures
absorbable 61
fast-absorbable 61
length 62
material 58
choice of 61
nonabsorbable 61
sinus formation 61
slowly absorbable 61
slowly nonabsorbable 61
technique 58, 61
Swiss cheese
metaphor 38
model 37
Symptomatic proximal venous thromboembolism 181, 182
Syncope 166
Systemic immune response 110
Systemic inflammation, signs of 124
Systemic venous drainage 157

T

Tachycardia 186
Tacrolimus 158
Tamoxifen 74-80, 83-85
Targeted biological therapy 110
Taselisib 82
Tear, development of 165
Temporary stoma 59
Tenderness 124
Thalassemia 120
Thermal ablation 104, 106
techniques for 106
Thermal injury 129
Thoracic aorta 167
Thoracic cavity 167

Thoracic endovascular aortic repair 167, 173
Thoracic stent graft 174
Thoraflex hybrid endoprosthesis 171
Thrombocytopaenia 75
Thromboembolic events 75
Tiredness 38, 40
Tissue
damage 180
fibrosis 131
peripheral 75, 76
specific effects 74
type plasminogen activator 180
Toremifene 74
Total intestinal aganglionosis 153
Total parenteral nutrition, use of 124
Tranexamic acid 179, 180, 182, 186, 187
mechanism of action of 180
perioperative 183
role of 179
use 184, 185
Transcutaneous vacuum-assisted needle excision 109
Transplant bowel resection 161
Transplant recipient, scientific registry of 151, 153
Transverse incision 60
Transversus abdominus 65
Trauma 180
abdominal 58
penetrating 145
sonography for 143
Traumatic injury 140, 142, 143
Triptorelin 83
Tube feeding formula 160
Tuberculosis 62
Tumour 73
ablation 103
cell necrosis 110
Typhoid 62

U

Ubiquitin-mediated proteasome 76
Ultra-short gut syndrome 154
Ultrasound 53, 86, 103, 124
scan 124
Umbilical cord 186
Upper rectum, intraperitoneal injury of 139

Uraemia 58
Urethral meatus 144
Uterine
    cancers 75
    fibroids 74, 75

V

Vacuum assisted needle excision 103, 109, 110
Vaginal bleeding 75
Vaginal discharge 75
Vaginal dryness 75
Vaginal symptoms 76
Valvular dysfunction 176
Vascular access 175
Vascular anastomoses 157
Vascular injury 132
Vascular reconstruction 156
Vascular surgery 163
Vasomotor symptoms 75, 76
Vasopressor support 125
Vein, hepatic 132, *155*
Venous thromboembolism 182, 183
Venous thrombosis 183
Ventilation 143
Veress needle insertion 131
Vertical traction device *65*
Vessel injury 131
    major 131

Visceral ischaemic time 174
Visceral malperfusion syndromes 167
Visceral oedema 65
Vorozole 80

W

Waste disposal 9
Waterless hand scrub 8
Weakness 166
Weight loss, sudden severe 124
White cell count, elevated 124, 125
World Health Organisation 4, 36
World Maternal Antifibrinolytic trial 180
Wound 58, 61
    dehiscence 60, 61, 63
    infection 58, 60, 64
    length 62
    pain 61
    penetrating 142, 145

X

X-ray 53

Z

Zoledronic acid 80